Silicone Hydrogels

For Butterworth-Heinemann:

Publishing Director: Caroline Makepeace
Development Editor: Kim Benson
Production Manager: Morven Dean
Design: George Ajayi

Silicone Hydrogels

continuous-wear contact lenses

SECOND EDITION

Edited by

D. Sweeney

Chief Executive Officer, Vision Cooperative Research Centre;
Associate Professor, School of Optometry and Vision Science,
The University of New South Wales, Sydney, Australia

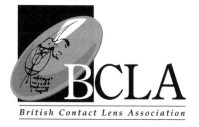

British Contact Lens Association

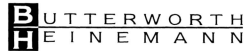

EDINBURGH LONDON NEW YORK OXFORD PHILADELPHIA ST LOUIS SYDNEY TORONTO 2004

BUTTERWORTH-HEINEMANN
An imprint of Elsevier Limited

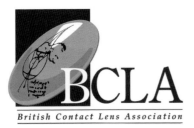

First edition 2000
Second edition 2004

ISBN 0 7506 8779 7

British Library Cataloguing in Publication Data
A catalogue record for this book is available from the British Library

Library of Congress Cataloging in Publication Data
A catalog record for this book is available from the Library of Congress

Note
Medical knowledge is constantly changing. As new information becomes available, changes in treatment, procedures, equipment and the use of drugs become necessary. The author/contributors and the publishers have taken great care to ensure that the information given in this text is accurate and up to date. However, readers are strongly advised to confirm that the information, especially with regard to drug usage, complies with the latest legislation and standards of practice.

The Publisher

your source for books,
journals and multimedia
in the health sciences
www.elsevierhealth.com

The
Publisher's
policy is to use
**paper manufactured
from sustainable forests**

Printed in China

Contents

Preface

There are approximately 100 million contact lens wearers worldwide, representing some 1.4% of the population and only 4% of the 2.4 billion spectacle wearers. To really compete with spectacles, contact lenses need to be simpler, more convenient and very, very comfortable. Patients are looking for safe, long-term elimination of the need for vision correction even to the point where many turn to invasive procedures such as refractive surgery as a means of providing a permanent answer to their vision correction needs. However, surveys have consistently shown that an overwhelming majority of contact lens wearers would prefer continuous wear lenses over refractive surgery, if the lenses were safe, effective and comfortable.

High Dk silicone hydrogel lenses were approved for 30-night continuous wear in Australia and Europe in 1999 and in the United States in 2001, and since then the market for these lenses has grown rapidly. In the middle of 2003, there were close to a million silicone hydrogel wearers worldwide. Fuelling this market growth in many countries is the return of practitioner confidence in recommending extended wear to their patients. Hypoxia-free contact lenses represent the first step in the development of a contact lens that will successfully rival spectacles in market popularity, and challenge refractive surgery for convenience.

One of the major hurdles in the development of an extended wear lens has been adequate oxygen permeability for overnight wear. In the 1980s, Holden and Mertz established that to match the overnight edema with no lens wear, measured at that time by Mertz to be 4%, contact lenses must have an oxygen transmissibility (Dk/t) of at least 87. If we use the more accepted La Hood figure for overnight edema without lenses as 3.2%, the Holden–Mertz equation predicts that a Dk/t of 125 would be needed for long-term edema free extended wear. High oxygen permeability has been extremely difficult to attain in a soft water-containing material because of the hydrophobicity of conventional materials made of silicone- and fluorocarbon-containing polymers. Although silicone elastomer lenses provided more than adequate oxygen, they were not successful because of the problems associated with comfort, poor wettability, deposits and lens binding.

High Dk silicone hydrogel lenses have the comfort, movement and wettability of conventional soft contact lenses with the additional and substantial benefits of eliminating the effects of hypoxia during sleep. Patients report that they have whiter eyes, and practitioners no longer see high levels of microcysts and other clinical signs of hypoxia. Microbial keratitis rates seem to have been reduced but we await the results of market surveillance and other studies to ascertain the magnitude of the reduction in risk of ocular infection.

This book provides the researcher and practitioner with the latest information on the development of silicone hydrogel materials. It also summarizes the eye's needs, the effects of eye closure, the control variables for tear exchange and the factors that drive the adverse responses that occur with extended wear. Practitioners can learn what to expect when they use these lenses in their practice. Many practice management tips are provided in the last chapters to help ensure an easy transition to the use of silicone hydrogel lenses.

In Chapter 1, Professor Brian Tighe provides an informative overview of the material developments that have occurred and the breakthroughs in technology achieved by Bausch and Lomb and CIBA Vision.

In Chapter 2, Professors Graeme Wilson, Dr Patrick Ladage and Dwight Cavanagh give a unique insight into the effects of contact lens wear on the anatomy and physiology of the ocular surface. In particular they discuss how extended wear might affect the shedding of epithelial cells, and the maintenance of normal epithelial homeostasis is reviewed.

Chapter 3 by Professor Ken Polse, Dr Clay Radke and colleagues focuses on the assessment of tear mixing and how tear mixing could be enhanced with silicone hydrogels.

Associate Professor Mark Willcox and fellow researchers discuss in Chapter 4 the changes that occur during lens wear which disrupt normal corneal homeostasis, and their effects on bacterial and other inflammatory mediators.

In Chapter 5, Drs Desmond Fonn and Noel Brennan review the state of research into corneal oxygenation by considering the basics of cellular physiology, techniques for assessing the corneal physiological response and the influence of silicone hydrogel lens wear on this response.

In Chapter 6, Associate Professor Deborah Sweeney and colleagues provide an account of the long-term clinical performance of silicone hydrogel lenses, including the subjective responses of patients and their ocular physiological responses.

In Chapter 7, my co-authors and I outline the adverse responses that can occur in extended wear and discuss which responses are likely to be seen with silicone hydrogels.

Finally in Chapter 8 Dr Noel Brennan and Chantal Coles detail many of the issues to be considered when using continuous wear and silicone hydrogels in your practice. Dr Anna-Karin Dahl adds her experience with the use of silicone hydrogels by many hundreds of patients in Scandinavia.

All indicators to date suggest that the issue of hypoxia and its side effects on corneal tissue have been eliminated. Patients enjoy the freedom of 30 days and nights of continuous wear. The convenience of this modality and the comfort and vision provided by the silicone hydrogels so far released on the market means that finally both patients and practitioners have convenient alternative to spectacles and surgery. Just how successful these materials will be in alleviating microbial keratitis will remain uncertain until the current studies have been completed. An increasing number of practitioners are now seeing high *Dk* silicone hydrogel lenses as the first choice lens for their patients irrespective of wear schedule, because these lenses offer superior metabolic health for the patient. Silicone hydrogel lenses represent a major step in the development of vision correction. With future generations of these products targeting anti-bacterial surfaces, even better biocompatibility and lenses designed for all prescriptions and age groups, the future of vision correction with contact lenses promises to be very exciting.

In many ways this book is a tribute to all those laboratory and clinical scientists who have contributed critical knowledge to achieving the Holy Grail of contact lenses, continuous wear, and to all those in the industry that have persevered with this particular vision.

This book is dedicated to three wonderful contributors to contact lenses who have passed away in recent years; Otto Wictherle, George Mertz and Jonathan Kersley and the European pioneers of extended wear contact lenses: John deCarle, David Clulow, Phillip Cordrey, Montague Ruben and Klaus Nilsson.

Brien A. Holden

Contributors' list

CHAPTER 1: SILICONE HYDROGELS: STRUCTURE, PROPERTIES AND BEHAVIOUR

Brian Tighe is Professor of Polymer Science at Aston University, Birmingham, UK and Director of Aston Biomaterials Research Unit; he is a member of the International Editorial Boards of *Journal of Biomaterials Science* and *Contact Lens and Anterior Eye*. Aston Biomaterials Research Unit is an interdisciplinary group of nine postgraduate and four postdoctoral researchers supported by a project coordinator working on a range of research activities that centre on the synthesis and behaviour of polymers primarily designed for biomedical applications including contact lenses. The group has produced over 400 publications of various types.

CHAPTER 2: THE EPITHELIUM IN EXTENDED WEAR

Dr Graeme Wilson completed his optometry training in Glasgow. He received an MSc from Manchester and a PhD from Berkeley. From 1971 to 1998 he was a Faculty member at the University of Alabama, and retired as Professor Emeritus. He is now Professor of Optometry at Indiana University. He has received the Max Shapero Memorial Award of the American Academy of Optometry and was the first optometrist to serve on the Program Planning Committee of the Cornea Section of the Association for Research in Vision and Ophthalmology (ARVO). He is currently President of the International Society for Contact Lens Research.

Dr Patrick Ladage is currently visiting research scientist at the College of Optometry, University of Houston, Texas. He received his optometric degree in 1995 from the Hogeschool van Utrecht, the Netherlands and his PhD on 'Corneal epithelial homeostasis during extended contact lens wear' in 2002 from the University of Houston. From 1998 to 2003 he worked at UT Southwestern Medical Center, Department of Ophthalmology under the supervision of H. Dwight Cavanagh MD PhD, studying the effects of silicone hydrogel lens wear in the human and rabbit. He is fellow of the American Academy of Optometry and a past William C. Ezell fellow of the American Optometric Foundation (AOF).

He was awarded the 2002–2003 Vistakon AOF research grant at the annual AAO meeting in San Diego to study the long-term effects of extended contact lens wear on the corneal epithelium.

H. Dwight Cavanagh is the W. Maxwell Thomas Chair, Professor and Vice-Chairperson of Ophthalmology, as well as Medical Director and Associate Dean for Clinical Services, Zale Lipshy University Hospital/University of Texas Southwestern Medical Center at Dallas. Dr Cavanagh has also served as a past president of the Contact Lens Association of Ophthalmologists (CLAO) and the Castroviejo Corneal Society (CCS), executive director of the ARVO, and as chair of the Visual Sciences A and the Neurosciences and Biobehavioral Sciences Study Sections of the National Institutes of Health. He is the recipient of Honor Recognition Awards from CLAO, CCS, ARVO and the American Academy of Ophthalmology. He was recently awarded an honorary fellowship by the American Academy of Optometry (2001); he has also been listed in the *Best Doctors in the U.S.* since 1979. Dr Cavanagh served a six-year term as Editor-in Chief of the journal *Cornea* (1989–1995), and currently serves as Editor-in Chief of *Eye & Contact Lens Journal* (formally *CLAO Journal*).

CHAPTER 3: TEAR MIXING UNDER SOFT CONTACT LENSES

Professor Clayton (Clay) J. Radke received his PhD degree in chemical engineering at the University of California, Berkeley, in 1971. After a two-year National Science Foundation Post-Doctoral Fellowship in physical chemistry at the University of Bristol, he joined the Faculty of Chemical Engineering at Pennsylvania State University. In 1975, he returned to the University of California, where he now holds Senior Professor positions in the Departments of Chemical Engineering and Vision Science, and Senior Scientist in the Earth Science Division of the Lawrence Berkeley National Laboratory. Dr Radke has garnered departmental, college and professional society teaching recognition including the campus-wide Distinguished Teaching Award at UCB in 1994. He is listed in *Who's Who in America* and was the 2003 winner of the American Chemical Society Award in Colloid Chemistry. Dr Radke has published close to 200 articles in surface science and technology.

Professor Kenneth A. Polse is Professor of Optometry and Vision Science at the University of California, Berkeley, School of Optometry. During his 30 years on the Berkeley faculty, Professor Polse has held several administrative and professional positions including Clinic Director (1975–1980), Associate Dean for Academic Affairs (1980–1984) and Associate Dean for Clinical Academic Affairs (1992–1995). Other professional roles include as Ad Hoc Reviewer to the National Institute of Health, Consultant to the National Eye Institute long-range program planning committee, President of the International Society for Contact Lens Research (1986–1988), Member of the American Optometric Association Council on Optometric Research (1988–1990), Chair of the Committee for Adverse Effects of Contact Lenses for the Committee on Vision, National Research Council (1988–1991), and Member of the National Advisory

Eye Council, NIH (1987–1991). He has received several honours, which include a Senior Fulbright Fellowship, two American Academy of Optometry Garland Clay Awards for most significant clinical publication in their journal (1984 and 1994) and the American Academy of Optometry Contact Lens Section Max Shapero Lectureship (1993). Professor Polse was the recipient of the University of California Morton D. Sarver Endowed Chair.

CHAPTER 4: INFLAMMATION AND INFECTION AND THE EFFECTS OF THE CLOSED EYE

Professor Mark Willcox is Director of Science and Core Capabilities at the Vision Cooperative Research Centre (Vision CRC), formerly the Cooperative Research Centre for Eye Research and Technology. He joined the group in 1993. His research areas include microbiology of the eye and oral cavity, ocular immunology, antimicrobial function of the tear film, dry eye and ocular mucin interactions of bacteria with host defence systems. In particular his interests centre on the effect of wearing contact lenses on all of these areas. He has published over 100 papers in journals, presented over 200 papers at national and international conferences and has two patents.

CHAPTER 5: CORNEAL HYPOXIA

Dr Noel A. Brennan codirects a Melbourne-based private research company. This consultancy specializes in preclinical assessment and development of contact lenses and ocular testing procedures, clinical trials and scientific writing. He has a Master's degree in Optometry, a PhD, is a Fellow of the American Academy of Optometry and a Councillor of the International Society of Contact Lens Research. He was formerly a Reader and Associate Professor in an Australian Optometry school. He also co-owns an optometry practice with a principal patient base of specialist contact lens fittings.

Desmond Fonn is a Professor and Director of the Centre for Contact Lens Research at the School of Optometry, University of Waterloo, Waterloo, Ontario, Canada. He is a graduate of the School of Optometry in Johannesburg, South Africa, and the University of New South Wales in Sydney, Australia, where he also served as a consultant for the Cornea and Contact Lens Research Unit. He is a fellow of the American Academy of Optometry and a diplomate of the Cornea and Contact Lens section, a member of the Canadian and Ontario Association of Optometrists, and of the Association for Research in Vision and Ophthalmology. He is the President Elect of the International Society for Contact Lens Research and a founding member of the International Association of Contact Lens Educators, in which he serves as Vice President. His research interests include the ocular response and symptomology of contact lens wear, extended wear, developments in contact lens materials, designs and disinfection systems. He has lectured extensively and published widely on these and other topics.

CHAPTER 6: CLINICAL PERFORMANCE OF SILICONE HYDROGEL LENSES

Deborah F. Sweeney is Associate Professor and Chief Executive Officer of the Vision Cooperative Research Centre, formerly the Cooperative Centre for Eye Research and Technology. Her major research area has been corneal physiology, and her work has been instrumental in developing an understanding of the physiology of the human cornea and the effects of contact lens wear on corneal function characteristics. Associate Professor Sweeney is also active in national and international optometric and ophthalmic organizations, including executive roles in the International Society for Contact Lens Research, the Keratoprosthesis (KPro) Study Group and the International Association of Contact Lens Educators.

CHAPTER 7: ADVERSE EVENTS AND INFECTIONS: WHICH ONES AND HOW MANY?

Padmaja Sankaridurg was awarded her Bachelor of Optometry from the Elite School of Optometry, Chennai, India in 1989 and in 1999 she gained her PhD degree from the University of New South Wales, Australia. After working for a number of years at the L.V. Prasad Eye Institute as the Chief of Contact Lens Services, she took up a position at the University of New South Wales, Australia and is now Senior Project Scientist at the Vision Cooperative Research Centre. Her research areas include myopia, contact lens induced infection and inflammation of the eye. She is a member of the International Society for Contact Lens Research, the Association for Research in Vision and Ophthalmology and the International Association of Contact Lens Educators.

Brien A. Holden is Scientia Professor of Optometry at the University of New South Wales (UNSW) and Deputy CEO of the Vision Cooperative Research Centre, formerly the Cooperative Research Centre for Eye Research and Technology. He is the author of over 200 refereed papers and 20 book chapters, and he holds two patents. He has held numerous academic, professional and university appointments, including as the President of the International Association of Contact Lens Educators and the International Society for Contact Lens Research, and currently as Chair of the International Centre for Eyecare Education. Professor Holden was awarded Honorary Doctor of Science degrees by the State University of New York in 1994, by the Pennsylvania College of Optometry in 1998, by the City University London in 1999 and by the University of Durban–Westville, South Africa, in 2002. Other awards include the Glenn A. Fry Award presented by the American Academy of Optometry in 1998, a British Contact Lens Association Medal in 1997, and a Special Recognition Award Medal from the Association for Research in Vision and Ophthalmology in 2002. Apart from these academic awards Professor Holden also received the Medal of the Order of Australia from the Australian government for contributions to eyecare research and education in 1997.

CHAPTER 8: SILICONE HYDROGELS IN PRIVATE PRACTICE

Dr M-L. Chantal Coles graduated from the New England College of Optometry in 1987. She has worked as a private practitioner in Canada and Australia and held a position as a Research Optometrist at the Centre for Contact Lens Research of the University of Waterloo for a period of three years. She moved to Australia in 1994 and cofounded two companies which specialize in vision research, clinical trials and industrial consulting. She is also co-owner of a private optometry practice in Melbourne.

Anna Karin Dahl is the Sales and Marketing Manager for Synoptik in Sweden. She completed her optometry degree in Borensberg, Linköping in 1990, followed by contact lens education at the Institute of Optometry in Stockholm, graduating in 1992. From 1992–2002 she worked as an optometrist at the Contacta eyewear chain in Sweden, responsible for contact lens development and education. She has been a member of the board in the Swedish Contact Lens Association (1997–2003); and is currently a member of the board of the Contact Lens Division of the Swedish Optometry Organisation. She has been involved in clinical studies for CIBA Vision, Bausch & Lomb and Johnson & Johnson, and over the last five years has focussed on the development of the silicone hydrogels segment in Sweden.

Chapter 1

Silicone hydrogels: structure, properties and behaviour

Brian Tighe

INTRODUCTION

The unique properties that polymers possess arise from the ability of certain atoms to link together to form stable bonds. Foremost among the atoms that can do this is carbon (C), which can link together with four other atoms either of its own kind or alternatively atoms of, for example, hydrogen (H), oxygen (O), nitrogen (N), sulphur (S) or chlorine (Cl). Silicone (Si) resembles carbon in this way to some extent, especially in its ability to link to carbon, hydrogen and oxygen. It is this property of carbon that forms the basis of what is called organic chemistry or the chemistry of carbon compounds. Most of the polymers that we encounter fall within the realm of organic chemistry, defined in this way. These polymers may be purely natural (such as cellulose), modified natural polymers (such as cellulose acetate) or completely synthetic (such as polymethyl methacrylate, PMMA). A much smaller family of polymers exists, based on silicone rather than carbon. Their properties differ somewhat from those of the carbon-based polymers and it is because of these differences that contact lenses based on silicone chemistry, whether rigid gas-permeable (RGP) lenses or hydrogels, are so important.

The single characteristic that unites both silicone-based and carbon-based polymers is the fact that, as the name (poly-mer) suggests, they are composed of many units linked together in long chains. Thus if we can imagine a molecule of oxygen and a molecule of water enlarged to the size of a tennis ball (the molecular size of water is very similar to that of oxygen), a molecule of polyethylene or PMMA on the same scale would be of similar cross-sectional diameter but something like 60 metres in length. It is the gigantic length of polymers (sometimes called macromolecules) in relation to their cross-sectional diameter that gives them their unique properties, such as toughness and elasticity.

The individual building blocks from which polymers are formed are termed 'monomers'. To indicate that a polymer contains more than one type of repeating monomer unit, for example when two different monomers are polymerized together, the term 'copolymer' is used. Thus by copolymerizing styrene monomer and methyl methacrylate monomer, a styrene–methyl methacrylate copolymer is obtained. The term 'copolymer' is a general one and can be used to describe polymers obtained from mixtures of more than two monomers. A further term that has become increasingly important in the field of contact lens materials is 'macromer'. A macromer, as the name suggests, is a large monomer which is formed by pre-assembly of structural units that will convey advantageous prop-- erties on the final polymer. It is the way in which these structural and functional groups interact with each other that governs the interaction of polymer chains and the resultant properties of the polymer itself.

Perhaps the best way of visualizing the way in which polymer chains arrange themselves is by taking several pieces of string to represent individual molecules. The most usual arrangement will be a random one in which the pieces of string are loosely entangled rather than being extended. It is the interaction and entanglement of the individual molecules in this way that give polymers their characteristic physical properties. By changing the chemical nature of the polymer chain and their arrangement together we can change the physical properties and thus obtain either flexible, elastomeric behaviour (like silicone rubber) or, at the other extreme, hard glassy behaviour (like PMMA). There is an important way in which a hard glassy polymer such as PMMA or polyvinyl chloride can be converted into a flexible material and that is by the incorporation of a 'plasticizer'. This is a mobile component, often an organic liquid having a high boiling point, that will act as an 'internal lubricant'. Its presence separates the polymer chains, and allows them to move more freely.

A good example is polyvinyl chloride, which in its unmodified state is a rigid glassy material and will be familiar as the clear corrugated roofing material used on car ports and similar domestic extensions. When a plasticizer is incorporated the material is converted into the flexible material used, for example, as 'vinyl' seat coverings in cars and general domestic applications. In these cases pigments and various processing aids will also have been added in order to enable the polymer to be produced in a variety of colours and textures. An almost identical principle is involved in the formation of hydrogel polymers. The structure of PMMA can be made more hydrophilic by the incorporation of hydroxyl groups. The simplest structure that can be made in this way is poly(2-hydroxyethyl methacrylate), or polyHEMA, which is obtained by polymerizing 2-hydroxyethyl methacrylate (HEMA) monomer: in the absence of water, polyHEMA is a hard glassy material which upon hydration is transformed into the familiar contact lens material.

It is simplest to regard hydrogels as 'washing line' polymers having a long (i.e. the 'washing line') backbone from which a variety of chemical groups may be suspended (the 'washing'). The function of the chemical groups in hydrogels is primarily to attract and bind water within the structure. Greater physical stability is achieved by fastening the washing lines together at intervals by the use of cross-links. Monomers used to achieve this attraction for water include *N*-vinyl pyrrolidone (widely used in Food and Drug Administration (FDA) Group II materials) and methacrylic acid (used in all FDA Group IV materials) in addition to HEMA (which is a component of many lens materials). In silicone hydrogels the same 'washing line' principle applies but here groups that contain silicone–oxygen bonds (silicones) are attached in order to increase oxygen permeability. Although the principle is fundamentally the same, a number of additional complexities are involved which form the basis of the questions to be addressed in the following sections.

SILICONE HYDROGELS AND OXYGEN PERMEABILITY

The understanding of contact lens behaviour, developed over many years, has established the importance of achieving adequate wettability, mechanical properties and oxygen permeability. The recognition of the outstanding oxygen permeability of silicone rubber has led to many very serious attempts to modify its wettability and indeed its mechanical properties in order that a commercially viable, clinically acceptable lens could be produced. Although that goal has not yet been achieved, the combination of some of the elements of the properties of silicone rubber with those of PMMA led to the current generation of highly oxygen-permeable RGP materials.

Similarly, once the synthetic problems had been overcome to a degree where comparisons could be made, it became clear that the incorporation of structural elements of silicone rubber into hydrogels produced a dramatic enhancement of oxygen transmission properties. This is illustrated schematically in Figure 1.1, which compares the oxygen permeability (Dk) of conventional hydrogels with typical values for a family of silicone-containing hydrogels. It is important to note that the permeability of these materials at water contents below 50 per cent is not dependent upon the water content and will be very dependent upon the precise composition of the non-aqueous part of the structure, which is not defined. It is, therefore, perfectly possible to make a series of silicone-containing hydrogels that have higher or lower permeabilities than those shown.

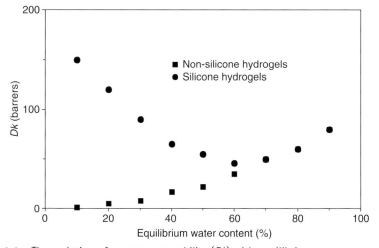

Figure 1.1   The variation of oxygen permeability (Dk) with equilibrium water content for conventional and silicone-containing hydrogels

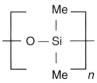

Figure 1.2   Structure of silicone rubber

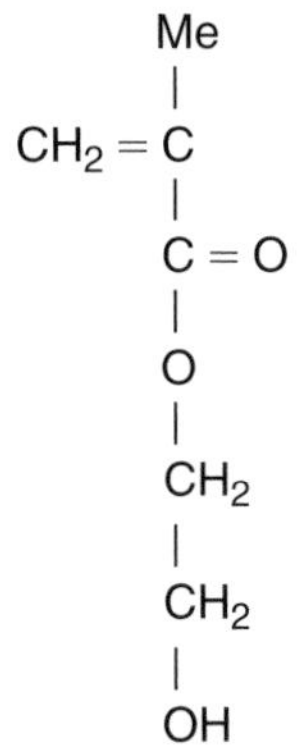

$$CH_2 = C$$

Me
|
CH₂ = C
|
C = O
|
O
|
CH₂
|
CH₂
|
OH

Figure 1.3   Structure of HEMA

The reason for the enhanced permeability is quite clear. The permeability (Dk) is a product of diffusion (D) and solubility (k). Oxygen is more soluble in water than it is in PMMA, but far more soluble in silicone rubber than it is in water. This is a property or function of the silicone–oxygen and silicone–carbon bonds that we find in silicone rubber (Figure 1.2).

In a conventional hydrogel the oxygen dissolves in, and is transported through, the aqueous phase. It has little affinity for, or solubility in, the carbon backbone polymer, which behaves rather like PMMA in the fact that it contributes little to the oxygen transport capability of the system. In the case of silicone-modified hydrogels, on the other hand, the water-borne transport is little affected (at higher water contents the transport behaviour of the two types of gel coincides) but the high solubility of oxygen in the silicone segments of the polymer causes the permeability to rise dramatically as the proportion of polymer in the gel increases (as the equilibrium water content decreases).

SILICONE HYDROGELS: UNDERLYING SYNTHETIC PROBLEMS

The initial question is this. How can we combine the elements of silicone rubber, shown in Figure 1.2, with those of a typical hydrogel-forming monomer such as HEMA (Figure 1.3) to form a copolymer that combines the properties of both?

The answer that springs to mind is to combine HEMA with the monomer that has been so successfully used in the preparation of RGP lens materials, commonly

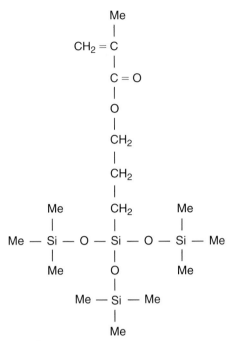

Figure 1.4   Structure of TRIS

referred to as TRIS (Figure 1.4). The method of polymer formation involves linking together, or polymerizing, the individual monomer units through the carbon–carbon double bond shown at the top of the structure.

Although this instinct is superficially right, there is one major difficulty. To combine hydrophobic TRIS with hydrophilic HEMA and then hydrate the product presents the same fundamental difficulty as trying to combine oil and water to form an optically clear product. To see how inventors, and in particular the contact lens companies, have addressed this and related problems it is useful to examine the patent literature.

One of the most widely pursued solutions to the problem of incompatibility in silicone-based hydrogels is illustrated in Figure 1.5.

Perhaps the earliest patent to propose this approach was granted to the Toyo Contact Lens Company in 1979, with Kyoichi Tanaka and four others as the named inventors (Tanaka et al., 1979). Their solution to the problem involves inserting a hydroxyl group into the section of the molecule arrowed in Figure 1.5 – simple in concept but less simple to achieve in practice. The structure developed by Tanaka is shown in Figure 1.6.

Tanaka describes the preparation of a copolymer suitable for use as soft contact lenses (SCLs) by copolymerizing this monomer with a hydrophilic monomer and a cross-linking agent. The patent states that an SCL made of the above copolymer has excellent oxygen permeability in spite of low water content and can be comfortably worn continuously long-term without a foreign body sensation and pain.

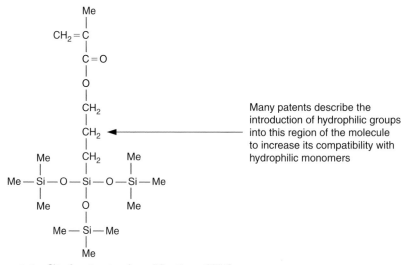

Many patents describe the introduction of hydrophilic groups into this region of the molecule to increase its compatibility with hydrophilic monomers

Figure 1.5   Site for structural modification of TRIS

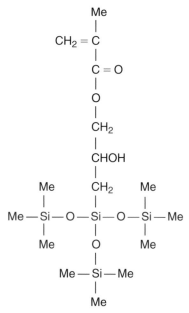

Figure 1.6   Tanaka's proposal for structural modification of TRIS

The fact that another 20 years elapsed before the widespread launch of silicone hydrogel contact lenses illustrates the point that the problems are more complex than might have been initially assumed. This conclusion is further supported by the fact that additional approaches have been regularly described in the patent literature of the 1980s and 1990s. It was not until the mid 1990s, however, that patents explicitly addressed the question of lens movement. This can be illustrated by reference to two approaches which have been harnessed in the development of the first commercially available silicone-based hydrogel lenses.

The first approach is the incorporation of fluorine, used principally because compounds based on the carbon–fluorine bond, rather than the carbon–hydrogen bond, have enhanced oxygen solubility. Fluorocarbon liquids dissolve so much oxygen that small mammals can survive (in terms of oxygen requirement) while totally immersed in them. One of the major fluorine-producing companies of the 1970s illustrated this fact with pictures of a mouse alive and breathing in a large measuring cylinder of fluorocarbon liquid. Happily, animals are no longer used in this way to support the advertising of medical products. The use of fluorine in contact lenses goes back to the same era and the period 1974–1984 saw several patents covering different types of fluorine-containing contact lenses. Of these, only the RGPs have been commercially successful.

The property enhancement of silicone hydrogels by the incorporation of fluorine was a logical extension of previous knowledge and clearly offered potential benefits. These benefits were principally seen in terms of the three basic criteria already mentioned: wettability, mechanical properties and oxygen permeability. This is illustrated by the background statement in this 1994 patent assigned to Bausch & Lomb (B&L; Künzler and Ozark, 1994):

> In the field of contact lenses, various factors must combine to yield a material that has appropriate characteristics. Oxygen permeability, wettability, material strength and stability are but a few of the factors which must be carefully balanced to achieve a useable contact lens. Since the cornea receives its oxygen supply exclusively from contact with the atmosphere, good oxygen permeability is a critical characteristic for any contact lens material. Wettability also is important in that, if the lens is not sufficiently wettable, it does not remain lubricated and therefore cannot be worn comfortably in the eye. The optimum contact lens would therefore, have both excellent oxygen permeability, and excellent tear fluid wettability.

The patent, entitled 'Fluorosilicone hydrogels', and one of Jay Künzler's many excellent contributions to the contact lens field, goes on to describe and disclose novel fluorosiloxane-containing monomers which are claimed to be especially useful for the preparation of contact lenses. The monomers are designed to improve the compatibility of TRIS-like monomers in hydrophilic monomers, thereby overcoming the problems outlined earlier. The approach is based on that illustrated in Figure 1.5 and involves attaching in the arrowed region 'a polar fluorinated side group having a hydrogen atom attached to a terminal difluoro-substituted carbon atom'. This reflects what has been the major thrust of most silicone hydrogel patents: the development of silicone-containing monomers that are sufficiently compatible with a range of hydrophilic monomers to enable hydrogels with water contents around 40 per cent and high loadings of silicone to be achieved. In this way a combination of adequate hydrophilicity and high oxygen permeability was sought.

The second approach is the development of macromer technology. Macromers, as previously stated, are large monomers formed by pre-assembly of structural units that are designed to bestow particular properties on the final polymer. This can be illustrated by a CIBA Vision (CIBA) patent entitled: 'Wettable, flexible, oxygen permeable contact lens containing block copolymer polysiloxane-poly-oxyalkylene backbone units and use thereof' with Robertson, Su, Goldenberg and Mueller as the named inventors (Robertson *et al.*, 1991). The title describes the nature of the invention very well. The principle involved is the construction of a macromer that contains, typically, hydrophilic polyethylene oxide segments and oxygen-permeable polysiloxane units. Polyethylene oxides, better known as poly-ethylene glycols or PEGs, are very hydrophilic materials widely used as compo-nents of surfactants, foodstuffs and various biomaterials. Their use in commercial contact lenses seems to be a logical step but has proved difficult to achieve. This patent provides an example of an alternative approach to that shown in Figure 1.5 but with the same ultimate objective, clearly stated in the body of the CIBA patent:

> This invention relates to ophthalmic devices, such as contact lenses and intraocular implants, and particularly contact lenses of a block copolymer con-taining polysiloxane and polyoxyalkylene oxide units possessing an advanta-geous blend of desirable properties including (a) high oxygen permeability, (b) good wettability, (c) flexibility, and (d) optical clarity in the ocular envi-ronment of use.

These two concepts, fluorine-containing silicone monomers and siloxy macro-mers, have been taken as examples of areas of development that underpin some aspects of current developments in commercial silicone hydrogel lens materials. They also illustrate a further point already alluded to. Until the mid 1990s the three paradigm properties against which the potential success of new contact lens materials was judged were wettability, mechanical behaviour and oxygen permeability. There were clearly other more or less obvious considerations such as optical clarity, cost, processibility, toxicity and deposit resistance. In terms of measurable physical properties that could be used (on the basis of acquired clinical experience) to predict minimum acceptable baseline performance of a material, however, reliance was inevitably placed upon measurement by appro-priate methods of its wetting properties, mechanical properties and oxygen permeability.

That situation lasted until the publication of an extensive CIBA patent that proposed a fourth type of property measurement which is linked to lens move-ment on the eye: hydraulic and ionic permeability. This patent (WO 96/31792), entitled 'Extended wear ophthalmic lens', was published on 10 October 1996, together with a group of related patents dealing with various aspects of the underlying chemistry. The patent is so extensive (124 pages) and raises such important issues that it is appropriate to assess it in some detail. It names some 20 inventors from around the world, representing a collaborative international team.

THE CIBA APPROACH: A BIPHASIC STRUCTURE THAT PROVIDES IONIC AND HYDRAULIC PERMEABILITY

The central invention of the CIBA patent is reflected in its first claim:

An ophthalmic lens having ophthalmically compatible inner and outer surfaces, said lens being suited to extended periods of wear in continuous, intimate contact with ocular tissue and ocular fluids, said lens comprising a polymeric material which has a high oxygen permeability and a high ion permeability, said polymeric material being formed from polymerizable materials comprising:

(a) at least one oxyperm polymerizable material and
(b) at least one ionoperm polymerizable material, wherein said lens allows oxygen permeation in an amount sufficient to maintain corneal health and wearer comfort during a period of extended, continuous contact with ocular tissue and ocular fluids, and wherein said lens allows ion or water permeation in an amount sufficient to enable the lens to move on the eye such that corneal health is not substantially harmed and wearer comfort is acceptable during a period of extended, continuous contact with ocular tissue and ocular fluids.

One far-reaching feature of this patent is that the first (and arguably the most important) claim describes a principle or method upon the basis of which successful extended-wear (EW) contact lenses may be designed; that is, the combination of adequate oxygen permeability and adequate ionic or hydraulic permeability. Much of the rest of the patent is concerned with a specific approach to the design of acceptable materials (the formation of biphasic structures) and with an appraisal of the link between ionic or hydraulic permeability and lens movement on the eye. These two topics must be dealt with separately.

THE CRUX OF THE INVENTION: BIPHASIC STRUCTURES WHICH MAY BE CO-CONTINUOUS

We now move to the principles involved in the improvements which, apparently, centre around the provision of both oxygen permeability and ion permeability in the lens together with a hydrophilic, non-lipophilic coating. More detailed descriptions provide for one oxyperm segment and one ionoperm segment or one oxygen transmission pathway and one ion transmission pathway.

The patent draws attention to the 'existence of a region of substantially uniform composition which is a distinct and physically separate portion of a heterogeneous polymeric material'.

More particularly, with respect to the polymeric components of a lens, two different types of phase, an ionoperm phase and an oxyperm phase, are described.

The picture that emerges is of a material that permits both oxygen and ions to permeate freely from the front to the back surface by means of two co-continuous phases. The water content range is subsequently defined as, desirably, 15–25 per cent and the type of material involved is thus best described as a biphasic hydrogel with co-continuous ionopermeable and oxygen-permeable phases. The term 'co-continuous' highlights an important (in contact lens terms) and novel element of the invention since biphasic polymers frequently consist of one phase in isolated regions or droplets, within a second continuous phase, the major component normally forming the continuous phase.

Since the preferred ranges defined for the oxygen-permeable component (60–85 per cent) are always greater than for the ionopermeable components (15–40 per cent), it is likely that the former component will always form a continuous phase. The invention contains a description of methods that enable the ionopermeable phase to exist as a co-continuous second phase rather than as an isolated region. The description of the chemical nature of the oxyperm and ionoperm phase constituents contains no surprises.

The oxyperm materials are described as monomers and macromers which are siloxane-containing, fluorine-containing or carbon–carbon triple bond-containing. These classes are all well known in the existing patent literature.

The ionoperm materials are simply hydrophilic monomers which are known in hydrogel production, together with PEG.

Since there is nothing novel in the broad description of the constituents of the invention, we are led to the conclusion that the novelty must rest in the morphology, which raises an important paradox. Conventional phase-separated materials have phases of different refractive indices and phase dimensions greater than the wavelength of light (ca. 500 nm), which results in scattering of light, opalescence and opacity. In the preferred embodiments of this invention, the existence of two co-continuous phases is coupled with optical clarity. How is this achieved? The possible existence of interphase regions (between the hydrophobic and hydrophilic phases) is offered as an explanation. There is no elaboration of this point but it seems likely that the minor phase, being hydrophilic, could be organized as a continuum ranging from water through to a hydrophilic polymer interphase region in such a way as to avoid the combination of phase structure and refractive index that would produce opacity. It is clear, however, that the achievement and identification of the co-continuous phases constitute the key step of the invention.

THE ACHIEVEMENT AND CONTROL OF POROSITY BY PHASE INVERSION

Although this patent contains a range of materials and different chemistries, the novelty of the invention lies in the polymerization methodology. The underlying principle of the invention can best be illustrated by taking two of the four example classes identified in the patent, each of which is based on a separate type of macromer. These two examples are characterized here as macromers A and B

Macromer A

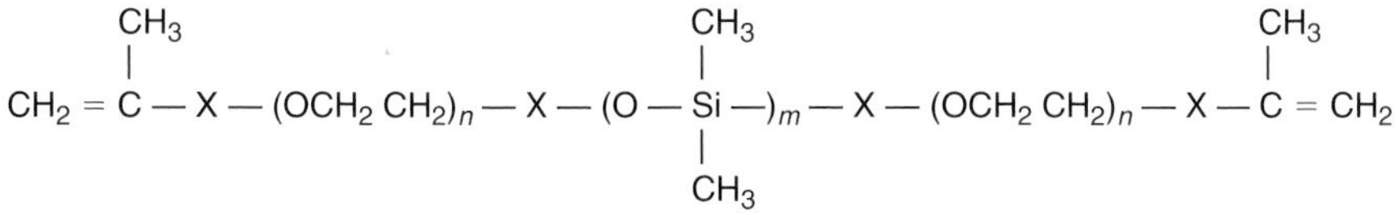

$$CH_2 = \underset{\underset{CH_3}{|}}{C} - X - (OCH_2\,CH_2)_n - X - (O - \underset{\underset{CH_3}{|}}{\overset{\overset{CH_3}{|}}{Si}} -)_m - X - (OCH_2\,CH_2)_n - X - \underset{\underset{CH_3}{|}}{C} = CH_2$$

(where n = 3 to 44, m = 25 to 40 and total molecular weight = 2000–10 000)

Figure 1.7   Example of siloxy-based polyether macromer

Macromer B

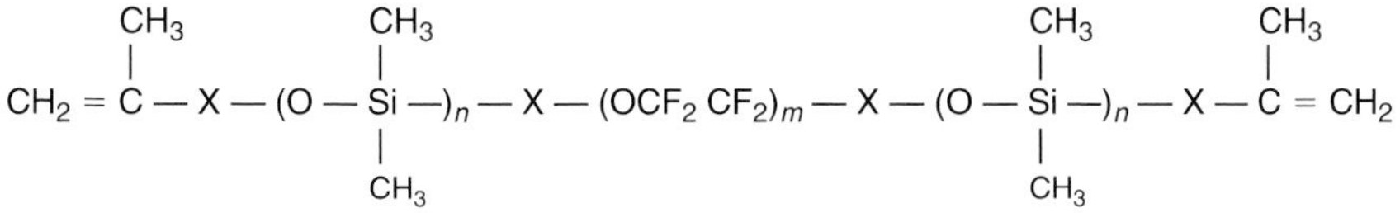

$$CH_2 = \underset{\underset{CH_3}{|}}{C} - X - (O - \underset{\underset{CH_3}{|}}{\overset{\overset{CH_3}{|}}{Si}} -)_n - X - (OCF_2\,CF_2)_m - X - (O - \underset{\underset{CH_3}{|}}{\overset{\overset{CH_3}{|}}{Si}} -)_n - X - \underset{\underset{CH_3}{|}}{C} = CH_2$$

(where n = 5 to 100, but especially 14 to 28, and m = 10 to 30)

Figure 1.8   Example of siloxy-based polyfluoroether macromer

and are illustrated in Figures 1.7 and 1.8. Each is consistent with our earlier description of macromers and consists of an assembly of segments having particular (i.e. hydrophilic or oxygen-permeable) properties. Each macromer contains carbon–carbon double bonds that enable it to be linked to other monomers.

The many compositions identified in the patent can be simplistically regarded as being formed from four components: a macromer (e.g. A or B) plus TRIS monomer (Figure 1.4), together with two 'solvents' (one of which is a hydrophilic monomer). The polymerization involves an increase in molecular weight coupled with network formation, together with a concurrent disappearance of one of the 'solvents' (usually N,N-dimethyl acrylamide). The resultant network is left as a swollen gel in the 'permanent' solvent (e.g. ethanol). This polymerization has all the features of a phase inversion process, such as those used to form porous (sometimes asymmetric) membranes commonly used in separation processes. In the most common phase inversion processes a mixture of solvents is evaporated from a polymer solution at differential rates. By control of the polymer precipitation and gelation process the microstructure of the resultant polymer is determined. In the process described here no evaporation occurs (if a closed mould is used) but the solvent properties change concurrently with the polymerization by conversion of N,N-dimethyl acrylamide monomer to matrix-bound copolymer. In conventional phase inversion processes the rate of solvent evaporation has a marked effect on the pore size and asymmetry of the product. Phase inversion processes involving polymerization (e.g. by interfacial techniques) are also well recognized.

The patent itself makes only a passing reference to the mechanism whereby ionic permeability is induced and controlled in these polymers. This reference draws attention to the common feature of the macromers, i.e. their ability to bring about microphase separation in polymerized solutions and hydrophilic monomers in appropriate proportions. The consequence of successful polymerization of this type is highlighted as the likely formation of porosity having dimensions in the region of 100 nm, reference also being made to the possible existence of an interphase region of distinct composition and structure. It is reasonable to comment that the patent has, no doubt for commercial reasons, been less explicit than it might have been in the exposition of the underlying principles of those features of the invention that underpin its success. It may be the intention to obscure a general principle that could be exploited by others with polymer structures that fall outside the scope of compositions claimed within the patent.

THE IONIC AND HYDRAULIC PERMEABILITY CRITERIA FOR LENS MOVEMENT

In addition to describing optically clear phase-separated materials which allow ionic transport and oxygen transport to take place through separate phases, the CIBA patent establishes criteria for on-eye lens movement. These are essentially 'threshold values'. They can be best understood by examining the way in which ionic transport and hydraulic transport relate to water content in conventional hydrogels. This is illustrated in Figure 1.9. Conventional hydrogels behave in some ways as though they consist of dynamically fluctuating water-filled pores, the size of which diminishes as the water content decreases. Because water and oxygen molecules are similar in size, their permeability behaviour has many similarities. As a result, the way in which the oxygen curve in Figure 1.9 varies with water content may be taken to represent the behaviour of water transport. On this basis Figure 1.9, for the remainder of the discussion, may be regarded as a representation of relative hydraulic and sodium ion transport through all classes of non-phase-separated hydrogels. It will be clear that sodium ion transport varies with water content in a quite different manner from the transport of water itself and is totally impeded at water contents below 20 per cent. This is because sodium requires a shell of water molecules around it and is unable to diffuse through low-water-content membranes.

This fact underpins the operating principle of desalination (reverse osmosis) membranes. These have a 'salt-rejecting' polymer skin which is modestly hydrophilic but with a water content below 20 per cent. This allows water to pass through under pressure, but 'rejects' sodium ions. In the case of silicone hydrogels with a homogeneous phase structure (i.e. not the biphasic materials described in the CIBA patent) the hydraulic permeability will follow the oxygen curve of conventional hydrogels, whereas the oxygen permeability increases with decreasing water content, as shown in Figure 1.1. This is because hydraulic permeability always takes place through the aqueous phase whereas, in silicone hydrogels, the transport of oxygen takes place predominantly through the silicone polymer phase.

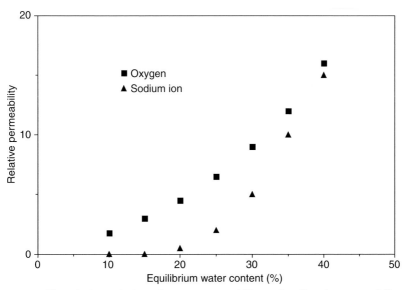

Figure 1.9   The relative variation of oxygen permeability and sodium ion permeability with equilibrium water content for conventional hydrogels

The patent goes on to describe and exemplify the limiting hydraulic and ionic permeabilities that have been observed to be necessary for lens movement on-eye. It will be obvious from Figure 1.9 that, as the water content increases, the difference between ionic and hydraulic permeability becomes unimportant. As the water content falls, however, it is the ionic permeability that becomes critical since the tear layer on both sides of the lens behaves as a dilute salt solution. The critical minimum sodium ion permeation value claimed in the patent to be necessary for lens movement ($0.2 \times 10^{-6}\,cm^2/s$) is very similar to the reported literature value for polyHEMA ($0.18 \times 10^{-6}\,cm^2/s$). The patent claims that the same minimum value for hydraulic permeability is required for lens movement ($0.2 \times 10^{-6}\,cm^2/s$), which is consistent with the analysis suggested here. It also indicates the value, as an interpretive tool of Figure 1.9, which is based on independent data obtained in these laboratories.

Independent data again confirm the logic of the observation that a minimum level of hydraulic permeability is necessary to maintain lens movement on the eye. Although the calculation is not appropriate here, it is a fairly straightforward matter to demonstrate that hydraulic flow through the lens is capable of maintaining the hydrodynamic boundary layer between lens and eye at adequate thickness to avoid hydrophobic binding. If the flow falls below a critical level, the coefficient of friction between lens and substrate rises rapidly. Parallel phenomena are observed in the development of hydrogel skin adhesives and articular joint liners.

Given that the critical minimum flow hypothesis provides a basis for understanding lens movement, how does it help in the design of silicone hydrogels for contact lens use? That question is perhaps best answered in the context of the two commercially available EW silicone hydrogel lenses, PureVision (B&L) and Focus Night & Day (CIBA).

THE NATURE AND PROPERTIES OF CURRENT COMMERCIAL MATERIALS

COMPOSITION

Given that over 20 years have elapsed since the publication of Tanaka's patent, it is reasonable to ask why silicone hydrogel lenses were not available much sooner. It is undoubtedly the case that commercial considerations and the clinical climate have much to do with this. On the other hand, we must not overlook the fact that there are many issues involved in the successful development of a new lens material other than those discussed here. Increasing silicone content may bring the benefit of increased oxygen permeability but it has attendant disadvantages. Decreased wettability, increased lipid interaction and accentuated lens binding all have to be overcome. This involves surface treatment, a notoriously difficult task with any silicone-based material. Added to this is the fact that lens fabrication and subsequent surface treatment have to be carried out on a commercially viable scale, at economic cost and with adequate quality assurance controls. Once the prototype process is finalized, clinical and regulatory approval work on the final product needs to be carried out at an acceptable level, bearing in mind the potential risks involved in unsupervised overnight wear. The time-scale and cost of such steps go far beyond the cost of laboratory experimentation to provide adequate minimum information for an initial patent filing and it would be naïve to underestimate the phenomenal costs that have been involved in bringing PureVision and Focus Night & Day to the marketplace.

Although apparently similar, significant differences exist between the two materials. PureVision is based on the enhancement of the compatibility principle that has underpinned B&L's extensive patent coverage and reflects increasingly sophisticated iterations of the approach shown in Figure 1.5. The PureVision material, balafilcon, derives from a 1997 patent entitled 'Vinyl carbonate and vinyl carbamate contact lens material monomers', which names Ronald Bambury and David Seelye as inventors (Bambury and Seelye, 1997). Inspection of the related application data shows that the original date of material filing was 1989 and that an equivalent Bambury and Seelye patent exists with a publication date of 1991 (US 5070215; Bambury and Seelye, 1991). The patent contains a detailed set of examples, including materials with properties similar to the commercial PureVision (balafilcon) lens. The novel monomer that is used in balafilcon involves replacing the CO–O link above the three carbon atoms in the arrowed section of Figure 1.10 with an O–CO–NH link and replacing the methyl group at the top of the molecule by a single hydrogen. This produces the vinyl carbamate derivative of TRIS, which is shown in Figure 1.10.

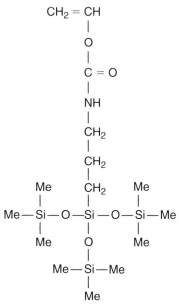

Figure 1.10   Vinyl carbamate derivative of TRIS proposed by Bambury and Seelye (1991) and Harvey (1985)

The material upon which PureVision is based then appears from the patent to be a substantially homogeneous copolymer of a vinyl carbamate derivative of TRIS with a water content of 35 per cent and a Dk of 110 barrers. The fact that it is said to have a water transport slightly (10 per cent) in excess of that of polyHEMA would put it above the critical minimum value of ionic and hydraulic permeability for lens movement on-eye. It is logical to expect that there is some degree of phase separation in the material to account for the fact that the water transport value corresponds to a water content of 40 per cent rather than 35 per cent. Physical evidence for this non-homogeneity of the structure has recently been presented (Lopez-Alemany *et al.*, 2002). In any event the chosen water content of 35 per cent gives optimal enhancement of oxygen permeability consistent with adequate water permeability to maintain lens movement on-eye. The critical nature of this balancing act can be appreciated by comparing the oxygen curve in Figure 1.1 with the sodium ion curve in Figure 1.9.

Although the B&L PureVision material appears to be quite distinct from CIBA's Focus Night & Day, the post-launch period has seen a battle between the two companies for intellectual property supremacy. Two significant aspects appear to have gone in favour of CIBA. The first is the extensive patent position, reviewed here, that identifies the need for ion permeability and the role of porous or biphasic structures in achieving a clinically acceptable level. The fact that PureVision has a level of undesigned inhomogeneity appears both to allow it to achieve acceptable on-eye mobility, and thereby to fall within the scope of the CIBA patent. The second point is equally adventitious. When CIBA acquired

Wessley-Jessen they also scooped up a tranche of intellectual property that had been accumulated in previous company mergers and takeovers. Among these emerged a patent granted to Sola almost 20 years ago that pre-dates the B&L Bambury and Seelye patent and covers the critical vinyl carbamate molecule (Figure 1.10) that forms the basis of Focus Night & Day. The Sola patent was granted in the USA and appears to have provided CIBA with the means of blocking American sales of PureVision (Harvey, 1985).

Focus Night & Day is somewhat simpler to describe, following the discussion of the 1996 CIBA patent in an earlier section. The material (lotrafilcon) is based on a fluoroether macromer of the general form shown in Figure 1.8 copolymerized with TRIS monomer and N,N-dimethyl acrylamide in the presence of a diluent. It is a fluoroether-based silicone hydrogel having a water content of 24 per cent and a Dk of 140 barrers. With a water content as low as 24 per cent it is clear from Figure 1.9 that neither sodium ion nor hydraulic permeability would approach that of polyHEMA if the structure were homogeneous. Because of the biphasic structure upon which the material is based and which allows oxygen and water permeability to be uncoupled, the hydraulic and ionic permeability of the material both exceed that of polyHEMA, and consequently the lens is reported to have adequate on-eye movement.

SURFACE MODIFICATION

One final difference between PureVision and Focus Night & Day lies in the surface treatment. Both are treated using gas plasma techniques but, whereas B&L have opted for plasma oxidation, CIBA have chosen to apply a plasma coating. In the former case, glassy islands are produced on the surface and on the latter a 25 nm thick, dense, high-refractive-index coating. Neither company has produced publicity material with illustrations of their relative surfaces, but pictures of the surfaces produced by an imaging technique called atomic force microscopy (AFM) have been shown at meetings.

The technique produces a 'relief map' of the surfaces at a scale that enables an area equivalent to a square with 50 μm (0.05 mm) sides to be visualized. If this very small area is imagined to be the size of a chessboard, the different physical nature of the surfaces of the two materials can be clearly seen. In the case of PureVision the glassy silicate islands would have about the size and distribution of the white squares – but being less regular in size and having a rounded rather than square appearance. The black squares correspond to the balafilcon substrate, illustrating that the silicate islands do not completely occlude the surface and so have only a limited effect on the permeability of the bulk material. The relative size of these areas (think of the 0.05 mm × 0.05 mm miniature chessboard) is so small that the wettability of the glassy silicate area 'bridges' over the hydrophobic balafilcon regions. Additionally the surface of the exposed balafilcon may also have been influenced to some extent by the plasma and thus be less hydrophobic than the bulk material. The 'island' structures are isolated rather than connected and thus allow the substrate to 'flex'. The depth of these islands appears to be between 10 and 50 nm, although it would be necessary to examine the data in much more detail to be sure of the limits. In summary, it represents a novel surface produced by oxidation of organic silicone in a TRIS-type molecule to inorganic silicate.

The surface of the Focus Night & Day lens has a quite different physical appearance. If we take the 0.05 mm × 0.05 mm miniature chessboard produced by AFM, the surface of this lens is chemically uniform – there is no distinctive appearance of islands, squares or other shaped regions. The surface has been uniformly coated with a new hydrophilic polymer, the thickness of which is said to be 25 nm. The polymer has been produced by making use of a gas plasma, as in the case of the B&L product, but here reactive precursors are fed into the plasma, which changes their structure and causes them to deposit as a polymer on the surface. The plasma produces hydrophilic end products but, in so doing, it changes the structure of the precursors, making precise characterization of the chemical structure of the final coating very difficult. This is a general feature of the technique, not a specific characteristic of the CIBA process. Although the structure of the coating is uniform, AFM does reveal one interesting physical feature of the surface. The 0.05 mm × 0.05 mm square appears to have a gently undulating surface in the form of curved diffuse ridges going from edge to edge of the square. These are insignificant in terms of any perceptible contribution to surface irregularities and seem to reflect the surface of tools used to produce the lens moulds. The height of the undulations is only a few nanometres.

A comparative summary of basic data relating to the properties of the two lens materials is shown in Tables 1.1 and 1.2; more detailed aspects of their behaviour in

Table 1.1   Summary of principal properties: B&L PureVision

Material name	Balafilcon
Water content	35%
Dk	110 barrers
Modulus	110 g/mm^2 (ca. 1.1 MPa)
Surface treatment	Plasma oxidation
Water transport	10% above pHEMA
Sodium transport	Not quoted (but cf. pHEMA)

Table 1.2   Summary of principal properties: CIBA Focus Night & Day

Material name	Lotrafilcon A
Water content	24%
Dk	140 barrers
Modulus	1.2 MPa
Surface treatment	25 nm plasma coating
Water transport	Not quoted (ca. 2 × pHEMA)
Sodium transport	Not quoted (ca. 2 × pHEMA)

comparison to that of conventional hydrogels are summarized in the following section. Various aspects of the scientific background relating to the development of these materials has been discussed by B&L and CIBA scientists (Künzler and Ozark, 1997; Alvord *et al.*, 1998; Grobe, 1999; Künzler, 1999; Nicolson and Vogt, 2001).

THE BEHAVIOUR OF SILICONE HYDROGEL MATERIALS: HOW DO THEY COMPARE TO CONVENTIONAL SOFT LENS POLYMERS?

WETTABILITY AND *IN VITRO* SPOILATION

There are several ways of measuring wettability, but perhaps the most generally valuable for contact lens materials is the dynamic contact angle technique, in which a sample of material is repeatedly and cyclically immersed in, and removed from, a test solution (usually saline or water). The reason that this technique is so valuable is that it reflects the break and re-formation of the tear film. Polymers, particularly hydrogels, undergo relatively rapid rotation around the atoms that link together to form the backbone. Using the analogy of the washing line, if the washing line with washing in place is completely immersed in water, the washing will be randomly arranged around the washing line and it will be quite difficult to see the continuous line. If the line and washing are removed from the water the washing will be drawn down by gravity, leaving the line much more exposed. With a hydrogel structure the same thing happens, but here the driving force is not gravity but the affinity for the functional groups on the hydrogel (the washing) for an aqueous environment. When covered by the tear film the polar water-loving groups surround the hydrophobic polymer backbone. When the tear film breaks and leaves the surface of the hydrogel exposed to air or to a deposited lipid layer (both of which are relatively hydrophobic) the polar groups turn away from the surface into the aqueous environment of the gel. This leaves a polymer surface with a structure that is more dominated by the relatively hydrophobic polymer backbone. The consequence of this change in the surface structure is that the intrinsic wettability of the polymer changes. This change is very effectively reflected in the change in contact angle as an aqueous layer advances over, and then recedes from, the surface. The advancing angle is designated as Θ_A, the receding contact angle is designated as Θ_R and the difference between them (the so-called contact angle hysteresis) is designated as Θ_H.

There is a range of values of Θ_A, Θ_R and Θ_H that have been found to correspond to minimum levels of clinical acceptability, and although values of around 70, 20 and 50, respectively, appear to be desirable, materials showing lower wettabilities (i.e. higher values of Θ_A and Θ_R) perform reasonably well. Packing solutions of conventional hydrogels frequently contain surface-active components to aid wettability and, by implication, initial comfort. All the values quoted here are measured in surfactant-free test solutions. Representative conventional hydrogel lenses of two FDA lens classes, Groups II and IV serve as useful controls and give values in the range Θ_A 80–90 degrees and Θ_R 30–45 degrees. It must be emphasized that wettability of unworn lenses, as determined by dynamic contact angle, is a necessary but not sufficient criterion for success. It is important that the material should retain its wettability (a) after spoilation by tear components and (b) under load in friction studies. Because individual patients exhibit wide differences in the nature and extent of the lens spoilation that they produce, *in vitro* tear models are often used to produce more uniform comparative spoilation of lens materials. This approach has been used to provide a comparison of the currently available silicone hydrogels (Franklin *et al.*, 2002).

The wettability of PureVision (B&L) before and after a period of 10 days' *in vitro* spoilation in a serum-based tear model is shown in Figure 1.11. Comparable results for Focus Night & Day (CIBA) are shown in Figure 1.12.

Results indicate that, although the two lenses have very similar receding contact angles (Θ_R), the advancing angles (Θ_A) are quite different. This is a reflection of the different surface treatments used by the two manufacturers. Focus Night & Day lenses are appreciably more wettable than PureVision lenses; the former show advancing contact angles of 80 degrees with a relatively low level of hysteresis (around 35 degrees) and no appreciable change after 10 days' spoilation. PureVision lenses show a higher advancing contact angle of 103 degrees and a high level of hysteresis of 65 degrees, with a slight increase in these values after 10 days' *in vitro* spoilation. Although both lenses have adequate wettability, Focus Night & Day material more closely approaches the wettability criteria defined by the '70–20–50' guideline outlined in the preceding introductory section. Neither material changes dramatically after spoilation, which is an important observation. Because of variations in individual tear chemistries, however, this does not imply that all patients will maintain adequate lens wettability throughout a given wear period.

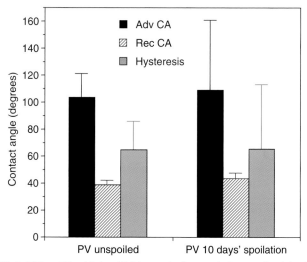

Figure 1.11 Wettability of PureVision (PV) lenses before and after 10 days' *in vitro* spoilation. Adv CA, advancing contact angle; Rec CA, receding contact angle

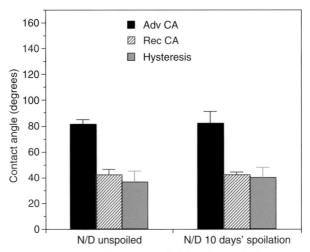

Figure 1.12 Wettability of Focus Night & Day (N/D) before and after 10 days' *in vitro* spoilation. Adv CA, advancing contact angle; Rec CA, receding contact angle

FRICTION AND BIOTRIBOLOGY

Biotribology is concerned with lubrication, friction and wear at biological interfaces. The frictional behaviour of surfaces follows a well-established pattern that links the coefficient of friction (resistance to movement) to a range of factors (e.g. load, rate) associated with the moving surfaces and the fluid that separates them. An important additional feature is the difference between the situation where the surfaces first start to move (so-called start-up or static friction) and when they are in motion (known as steady state or dynamic friction).

The study of the biotribology of other body sites provides a sound basis for understanding the behaviour of the lens-wearing eye. The lubrication of the normal eye involves both aqueous and non-aqueous species (proteins, mucins, lipids, etc.) and mechanisms that are common to other body sites, such as articulating joints and lung alveoli. The contact lens influences these lubrication mechanisms, and when lubrication breaks down complications inevitably follow. In the *in vivo* situation, lid movement over the lens surface induces both movement of the lens on the cornea and transfer of shear forces to the ocular surface. Although different contact lens materials show frictional differences, especially at start-up, the presence and nature of the hydrodynamic lubricating layer is the single most important factor.

Because the retention of a liquid (hydrodynamic) layer is vital to the normal lens lubrication mechanism, it is clear that lens wettability is a necessary but not sufficient surface property criterion. Whereas measurement of advancing and receding contact angles provides information on the stability of the intrinsic wettability of the surface layer, measurement of the coefficient of friction under eyelid load gives an indication of the stability of the wetting layer during the blink. For conventional hydrogel lenses it has been demonstrated that when this wetting

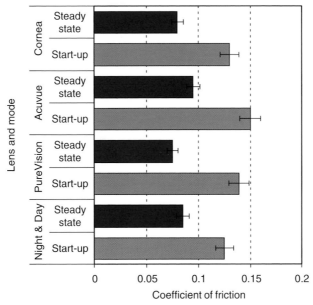

Figure 1.13   Comparative frictional behaviour of PureVision, Focus Night & Day, Acuvue and human cornea: comparison of start–up and steady state values of the coefficient of friction under eyelid load

layer (e.g. the tear film) is intact the frictional behaviour of the cornea and hydrogel lenses is very similar. Figure 1.13 shows values of start-up and steady state friction for the human cornea, Acuvue, Focus Night & Day and PureVision (Franklin *et al.*, 2002; Lydon *et al.*, 2002a).

These studies illustrate the *in vitro* behaviour of unworn lenses and provide further evidence of the sustained wettability of both Focus Night & Day and PureVision. Some deterioration in lubrication will occur, however, as a function of changes that occur during wear, such as lipid deposition and front surface dehydration. Both of these factors are patient-dependent and studies are in place to measure and monitor these factors. Changes in lubrication may well enable a link to be made between lid movement and clinically observable phenomena such as end-of-day discomfort, contact lens-induced papillary conjunctivitis (CLPC), mucin balls, corneal erosions and superior epithelial arcuate lesions (SEALs). Studies of ocular biotribology provide an important route to the understanding of these phenomena in terms of the surface and mechanical properties of the lens and the behaviour of the lid and tear film.

IN VIVO SPOILATION

The importance of the irreversible interaction of tear components with SCLs has long been recognized. The term 'spoilation' (not spoilation) was notably used by Montague Ruben in his 1970s book *Soft Contact Lenses: Clinical and Applied Technology* (Ruben, 1978).

At the time, the term was taken to encompass 'physical and chemical changes in the nature of the SCL and various extraneous deposits which may cause impairment of alteration in the optical property of the lens or produce symptoms of discomfort/intolerance in the wearer'.

Two of the most significant variables in the development of spoilation are length of wear and individual patient tear chemistry. With the advent of daily disposable and frequent-replacement wear regimes, length of wear is now much more carefully controlled and provides a means of countering the problems encountered by heavy depositors.

There remains the question of lens material. It is well recognized that FDA Group IV materials such as etafilcon (e.g. Acuvue) and vifilcon (e.g. Focus Monthlies) carry a negative ionic charge and attract the positively charged protein lysozyme. Although these materials, particularly etafilcon, absorb large quantities of lysozyme (around $1000\,\mu g$ per lens), the protein, which is an effective antibacterial agent, retains its biological activity and does not generate adverse clinical reaction. On the other, those FDA Group II materials that contain the monomer N-vinyl pyrrolidone (NVP) absorb more lipid than do other conventional soft lens materials (Maissa et al., 1998; Tighe and Franklin, 1999). Since many Group II materials are based on NVP, a belief grew up that higher-water-content materials are more susceptible to spoilation when in fact it is the presence of NVP rather than the water content per se that is responsible. In the short term, moderate levels of lipid deposition on contact lenses are well tolerated. As time progresses, however, levels of lipid continue to rise and the lipid deposits become progressively more insoluble and hydrophobic. Because silicone polymers tend to be hydrophobic and lipophilic, great interest attaches to the relative susceptibility to protein and lipid spoilation of silicone hydrogels.

The problem of patient variability has been mentioned and to some extent the use of an appropriate artificial tear solution can help to establish relative susceptibility of different materials to deposition (as in Figures 1.11 and 1.12). There is, however, no substitute for the examination of ex vivo lenses using appropriately sensitive analytical techniques. Before examining the results of such studies, it is important to recognize their relative value and validity.

Most comparative studies of the extent of deposition of proteins and lipids are carried out by first extracting the deposited components and then carrying out the appropriate analysis on the extract. Unfortunately, such extractions are never quantitative and there will always be a level of non-extractable material – particularly protein. Paradoxically, the lysozyme absorbed into the matrix of Group IV lenses is the most susceptible to removal and here the problem of quantitation is different. Unless the lysozyme in the storage solution used to contain the lens after removal from the eye is assayed the calculation of absorbed lysozyme will be incomplete, because leaching from the lens begins immediately it is placed in the storage vial. Similarly, extraction of lipid from lenses is a prolonged and somewhat tedious process which is extremely difficult to carry through to completion. The net result of these extraction difficulties is that amounts of absorbed tear components determined by extraction are invariably underestimated. The underestimate becomes relatively less significant as the amount of deposited material

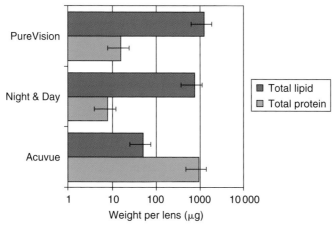

Figure 1.14 Total protein and lipid deposition on hydrogel lenses during EW: PureVision (30 nights), Focus Night & Day (30 nights) and Acuvue (seven nights)

increases and most critical in cases where the lens has relatively low levels of deposit.

An alternative and complementary technique is to assay the amount of protein and lipid deposited on the surface of the material. This can be done non-destructively, allowing an extraction process to be subsequently used on the same lens. The additional advantage of a surface assay carried out while the lens is fully hydrated (in contrast to techniques that work at high vacuum) is that the deposited components that make contact with ocular tissues are analysed, rather than those that have diffused into the lens matrix and is thus, arguably, less influential in causing adverse responses. Despite these apparent advantages and the fact that anterior and posterior surfaces can be examined separately, surface assays have to be interpreted with some caution. Although they provide an excellent basis for relative comparison, the method of detection (usually fluorescence) is not uniformly sensitive to all chemical species, which makes absolute quantitation difficult since there is considerable patient-to-patient variability, for example, in lipid composition.

Taken together, extraction-based and surface assays provide an excellent overview of the deposition behaviour of different lens materials across groups of patients. Figures 1.14 and 1.15 and the subsequent conclusions have been compiled from results obtained in these laboratories and those quoted by other workers (McKenney *et al.*, 1998; Jones *et al.*, 2001; Silicone Hydrogels Website, 2001; Franklin and Tighe, 2002; Franklin *et al.*, 2002; Senchyna *et al.*, 2002).

From these and related results it is possible to reach a series of conclusions:

- Both protein and lipid deposition are patient-dependent and time-dependent. For all but a minority of patients studied there was little significant change in surface deposition levels between 7 and 30 days EW (Acuvue lenses were worn for only seven days).

- Lipid deposition was much more patient-dependent than was protein deposition. For both components, where significant levels of left-to-right eye variation

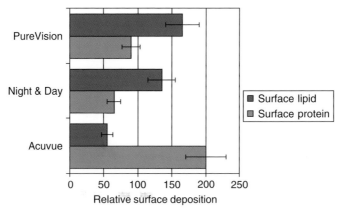

Figure 1.15   Relative levels of surface protein and lipid deposition on hydrogel lenses during EW: PureVision (30 nights), Focus Night & Day (30 nights) and Acuvue (seven nights)

and front-to-back surface variation were observed, these were patient-dependent rather than systematic.

- Levels of protein deposition were lowest on Focus Night & Day; both silicone hydrogel lenses showed relatively low levels of protein deposition (i.e. less than conventional FDA Groups I and II materials). Direct comparison with the much higher protein levels associated with Acuvue is misleading since these are produced by the reversible diffusion of lysozyme into the lens matrix.

- Although surface lipid levels of lipid for most patients do not increase dramatically with time, there is a progressive diffusion of lipid into the bulk (matrix) of the silicone hydrogel lenses. Both surface and bulk lipid levels are measurably and significantly higher on PureVision than on Focus Night & Day. Although lipid levels are much higher than those on Acuvue, they are lower than those encountered on many NVP-containing FDA Group II materials.

MECHANICAL PROPERTIES

The mechanical behaviour of different contact lens materials may be characterized by simple tensile tests which enable the tensile modulus (stiffness) and tensile strength to be determined. Such tests are routinely used by manufacturers to characterize materials (Tables 1.1 and 1.2) and involve the gradual application of a force in tension. In the *in vivo* situation, lid movement over the lens surface induces both movement of the lens on the cornea and transfer of shear forces to the ocular surface. The ability to model the transfer of eyelid forces through the lens to the cornea is an important key to the more complete understanding of contact lens–tissue interactions. One aspect of this is an understanding of the way in which the mechanical properties of the lens are affected by the rapidity of the transient eyelid motion.

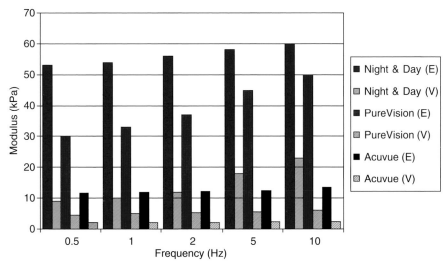

Figure 1.16 Oscillatory dynamic mechanical testing of PureVision, Focus Night & Day, Acuvue lenses as a function of frequency: variation in elastic (E) and viscous (V) components of the modulus

Some insight into the behaviour of the lens materials under these conditions is gained from measuring the so-called dynamic mechanical properties under variable cyclic load. The dynamic method is more similar to deformation processes found in nature, such as flexing muscles or blinking. The mechanical properties of polymer-based materials are not simple; they reflect the viscoelastic nature of these materials, and are represented by an elastic and a viscous flow component. If we are to understand and match the behaviour of natural tissue in use, it is important to measure these components separately, which are referred to as the storage and loss modulus, as a function of time.

Dynamic mechanical properties of contact lenses are conveniently measured in oscillation using a parallel plate set-up. Samples are typically subjected to frequencies between 0.5 and 20 Hz. The higher frequencies are intended to mimic the frequency that the cornea or a contact lens would be subjected to during blinking.

Such techniques enable the elastic component of the modulus and the viscous component of the modulus to be separately identified. The elastic component, as the name suggests, describes the extent to which the lens material behaves as an ideal elastic solid. A rubber band would be an example of a material with a high proportion of elastic behaviour. The viscous component describes the extent to which the material dissipates energy that is put into it through permanent deformation or flow. Water is an example of a material that has no effective elastic behaviour but would undergo flow with only modest resistance when a force is applied to it. Hydrogel polymers show behaviour that is intermediate between that of water and an elastic band. Use of dynamic mechanical testing will tell us whether silicone hydrogels are substantially more elastic than conventional hydrogels. Figure 1.16 compares the magnitude of the viscous and elastic components of

Acuvue, Focus Night & Day and PureVision (Franklin *et al.*, 2002; Lydon *et al.*, 2002b).

It is immediately apparent that the dynamic mechanical properties of the two lens materials are not only significantly different from each other, particularly at higher frequencies, but also are greatly different from the conventional hydrogel material. One interesting manifestation of this difference between silicone hydrogels and conventional hydrogels is that the silicone materials become stiffer at increasing shear rate. This means, for example, that the materials show greater stiffness at deformation rates characteristic of the blink cycle than under the deformation encountered during handling. The stiffness of Focus Night & Day is measurably greater than that of PureVision, although the difference reduces as the frequency of deformation increases.

The characteristic combination of viscous and elastic components in a given material will change, then, in different ways depending on the 'speed' at which it is deformed. The behaviour of Acuvue, for example, changes little as the rate of oscillation is increased. We can deduce that its elastic behaviour does not change under the influence of eyelid movement. Both of the other materials do change, however, and it appears that PureVision acquires a noticeably greater level of elastic behaviour under the influence of eyelid movement, whereas Focus Night & Day, which is significantly stiffer that PureVision at low frequency, shows a steady increase in both its elastic and viscous components in moving from a low deformation rate to the sort of deformation encountered in the anterior eye.

It does seem clear that the combined effect of these mechanical property effects, together with the less than ideal wetting behaviour – particularly the high hysteresis – and the recognized importance and compromised nature of the post-lens tear film, is responsible for the observed back-surface complications, such as SEALs, corneal erosions and CLPC.

The first-generation silicone hydrogels have provided a clinical spearhead and brought a wealth of experimental raw material to the study of contact lens behaviour. It is logical to expect developments to this important class of materials that will enhance their performance and minimize patient problems.

REFERENCES

Alvord, L., Court, J., Davis, T. *et al.* (1998) Oxygen permeability of a new type of high *Dk* soft contact lens material. *Optom. Vis. Sci.*, **75**, 30–36

Bambury, R. E. and Seelye, D. (1991) Vinyl carbonate and vinyl carbamate contact lens material monomers. US Patent 5070215

Bambury, R. E. and Seelye, D. (1997) Vinyl carbonate and vinyl carbamate contact lens material monomers. US Patent 5610252

Franklin, V. J. and Tighe, B. J. (2002) Spoilation profiles of two extended wear hydrogel lenses. *Cont. Lens Ant. Eye*, **25**, 34

Franklin, V. J., Tonge, S. R., Lydon, F. J. and Tighe, B. J. (2002) Silicone hydrogels: a comparative study of surface and mechanical properties. *Cont. Lens Ant. Eye*, **26**, 210

Greisser, H. J., Laycock, B. P., Papaspiliotopoulos, E., Ho, A. *et al.* (1996) Extended wear ophthalmic lens. WO 96/31792

Grobe, G. L. (1999) Surface engineering aspects of silicone-hydrogel lenses. *Cont. Lens Spectrum* (suppl.) August

Harvey, T. B. (1985) Hydrophilic siloxane monomers and dimers for contact lens materials and contact lenses fabricated therefrom. US Patent 4711943

Jones, L., Senchyna, M., Louie, D. and Schickler, J. (2001) A comparative evaluation of lysozyme and lipid deposition on etafilcon, balafilcon and lotrafilcon contact lens materials. *Invest. Ophthalmol. Vis. Sci.*, **42**(s593), 3186

Künzler, J. F. (1999) Silicone-based hydrogels for contact lens application. *Cont. Lens Spectrum* (suppl.) August

Künzler, J. and Ozark, R. (1994) Fluorosilicone hydrogels. US Patent 5321108

Künzler, J. and Ozark, R. (1997) Methacrylate-capped fluoro side chain siloxanes: synthesis, characterization and their use in the design of oxygen-permeable hydrogels. *J. Appl. Polymer Sci.*, **65**, 1081–1089

Lopez-Alemany, A., Compan, V. and Refojo, M. F. (2002) Porous structure of Purevision versus Focus Night&Day and conventional hydrogel contact lenses. *J. Biomed. Mater. Res.*, **63**, 319–325

Lydon, F., Benning, B., Young, R. and Tighe, B. J. (2002a) Frictional behaviour of contact lenses and ophthalmic solutions: measurement and clinical consequences. *Cont. Lens Ant. Eye*, **25**, 35

Lydon, F., Tighe, B. J. and Young, R. (2002b) Techniques for the study of physico-chemical properties of corneal tissues and synthetic hydrogel substitutes. *Cont. Lens Ant. Eye*, **25**, 35

Maissa, C., Franklin, V. and Tighe, B. J. (1998) Influence of contact lens material surface characteristics and replacement frequency on protein and lipid deposition. *Optom. Vis. Sci.*, **75**, 697–705

McKenney, C., Becker, N., Thomas, S. *et al.* (1998) Lens deposits with a high *Dk* hydrophilic soft lens. *Optom. Vis. Sci.*, **75**, 276

Nicolson, P. C. and Vogt, J. (2001) Soft contact lens polymers: an evolution. *Biomaterials*, **22**, 3273–3283

Robertson, J. R., Su, K. C., Goldenberg, M. S. and Mueller, K. F. (1991) Wettable, flexible, oxygen permeable contact lens containing block copolymer polysiloxane-polyoxyalkylene backbone units and use thereof. US Patent 5070169

Ruben, M. (Ed.) (1978) *Soft Contact Lenses: Clinical and Applied Technology.* Wiley, New York, pp. 299–344

Senchyna, M., Jones, L., Louie, D. *et al.* (2002) Optimization of methodologies to characterize lysozyme deposition found on balafilcon and etafilcon contact lens materials. *Invest. Ophthalmol. Vis. Sci.*, ARVO abstract, 3082

Silicone Hydrogels (2001) Website: www.siliconehydrogels.org

Tanaka, K., Takahashi, K., Kanada, M., *et al.* (1979) Copolymer for soft contact lens, its preparation and soft contact lens made therefrom. US Patent 4139513

Tighe, B. J. and Franklin, V. J. (1999) Lens deposition and spoilation. In *The Eye in Contact Lens Wear* (ed. J. Larke). Butterworth-Heinemann, Oxford, Ch. 4

Chapter **2**

The epithelium in extended wear

Graeme Wilson, Patrick M. Ladage and
H. Dwight Cavanagh

INTRODUCTION

When the eye is open, the central cornea is remote from blood vessels. This isolation is compensated for by glands that use tears to deliver their secretions to the corneal surface. During sleep the epithelium of the cornea is in intimate contact with the epithelium of the back of the lid and thus has access to the capillaries of the palpebral conjunctiva. Transfer of substances is assisted by movements of the eye and lids. Part of the challenge of extended wear (EW) is that the lens interferes with this transfer because it continuously isolates the cornea both from tears and from the palpebral conjunctiva.

This chapter describes and enlarges upon the challenges EW presents to the ocular surface epithelia. The emphasis is on the corneal epithelium, with particular attention to how EW might affect the shedding of epithelial cells and maintenance of normal epithelial homeostasis.

THE CORNEAL EPITHELIUM

To understand the way cells might accumulate under an EW lens over a period of weeks it is useful to look at the migratory path of cells in the corneal epithelium and to enquire if there are homeostatic mechanisms to control the accumulation of cellular debris under the lens.

CELL MIGRATION AND MITOSIS

The basal cells of the corneal epithelium arise from stem cells at the limbus and migrate towards the centre of the cornea (Figure 2.1). This centripetal migration of epithelial cells from the limbus is very slow, so that cells take months to reach the centre of the cornea. Migration of the epithelium takes place mainly as a unit with

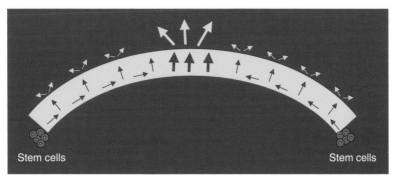

Figure 2.1   The migratory path of corneal epithelial cells from their origin at the limbus (stem cells) to shedding at the corneal surface

the basal cell layer, the overlying layers, epithelial nerves and possibly Langerhans cells all moving together (Auran *et al.*, 1995). As basal cells migrate they divide and, after a variable number of mitotic divisions, they move vertically towards the epithelial surface. Movement towards the surface is accompanied by differentiation, which includes loss of ability to divide, a gradual adoption of a squamous morphology and the development of a glycocalyx in cells approaching the surface. Over 40 years ago it was observed that some cells were sloughed three to four days after mitosis in the basal layer (Hanna and O'Brien, 1960). This gave rise to the idea that the whole corneal epithelium was replaced every three to four days. This logic is faulty for at least two reasons:

1. Not all cells move towards the surface after mitosis. Some might remain in the basal layer for further rounds of cell division (Beebe and Masters, 1996). Also, it has not been shown that all cells in the basal epithelium enter mitosis at frequent intervals and the regeneration time of the whole epithelium will depend on the cell cycle times of all cells in the basal cell population (Haaskjold *et al.*, 1989a). The cell cycle time includes the period between bursts of mitotic activity when the cell is quiescent.

2. Because it takes months for epithelial microcysts to be washed out of the cornea (Holden *et al.*, 1985) it must be assumed that there are structures in the basal layer which are not part of the replication pool of cells. For example, some immature Langerhans cells are present in the peripheral cornea although other immune system cells such as T cells, B cells, plasma cells, neutrophils and mast cells, which are present in the normal conjunctiva, are absent or rare in the cornea (Chandler, 1996).

Thus we do not know the regeneration time of the whole epithelium, even under normal circumstances. The idea of finding a single turnover time or replacement time for the epithelium is probably not useful.

Mitosis has a circadian rhythm, with greatest mitotic activity occurring early in the day (Fogle *et al.*, 1980; Haaskjold *et al.*, 1989b). It is likely that mitosis is under

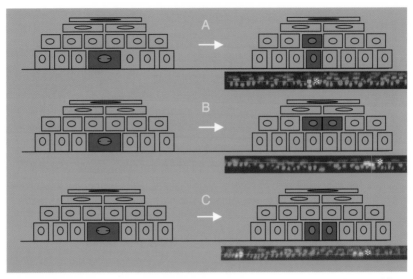

Figure 2.2 Schematic illustrations and stained rabbit corneal sections with propidium iodide and BrdU (*) show three possibilities open to the offspring of mitosis in the basal layer (Beebe and Masters, 1996). Option A is the least likely. The two daughter cells either migrate together to the corneal surface (Option B) or remain in the basal layer (Option C) (photographs by Dr Patrick M. Ladage)

some kind of central control as the two eyes appear to be synchronized. The mitotic rate can be reduced by a contact lens, which renders the epithelium hypoxic. Not all regions of the corneal epithelium contain cells of the same age and proliferative potential. For example, mitotic rate is higher in cells in the periphery of the cornea than in cells in the centre (Ebato *et al.*, 1988; Haaskjold *et al.*, 1990; Lehrer *et al.*, 1998; Ren *et al.*, 1999a; Ladage *et al.*, 2001a), and samples of peripheral epithelial cells migrate more rapidly in organ culture than do samples of central epithelial cells (Cameron *et al.*, 1989).

Following mitosis, a point of decision is reached for the two daughter cells. An obvious move in the interest of maintaining a constant number of cells in the epithelium would be for one daughter to remain in the basal layer and for the other to migrate to the surface to be shed into the tears (Figure 2.2). Thus one would leave and one would remain and the total number of cells would be unchanged. Recent research has shown, however, that the majority of paired daughter cells do not separate, but undergo terminal differentiation and move upward to be shed together from the corneal surface (Beebe and Masters, 1996 (rat); Ren *et al.*, 1999a; Ladage, 2002 (rabbit)). The distribution of mitotic activity of corneal epithelial cells is shown in the open and closed rabbit eye in Figure 2.3. The limbal area shows very low mitosis, corresponding to the location of stem cells. The proliferation rate of the corneal epithelium is the highest in the far periphery. Several recent studies have examined the effect of overnight contact lens wear on this normal proliferation process. Ren *et al.* (1999a) and Ladage *et al.* (2001a, 2003a) have shown that all contact lens wear (rigid gas-permeable (RGP),

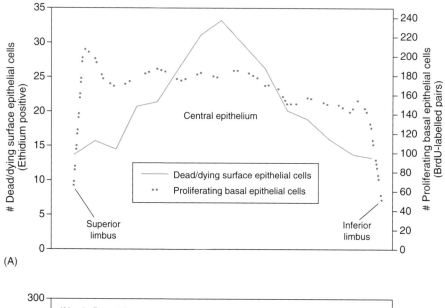

(A)

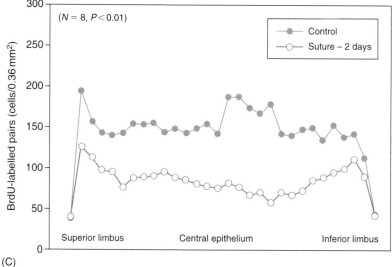

(C)

Figure 2.3   (A) Compilation graph showing the rates of basal cell proliferation (left *y*-axis) and surface cell death (right *y*-axis) from superior to inferior in the rabbit corneal and limbal epithelium. Note the regional differences: in the centre of the cornea most cells are dead/dying, while cell division occurs mostly in the far peripheral cornea. The limbus, by contrast, has a low epithelial cell division and surface cell death rate (Ladage, 2002). (B) Live/dead staining after prolonged eyelid closure (sutured) (Yamamoto *et al.*, 2002). (C) Proliferation rate of basal cells after prolonged eyelid closure (Ladage, 2002). (D) Annexin V staining after prolonged eyelid closure (Li *et al.*, 2002)

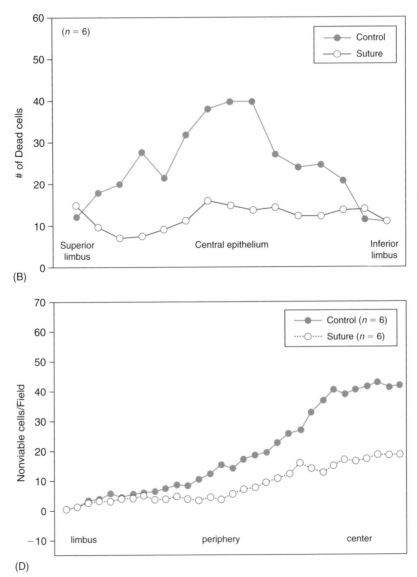

(B)

(D)

Figure 2.3 *Continued*

hydrogel (H) or silicone hydrogel (SiH)) depresses central corneal epithelial basal cell proliferation. This effect seems to be mediated in part by lens oxygen transmissibility: low O_2 transmission > hyper-O_2-transmitting SiH lenses. The process of orderly terminal differentiation and upward vertical migration of paired basal cells is also suppressed by contact lens wear (Ladage *et al.*, 2003b). Taken together, with contact lens-mediated suppression of surface corneal epithelial cell shedding, these observations in the animal model predict that contact lens wear will slow the overall process of normal corneal epithelial homeostasis. Basal cell proliferation/vertical migration, plus surface cell shedding loss, equals constant epithelial layer thickness. These effects have been demonstrated in recent long-term human clinical trials of EW, which have shown: (1) decreased epithelial layer thickness in the central cornea; (2) decreased corneal epithelial surface cell shedding; and (3) increased corneal surface cell size taken as a confirmation of longer surface residence time, i.e. correlates with decreased shedding rate (Ren *et al.*, 1999b, 2002). These trials have also demonstrated: (1) both lens type and lens oxygen transmission effects – RGP > H > SiH and lower O_2 > hyper-O_2 RGP or SiH lenses; and (2) adaptive effects over time with attempted physiological recovery during prolonged EW to return to pre-lens surface shedding and thickness values. These results are shown in Figures 2.4 and 2.5.

CELL SHEDDING

After the daughters have lost their attachment to the basement membrane they can no longer divide and are committed to being exfoliated from the surface in a few days (Beebe and Masters, 1996). At any position on the cornea, the most mature cells are on the surface. These are referred to as terminally differentiated cells. However, as shown in Figure 2.1, it is clear that terminally differentiated cells reach this position along path lengths from the stem cells that are very different. The most travelled (and probably oldest) epithelial cells will be located in the central cornea. In support of this, more dead cells have been reported on the central epithelial surface than on the peripheral surface (Ren and Wilson, 1996a; Yamamoto *et al.*, 2002).

Attempts have been made to find a quantitative relationship between the rate at which cells are shed and the number of dead cells on the corneal surface. There are fluorescent labels which can be used to identify dying cells, such as the two terminally differentiated cells shown in Figure 2.6. It can be seen that the normal surface has a large number of living cells (green) and fewer dead cells (red). It has been estimated that after washing the surface, between 1 per cent (Ren and Wilson, 1996a) and 20 per cent (Jester *et al.*, 1998) of cells on the surface are dead. In support of the death–shedding relation, the number of dead cells on the surface increases when the eye is exposed to surfactants and the increase in dead cells is accompanied by epithelial thinning (Jester *et al.*, 1998). Epithelial thinning is taken as an indication that a large number of cells have been lost. However, under normal circumstances, a relationship between the number of dying cells on the surface and the rate at which cells are shed has not yet been established (Ren and Wilson, 1997).

Recent quantitative estimates have been reported for the number and distribution of 'dead/dying' surface corneal epithelial cells in both human (Yamamoto *et al.*, 2001a) and rabbit (Yamamoto *et al.*, 2001b, 2001c, 2002; Li *et al.*, 2002) surface corneal cells. Collectively these quantitative whole-mount studies have demonstrated a central peak of dead/dying surface corneal epithelial cells by TUNEL, Annexin V and live–dead assays in the normal cornea (open eye; Figure 2.3). The oxygen-related pro-survival protein Bcl-2 appears to regulate this process. There are no Bcl-2-positive epithelial surface cells that are simultaneously TUNEL-positive

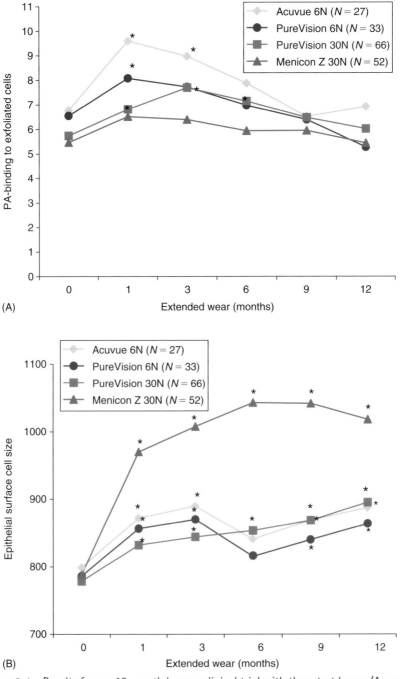

Figure 2.4   Results from a 12-month human clinical trial with three test lenses (Acuvue, PureVision or Menicon Z) following six or 30 nights' EW. Four outcome measures were studied: (A) *P. aeruginosa* binding to exfoliated corneal epithelial surface cells; (B) corneal epithelial thickness; (C) corneal epithelial surface cell size; (D) corneal epithelial surface exfoliation rates (Ren *et al.*, 2002)

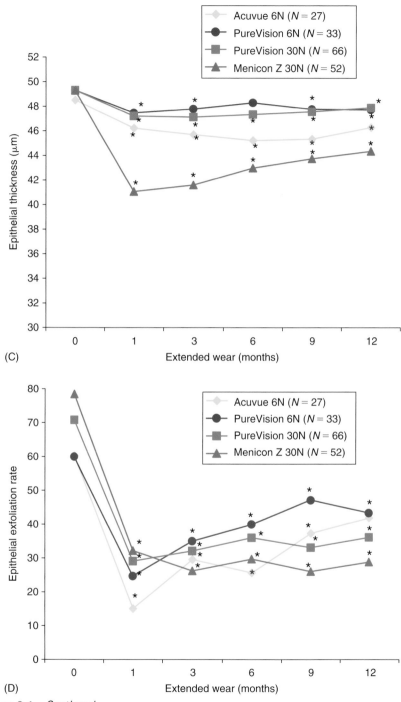

Figure 2.4   *Continued*

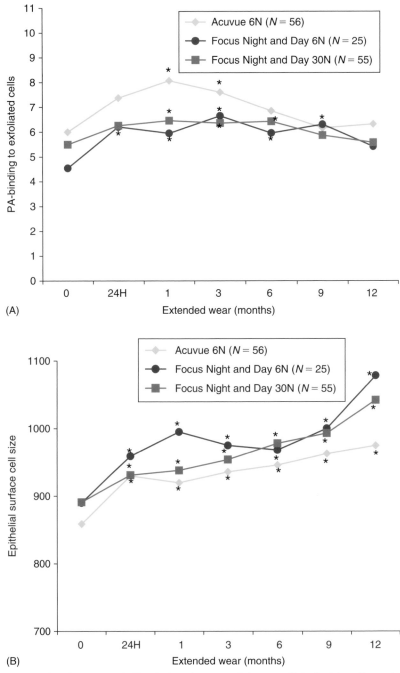

Figure 2.5   Results from a similar designed 12-month human clinical trial as Figure 2.4 with two test lenses (Acuvue, Focus Night & Day) following six or 30 nights' EW. Four outcome measures were studied: (A) *P. aeruginosa* to exfoliated corneal epithelial surface cells; (B) corneal epithelial thickness; (C) corneal epithelial surface cell size; (D) corneal epithelial surface exfoliation rates (Cavanagh *et al.*, 2002)

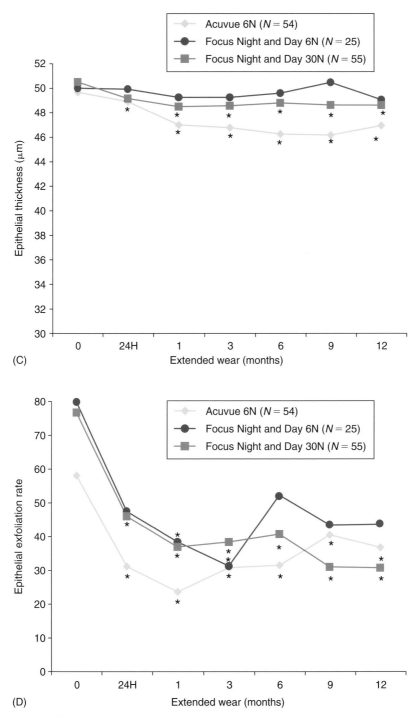

Figure 2.5   *Continued*

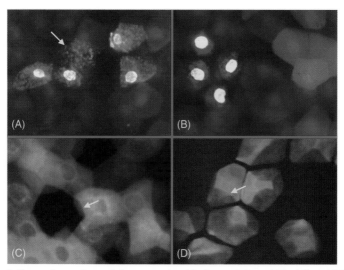

Figure 2.6   Cells on the surface of the corneal epithelium of the rabbit. (A) and (B) are stained with calcein and ethidium homodimer. The nuclei of dead cells fluoresce red and living cells fluoresce green. Dead cells show red staining of the nucleus and punctate staining of the cytoplasm; (C) and (D) show cells stained with rose bengal. The arrows identify the images of cell ghosts which have failed to take up stain in the same way as underlying nucleated cells (photomicrographs by Dr David H. Ren)

(Yamamoto *et al.*, 2001a, 2001b, 2001c) in the human (eye bank cornea *in vitro*) or the *in vivo* rabbit model. Both eyelid closure and all contact lens wear cause Bcl-2 expression (pro-survival) to persist in the nuclei of the epithelial surface cells, correspondingly decreasing the number of dead/dying surface cells (TUNEL, Annexin V or live–dead positive). Thus, the disappearance of Bcl-2 expression in central surface corneal epithelial cells appears to be a prerequisite for normal apoptotic cell shedding to occur (Figure 2.7). Based on an average number of 151 ± 17 superficial epithelial cells covering 3.0 mm of the central human cornea in each tissue section, approximately 4.3 per cent of surface cells in the cornea show loss of Bcl-2 immunostaining and 2.5 per cent of surface cells show DNA fragmentation identified by TUNEL labelling (Yamamoto *et al.*, 2001a). Even taking into account differences in species and post-mortem handling, the amount of TUNEL-positive labelling in the *ex vivo* human cornea is still quite consistent with that identified for the *in vitro* rabbit cornea (Ren and Wilson, 1996a). The 2:1 ratio of Bcl-2 negative and TUNEL-positive surface epithelial cells *in situ* also matches that found for human exfoliated corneal epithelial cells *in vivo*. Estil and Wilson (2000) found that only 57 per cent of shed cells showed TUNEL-positive labelling. Although this latter investigation postulated the existence of a non-apoptotic pathway to explain the pressure of a population of TUNEL-negative shed cells, the persistence of Bcl-2 expression in superficial surface corneal epithelial cells suggests that DNA fragmentation is downstream of initial events leading to cell shedding for which loss of nuclear Bcl-2 is a precondition.

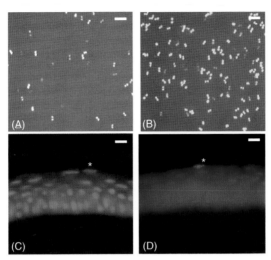

Figure 2.7 (A) BrdU labelling (= proliferation) of the central corneal epithelium following short-term low-*Dk* RGP lens wear versus (B) a control cornea; (C) Bcl-2 is expressed in all nuclei of the corneal epithelium with the exception of isolated surface cells (*) prior to apoptotic exfoliation; (D) TUNEL labelling (*) shows a surface epithelial cell undergoing apoptosis (photographs by Dr Patrick M. Ladage and Kazuaki Yamamoto). Scale bar = 10 µm

SURFACE CELL TYPES

Contact lens cytology

Staining of cells using fluorescent microscopy techniques in which cells can be viewed immediately and do not have to be fixed suggests that there might be several later changes which occur in cells as they sit on the corneal surface. An easy way of collecting cells is by using a soft contact lens in which cells are irrigated from the lens after it has been removed from the eye (Figure 2.8). The technique is known as contact lens cytology (CLC). Cells collected in this way have the same appearance as cells irrigated from the pre-corneal film with a corneal irrigating chamber (Figure 2.8). In Figure 2.9 cells are shown which have progressed beyond the point of having an intact nucleus. These cell-like structures have the cytoplasmic character of squamous epithelial cells but lack a nucleus. They are referred to as cell ghosts. Unfortunately they are similar in appearance to keratinized skin cells; therefore, much caution has been shown by experimenters in declaring that they arise from the cornea. However, a model has been presented which suggests that cell ghosts are a late stage of terminal differentiation of corneal epithelial cells (Estil and Wilson, 2000).

Investigators observing the human cornea with specular microscopy have described the size of cells on the epithelial surface using both cell area and cell length. The mean cell area has a reported range of 355–850 µm^2 (Nelson *et al.*, 1983; Mathers and Lemp, 1992; Barr and Testa, 1994). Cell length has been reported at 20–75 µm (Lohman *et al.*, 1982). Using cells removed from the back

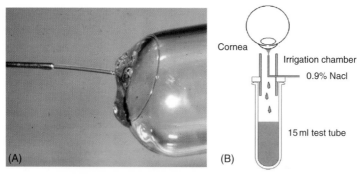

Figure 2.8   (A) The technique of CLC in which cells are irrigated from a hydrogel lens after removal from the eye. In this case cells are being collected from only the back surface of the lens. (B) The eye irrigation chamber to collect epithelial cells in a tube as developed by Dr G. Wilson and revised by Ren *et al.* (1999a)

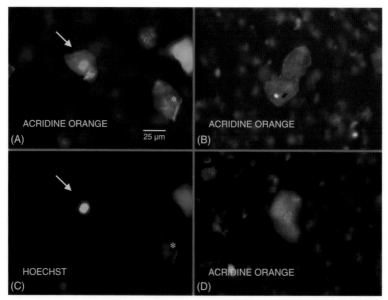

Figure 2.9   Nucleated cells and cell ghosts collected by CLC. (A) and (C) show the same preparation which has been stained with both acridine orange and Hoechst. The arrows show the nucleus of the same cell, which stains blue with Hoechst in (C) and green with acridine orange in (A). A cell ghost is shown with an asterisk (*). Cell ghosts are also shown in (B) and (D) (photomicrographs by Dr Salih Al Oliky)

surface of a contact lens (CLC), a mean of $35.3 \pm 5.1\,\mu m$ has been reported for cell length from normal eyes (Laurent and Wilson, 1997), corresponding to a mean cell area of $670\,\mu m^2$. Similar sizes have been found using scanning electron microscopy (SEM). The size of cells on the surface varies with a number of factors. There is a decrease in cell size (μm^2) when the relative percentage of dead cells increases (Jester *et al.*, 1998). In EW the size of corneal surface cells increases with the wearing time (Tsubota *et al.*, 1996). A summary of cell size in normal, daily wear (DW) and dry eye is shown in Figure 2.10.

In vivo confocal microscopy

In vivo confocal microscopy is a new imaging technique that allows non-invasive measurement of sizes of corneal epithelial cells within individual corneal epithelial layers (three-dimensional viewing in depth versus flat two-dimensional surface viewing afforded by specular microscopy and SEM). The normal rabbit or human corneal epithelium demonstrates five to seven cell layers, with the outer three characterized by flattened and elongated cells. The most superficial central surface cells (pre-desquamation) are the largest ($903 \pm 15\ \mu m^2$, human) and $1502 \pm 237\ \mu m^2$, rabbit), which corresponds to the mean cell size of desquamated cells in the tear film ($875 \pm 117\ \mu m^2$, human, and $1436 \pm 286\ \mu m^2$, rabbit; Ren *et al.*, 1997). Figures 2.4 and 2.5 show the results of increased changes in corneal epithelial surface cell size measured by *in vivo* confocal microscopy following prolonged EW in recent clinical trials (Cavanagh *et al.*, 2002; Ren *et al.*, 2002). In these long-term wearing studies, surface cell size increases are dependent upon lens type (RGP > H = SiH). Adaptation with a trend towards a return to pre-lens surface cell size is also demonstrated (Figures 2.4 and 2.5).

BARRIER FUNCTION

The corneal and conjunctival epithelia must maintain a barrier to protect the deeper and more vulnerable layers of cells. Tight junctions, and the membranes of the cells which make them, provide this permeability barrier between the interior of the epithelium and the outside world. It can be disrupted easily by trauma, by preservatives (Bernal and Ubels, 1991; Ubels, 1998) and by inadequate oxygen transmissibility (Ichijima *et al.*, 1999). Techniques have been developed for studying permeability in humans (McNamara *et al.*, 1997), and it has been found that EW does cause an increase in permeability (McNamara *et al.*, 1998a).

Squamous cells with tight junctions are polarized in the sense that the membranes on the two sides of the cell are different. Proteins in the cell membrane facing the pre-corneal tears are better able to defend the cell against bacterial attack than those on the side which faces the wing cells. Some proteins in the cell membrane cannot migrate past the tight junctions, so they remain facing the deeper wing cells and are not exposed to the pre-corneal tears. Some of these proteins are vulnerable to bacterial attachment (lectins) and remain hidden when surface cell tight junctions are intact. Recently, however, it has been shown in both the rabbit model and human clinical studies in both DW and EW that lens oxygen transmission can regulate specific lectin binding sites to *Pseudomonas aeruginosa* (Imayasu *et al.*, 1994; Ren *et al.*, 1999b; Ladage *et al.*, 2001b; Ren *et al.*, 2002, Cavanagh *et al.*, 2002). Specifically, DW or EW of either RGP or SiH lenses which are composed of novel hyper-oxygen-transmitting materials either do not increase

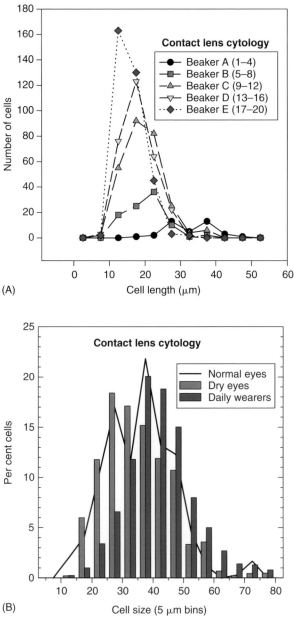

Figure 2.10   (A) The size of cells collected when a hydrogel lens is removed repeatedly from the eye (Primo, 1997). All the cells from the first four removals were irrigated into Beaker A (collections 1–4), and all the cells from the last four removal into Beaker E (collections 17–20). (B) The size of cells collected by CLC from three different categories of patients: diagnosed dry eye, daily contact lens wearers and normal non-contact lens wearers (normals). The data are collated from three different studies (Laurent and Wilson, 1997; Wilson and Laurent, 1998; Wilson et al., 1998). Contact lens wearers tend to have larger cells than normal, and dry eye patients tend to have smaller cells than normal

lens-related *P. aeruginosa* binding over pre-lens baseline control values or promote significantly less *P. aeruginosa* binding *in vivo* than wear of conventional hydrogel counterparts (Figures 2.4 and 2.5; Ladage *et al.*, 2001a; Ren *et al.*, 2002; Cavanagh *et al.*, 2002). Taken together, these data suggest that wear of these hyper-oxygen lenses should be accompanied by a lessened risk for the development of microbial keratitis. It is worth noting, however, that at least under *in vitro* laboratory conditions (incubation of a solution of *P. aeruginosa* with isolated corneas or corneal epithelial cell cultures) there are strains of *P. aeruginosa* which can attack the corneal epithelial cells by directly entering the cell without the prerequisite of initial attachments (Zaidi *et al.*, 1996; Fleiszig *et al.*, 1998). Hence, even a normal epithelium may be susceptible to invasion by some bacterial strains. At this stage we do not yet have a completely clear idea of all the ways in which microbial keratitis may be initiated by invading bacteria. Furthermore, there are strains of *P. aeruginosa* that attack the epithelium by directly entering the cell rather than evading the barrier of the cell membrane (Zaidi *et al.*, 1996; Fleiszig *et al.*, 1998). Hence an epithelium with intact tight junctions can still be invaded by some bacterial strains. However, it might be that shedding cells should capture bacteria, like fly paper, so that harmful organisms can be transported away from the corneal surface. Arguments can be mustered in both directions: either that capture of *Pseudomonas* by shedding cells is protective (fly paper), or that it is harmful (indicative of invasion of the surface epithelium). At this stage we do not have a complete understanding of the mechanisms by which the epithelium is invaded by bacteria which cause microbial keratitis under *in vivo* conditions.

THE SHEDDING RATE

The rate at which cells detach from the surface of the corneal epithelium in relation to the rate at which they can be transported away could determine the success of EW. Thus it is of some consequence to examine what is known about the rate at which cells are shed from the surface. There are obviously a number of factors at the surface that could alter the rate at which cells leave. Attention is directed to several factors in tears which are known to change and which might affect the shedding rate:

1. Osmolality

When the osmolality is very high or very low, the shedding rate is increased (Wilson, 1996). However, in near physiological conditions (260–350 mOsm/kg) osmolality changes do not cause increased shedding. Any osmolality changes occurring in EW will be well within this range.

2. Hypoxia

Many physiological effects of hypoxia in contact lens wear have been studied but the interest in relation to cell shedding is recent. When the rabbit cornea was bathed with a solution containing no oxygen there was an immediate reduction in the shedding of cells from the epithelium. Over the first hour of hypoxia the shedding rate was less than half that of the control (Wilson, 1994). After about two hours there was no difference in shedding rate between a hypoxic cornea and a control. In human subjects wearing nitrogen goggles over a period of 6 hours, the total effect was a reduction in shedding over that time period (Ren *et al.*, 1999c). Thus there is agreement among authors that hypoxia can reduce shedding rate in the short term. What happens over a period of anoxia greater than six hours or even several days is complicated by other factors such as the nocturnal environment and circadian effects.

In the long run shedding rate affects the thickness of the epithelium, which depends on the balance between cell loss and cell production. Even with lenses of high oxygen transmissibility ($Dk/L = 95$), the epithelium thins (Ren *et al.*, 1999b). Recent human clinical studies have shown a decrease in surface cell shedding in both DW and EW (Ren *et al.*, 1999b, 2002; Ladage *et al.*, 2001a; Cavanagh *et al.*, 2002), which suggests a slowdown in epithelial turnover. This decrease in corneal surface cell shedding is accompanied by a concomitant suppression of basal cell mitosis, which is regulated, in part, by lens oxygen transmission (Ladage *et al.*, 2002).

3. Toxic exposure

Preservatives such as benzalkonium chloride and surfactants (Jester *et al.*, 1998) increase the shedding rate, as does exposure to suprathreshold ultraviolet radiation (Ren and Wilson, 1994).

4. Small ions

Any contact lens is a barrier to the traffic of cells and large molecules between the epithelial surface and tears, but small molecules which can diffuse through a lens will not be withheld from the ocular surface. Potassium and calcium have been shown to have a role in the maintenance of the epithelium (Bachman and Wilson, 1985) and could affect shedding rates. Potassium has been included in irrigating solutions and tear supplements for this reason. Incubation of cells in low-calcium solutions leads to detachment of cells (Wang *et al.*, 1993). When tight junctions are affected by ionic deficiency they are reassembled deeper in the wing cells (Wolosin and Chen, 1993). Thus there is no evidence that inaccessibility to small ions is a problem with contact lenses.

5. Shear forces

A major change that the epithelium experiences during EW is the prolonged absence of a shearing force removing cells from the surface. The data giving credence to the existence of this force come from a number of different experiments. These are described in some detail as it is likely that cell shedding and corneal surface stagnation will become of increasing importance in EW.

Some effort has been directed at defining a constant set of conditions for the measurement of shedding rate so that there would be some standard against which other rates could be compared (Ren and Wilson, 1996b). It was found that mechanical forces applied to the surface played a significant part in the rate cells were collected (Ren and Wilson, 1996b). This led to the idea that the shear force of the lids during blinking is the main factor outside the epithelium which causes cells to be removed. It is not possible in the human eye to remove this factor completely, so an experiment was performed in an excised rabbit cornea which could be maintained in an environment that was free from shear forces (Ren and Wilson, 1997). A clear difference was found between a static surface and a surface perturbed by a solution in motion. The static surface had a shedding rate of 7 cells/min per cornea, while the perturbed surface had an average shedding rate of 54 cells/min per cornea. However, even in unperturbed corneas, shedding rates up to 400 cells/min per cornea have been reported. In general, the lowest shedding rates occurred when minimal shear force was applied to the surface. The term 'spontaneous shedding rate' has been coined to describe the rate at which cells are presumed to leave the surface in the absence of any shear force (Ren and Wilson, 1996b).

The question arises of whether these results are applicable to the human eye. The answer was provided by subjecting the human cornea to differences in shear force. The shear force was provided by removing a hydrogel lens 20 times from the eye (Wilson and Primo, 1997). Cells removed from the lenses had the appearance shown in Figure 2.6. The number of nucleated cells was counted and measured for size. In Figure 2.10 it is seen that more and more cells are collected with each removal. In this experiment an additional effect was revealed which had been predicted from earlier experiments on rabbit eyes (Ren and Wilson, 1997); as more cells are shed from the cornea they become smaller in size. Interestingly, a similar effect has been reported when a surfactant is applied to the eye (Jester et al., 1998). The general rule emerging from these experiments is that when the surface is irritated the number of cells shed increases and the cells decrease in size. How can this be explained? The first possibility is that surface cells are being removed by the lens (or by the surfactant) and smaller underlying cells are being uncovered and then being shed. However, in the case of the contact lens experiment, when the number of cells lost from the surface is considered in the context of the total number of cells available on the surface, the numbers do not add up. Not enough cells have been removed to reach the wing cells, and such a massive loss of cells would inevitably be accompanied by greater discomfort than subjects experienced. A second possibility is that CLC is removing select groups of cells: initially it removes the larger cells, and then later it removes the smaller cells in the group that are ready to shed. A third possibility is that apoptosis has been invoked as a protective mechanism (Ren and Wilson, 1996a). Apoptosis (programmed cell death) occurs in many tissues and describes a form of cell death that does not produce a destructive inflammatory response. Apoptosis is quite distinct from necrosis, in which the chaotic dissolution of the cell initiates an inflammatory response which can in itself cause damage to healthy cells. Apoptosis is an orderly mechanism for removing cells that are no longer useful. Whether this change in cell size is an apoptotic process, or simply due to selection of smaller cells from the epithelial surface, has yet to be determined.

Stratified epithelia are designed to withstand friction, and have well-defined programmes to deal with mechanical excesses. In the case of the fingers and palms, the epithelium increases the number of stratified layers as a protective mechanism. If this long-term response is overwhelmed, a blister is formed between the layers of the skin as a short-term defence. In the case of the cornea, the shedding of more and smaller cells appears to be its programmed response to mechanical friction. It also seems likely that, analogous to the squames on the surface of the skin, more cells which have lost their nuclei are laid down on the surface of the epithelium as a sacrificial first line. There has been considerable reluctance to admit the presence of these netherworld structures or cell ghosts on the surface of the cornea. However, the evidence is accumulating that ghosts on the surface of the epithelium are real and they must be included in models of the pre-corneal film (Estil and Wilson, 1998). A model for the formation of cell ghosts is shown in Figure 2.11. It is possible that the progression of a living cell on the surface from a terminally differentiated cell to cell ghost is a specialized form of apoptosis.

The above results suggest that the shear force exerted on the normal eye by the lids may have a profound effect on the rate cells are removed from the surface. If, however, cells are collected from three different groups of normal, dry eye and extended-lens-wearing subjects using CLC (Wilson and Laurent, 1998), the results suggest that lid shear force can be an important determinant of shedding rate.

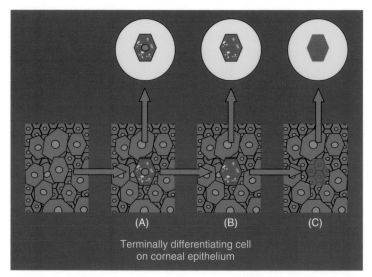

Figure 2.11   A model that explains how cell ghosts can be formed at the epithelial surface. The yellow circles show the appearance of dying cells after they have been collected on a contact lens and visualized using fluorescence microscopy. A cell progresses from a typical viable cell on the surface (far left), to a dying cell with a nucleus (A), to a cell ghost with no nucleus and some enzyme activity in the cytoplasm (B), to a cell ghost in its final stage (C)

As shown in Figure 2.10, dry-eye subjects tend to have smaller cells, while overnight lens wear increases corneal surface epithelial cell size (Cavanagh *et al.*, 2002; Ren *et al.*, 2002). When the ability of different hydrogel lenses to remove cells from the cornea was measured using CLC, there were no differences among the three lens types tested (Wilson *et al.*, 1998). When the normal rabbit eye is closed, however, cell surface death and presumably shedding are decreased (Li *et al.*, 2002; Yamamoto *et al.*, 2001c). Overnight contact lens wear mimics eyelid closure (no lid shear force) and also decreases surface cell death and shedding (Yamamoto *et al.*, 2001a; Li *et al.*, 2002; Ren *et al.*, 2002; Cavanagh *et al.*, 2002). In this regard, the contact lens may shield the corneal surface from the effect(s) of lid shear forces, resulting in decreased surface cell death and shedding.

6.   Tear replenishment

The rate at which cells are lost from the epithelium is affected by the presence of a contact lens. Although the loss of cells from the epithelium itself is reduced, cells accumulate beneath the lens as a result of the relatively low rate of tear exchange. This stagnation could be problematic from two points of view. Firstly, it might in some way be unhealthy for the epithelium to have the shedding of cells reduced. Secondly, the stagnation of cells on the surface facilitates invasion by foreign organisms. Under either of these circumstances, removal of these cells is crucial. The issue becomes not whether they are attached or unattached to the surface, but whether they have been removed. Thus the rate of replenishment of tears beneath the lens could be the crucial issue. It has long been known that hard lenses pump faster than soft lenses. Fluorometric methods are available to make these measurements (McNamara *et al.*, 1998b). Whether SiH lenses are better or worse than other lenses in this respect can be determined (Chapter 3).

THE PRE-CORNEAL FILM

The corneal surface is the interface between the eye and the outside world. Interfaces are regions where order is often challenged, so it is important to understand how the corneal surface functions even before a contact lens is in place. Classical textbooks on ocular anatomy reveal the cornea as a structure terminating with the squamous cells of the corneal epithelium. The pre-corneal film cannot be visualized using traditional light microscopy because the epithelial surface is washed with fixatives. In such images the surface of corneal cells contains microplicae and the nucleus is visible (Beuerman and Pedroza, 1996). Traditional electron microscopy and light microscopy show a surface that is missing components which are present in the pre-corneal film of the living eye. However, rapid cryofixation reveals the presence of these structures and suggests that not all superficial cells have microplicae and that they are lacking other organelles. Although the aged epithelial cells lacked microplicae, the tear film remained on them (Chen *et al.*, 1995). This finding does not support the belief that microplicae are essential for an intact, overlying pre-corneal film. The tear layer is thicker on the normally dense surface cells, which are well attached to the underlying layers, and thinner on the low-density cells, which are not well attached (Chen *et al.*, 1995). This observation is at odds with the belief that the pre-corneal film is of even thickness. There are no maps of the thickness of the pre-corneal film so any statements regarding variations in thickness of the pre-corneal film must be speculative at this stage.

Each corneal structure, from posterior to anterior, contributes to the eventual smoothness of the surface. The final optical interface between air and eye is the lipid layer, which is the smoothest of all the surfaces. It disperses over the aqueous component of the tears at each blink and is anchored at the orifices of the meibomian glands above and below. It does not take part in the flow of tears from lateral canthus to punctum. Debris and desquamated cells flow along the lacrimal river but beneath the lipid layer. At each blink the smooth surface of the squamous cells of the marginal conjunctiva and the secretions of the conjunctival glands are drawn over the surface of the corneal epithelium. It was suggested, many years ago, that blinking rubbed conjunctival secretion into the corneal epithelium to form the deepest layer of the pre-corneal film (Wolff, 1976).

Beneath the pre-corneal film a substructure is provided by tight junctions which draw the living squamous cells together over the deeper epithelial cells. One can speculate that this tension is aided at the limbus by the rete pegs of epithelial cells which dip down and anchor into the episclera (Bron *et al.*, 1985), so that the epithelial surface is like a tent held down by peripheral guy lines staked into stable ground. Shedding cells must break through this canopy as they move from the epithelial compartment to the aqueous compartment of the pre-corneal film. A cell is thick enough to contribute significantly to the thickness of the tears. However, electron microscopy of the pre-corneal film shows that the aqueous component becomes thinner when a cell enters it. In this way the smoothness of the lipid layer is maintained (Chen *et al.*, 1997). Finally, the lipid layer reduces irregularities in the surface of the pre-corneal film and presents a smooth surface to incident light.

BLINKING

Blinking removes debris from the pre-corneal film and maintains the corneal surface in a condition which sustains acute vision. Most of the lid activity of blinking is accomplished by the upper lid. The downward movement is accomplished with a quickly accelerating motion followed by a much slower return (Doane, 1980). These movements have different functions. The slow retraction of the lids might have some action in reconstituting the pre-corneal film, which would not be accomplished with a fast movement. The rapid downward movement of the upper lid sweeps the surface clean like a squeegee and deposits debris in the marginal tear strip, in which it will be conveyed to the puncta. However, masses of dead cells have been observed piled up on the marginal conjunctiva (Doughty, 1997). Thus, when the ebb and flow of the marginal tear strip fail to carry detritus into the puncta, the marginal conjunctiva becomes the beach upon which the flotsam and jetsam of the ocular surface are cast by the pounding of the lids.

THE CONJUNCTIVAL EPITHELIUM

Most of the early effort in studying the biological effect of contact lenses on the eye was directed towards the cornea. However, papillary conjunctivitis associated with contact lens wear attracted the attention of clinicians and researchers to the palpebral conjunctiva (for a review see Efron, 1997). It is now clear that because of the differences in morphology, function and immunology all regions of the conjunctiva must be considered.

The conjunctival epithelium was once viewed as being interchangeable with the corneal epithelium, but detailed research revealed that it has a distinct lineage with a separate anatomical origin. The corneal epithelium arises from stem cells in the limbus and the conjunctival epithelium arises from stem cells in the fornices (Wei *et al.*, 1993, 1995). Conjunctival cells migrate from the fornical stem cells by two routes. One route takes them from the fornix to the bulbar conjunctiva and towards the limbus and the other to the palpebral conjunctiva and towards the margins of the lids. Recent evidence suggests that there may be another population of stem cells at the lid margin.

MUCUS

The tears over the conjunctiva are derived not just from the lacrimal gland but also from the secretions of the goblet cells and of the epithelial cells themselves. The conjunctiva expresses surface antigens, adhesion molecules and cytokines (Hingorani *et al.*, 1998). Inflammatory cells in the conjunctiva also patrol the ocular surface (Begley *et al.*, 1998) and cytokines are present in the tears.

Goblet cells share the same progenitor as other cells of the conjunctiva and, therefore, are part of the conjunctival lineage (Wei *et al.*, 1996). Goblet cells can be sampled and counted using impression cytology. Reports generally describe the bulbar conjunctiva because it is readily accessible. However, goblet cells and many other accessory lacrimal glands enjoy a ubiquitous distribution over the entire conjunctiva, including the tarsal portion of the palpebral conjunctiva (Bergmanson *et al.*, 1999). The secretions of goblet cells are mucin molecules which, in a hydrated form, become important structural and functional components of the pre-ocular tears (Inatomi *et al.*, 1996). There are nine distinct mucins, numbered MUC1 to MUC8, with two MUC5 mucins. MUC1 is a membrane-spanning mucin which, as a result of its long extended structure, can extend beyond the glycocalyx and possibly prevent bacterial adherence to the surface (Inatomi *et al.*, 1995). MUC1 appears to be associated with the cell membrane of both the conjunctiva and the cornea (Inatomi *et al.*, 1995) but doubt has been expressed about its presence in the corneal epithelium (Jumblatt *et al.*, 1999). One of the MUC5 mucins (MUC5AC) has been isolated from tears using Schirmer strips (Jumblatt *et al.*, 1999) but tears collected specifically from the pre-corneal film have not been tested. It has been suggested that the entire ocular surface epithelium produces mucins for the tear film (Watanabe *et al.*, 1995). In gastro-intestinal and respiratory tissues, where mucins have been most studied, they function as buffers, antioxidants and inhibitors of bacterial adhesion. However, the roles of specific mucins in mediating these effects are not fully understood in the cornea or elsewhere (Jumblatt *et al.*, 1999). There is some evidence that the glycocalyx is not evenly distributed over the surface of corneal epithelial cells and may be present in subsurface cells (Chen *et al.*, 1995, 1997). Changes in the corneal glycocalyx layer physically and biochemically have been reported, which are greatest when the Dk/L of the contact lenses is low (Latkovic and Nilsson, 1997).

There is an abundance of growth factors in the ocular surface tears which regulate cell proliferation and differentiation (You *et al.*, 1999). Their influences are complex, with the current explosion in molecular biology ensuring they will become even more so.

SHEDDING

The shedding of conjunctival cells has not attracted the same attention as the corneal epithelium. Unlike the cornea, the conjunctiva does not have a uniform number of cellular layers and may be as thin as two layers in some regions (Gipson, 1994). Cells of the conjunctival epithelium are less squamous than cells of the cornea and probably do not shed as readily. For example, desquamating cells are hard to locate on the tarsal conjunctiva with the electron microscope (Doughty, 1997) and the structure of most of the conjunctival epithelium suggests that it does not have the same high shedding rate as the cornea. The bulbar conjunctiva has cells with a small surface area. The general belief is that epithelia with high shedding rates have squamous cells on their surfaces. Skin has such a structure and, in regions of high friction, has many layers of stratified cells. Such cells serve to protect the underlying epithelium, as very little change is wrought upon underlying cells when they leave the surface. There has been a suggestion that the shedding of cells from the conjunctiva might occur at the marginal conjunctiva at the edge of the lids where cells are relatively squamous (Doughty and Panju, 1995; Greiner *et al.*, 1997). However, this could also be an accumulation of corneal cells which have been swept from the corneal epithelium during blinking.

BULBAR CONJUNCTIVA

Changes in cells in contact lens wear occur in the bulbar conjunctiva (Aragona *et al.*, 1998), including increased keratinization, snake-shaped nuclear material, increased inflammatory cells and reduced nucleus-to-cytoplasm ratios. There are differences in goblet cell counts and nucleus-to-cytoplasm ratio between RGP lenses and hydrogel lenses. Some studies reported that all patients showed squamous metaplasia (Knop and Brewitt, 1992). Squamous metaplasia is an enlargement of the cell cytoplasm, which is abnormal in conjunctival cells. Such enlargement is normal in the corneal epithelium as part of the mechanism to reduce stress on the surface and present a barrier of sacrificial cells which can be sheared from the surface without affecting the stability of the tissue.

In soft lens wear snake-like chromatin has been demonstrated throughout the whole bulbar conjunctiva (Knop and Brewitt, 1992), although these changes appear first in the upper bulbar conjunctiva, as this is the conjunctival region which is most exposed to excursions of the lens off the cornea (Knop and Brewitt, 1992). Similar changes have been reported in RGP wear (Adar *et al.*, 1997). Thus contact lens wear places stress on the conjunctiva. Dry eye also places stress on the conjunctiva and so it is not surprising that contact lens overwear can have similar symptoms (Knop and Brewitt, 1992).

PALPEBRAL CONJUNCTIVA

As evidence of regional differences in epithelial response, the force of rubbing the ocular surface through the lids produces very different effects on the tarsal conjunctival epithelium compared with the corneal epithelium (Greiner *et al.*, 1997). When rubbing the eye with the palm against the closed lid, the upper tarsal conjunctiva is brought in contact with the cornea forcibly. Stratified cuboidal epithelium is not usually subjected to such friction. The upper tarsal conjunctiva showed evidence of disrupted surface cells, characterized by superficial epithelial cells assuming a spheroidal shape. In the corneal epithelium an increase in exfoliating cells was observed but disappeared after four hours. Stratified squamous epithelia are designed to withstand friction by means of their multilayered squamoid cells (Greiner *et al.*, 1997).

The well-being of the ocular surface requires normality in all of its components (Liotet *et al.*, 1987; Versura *et al.*, 1999), each of which can change independent of the others. Thus, the ocular surface is a functional unit represented by the corneal and conjunctival epithelia, the tear film and other structures (Versura *et al.*, 1999). The privileged immune status of the cornea is due to the delegation of its needs to the conjunctiva, which contains an abundance of lymphoid tissue (Chodosh *et al.*, 1998). Conjunctival inflammation can be tolerated because the optical requirements are less demanding than those of the cornea. Whenever one of the components changes its functional, physical or chemical characteristics, equilibrium with the others can also change and the final result is symptoms of ocular discomfort and signs of subclinical inflammation or cytological changes (Tseng *et al.*, 1984; Versura *et al.*, 1999). Any one of these can be a precursor of more serious conditions.

CONCLUDING POSTSCRIPT

Thanks to this new generation of hyper-oxygen-transmissible soft lens materials, the hypoxic era during hydrogel lens wear is drawing to an end. The high levels of oxygen available to individual epithelial cells during SiH lens wear should benefit the overall health of the corneal epithelium and hopefully lead to a reduction of the corneal infection rate.

We can look back over the past 50 years as a time of extraordinary success. Problems were identified and solved and we now move to the next era. Yet, SiH lens wear may still face certain challenges from several directions:

1. Is the epithelium compromised in some way by a slowing down in shedding and mitosis? The epithelium appears to be capable of regulating cell production and loss under a variety of conditions. Is the physical presence of the lens one of these conditions?

2. Should tear exchange beneath a lens be increased? If mucus from goblet cells is an important part of the protective mechanism of the pre-corneal tears, will the susceptibility to infections be increased by the prolonged functional isolation of the corneal epithelium in EW? More exchange would allow more mucus and immune system components under the lens and more flushing of cellular debris and bacteria.

REFERENCES

Adar, S., Kanpolat, A., Surucu, S. and Ucakhan, O. O. (1997) Conjunctival impression cytology in patients wearing contact lenses. *Cornea*, **16**, 289–294

Aragona, P., Ferreri, G., Micali, A. and Puzzolo, D. (1998) Morphological changes of the conjunctival epithelium in contact lens wearers evaluated by impression cytology. *Eye*, **12**, 461–466

Auran, J., Koester, C., Kleiman, N. J. *et al.* (1995) Scanning slit confocal microscopic observation of cell morphology and movement within the normal human anterior cornea. *Ophthalmology*, **102**, 33–41

Bachman, W. and Wilson, G. (1985) Essential ions for maintenance of the corneal epithelial surface. *Invest. Ophthalmol. Vis. Sci.*, **26**, 1484–1488

Barr, J. T. and Testa, L. M. (1994) Corneal epithelium 3 and 9 o'clock staining studied with the specular microscope. *Int. Cont. Lens Clin.*, **21**(May/June), 105–111

Beebe, D. C. and Masters, B. (1996) Cell lineage and the differentiation of corneal epithelial cells. *Invest. Ophthalmol. Vis. Sci.*, **37**, 1815–1825

Begley, C., Zhou, J. and Wilson, G. (1998) Characterization of cells shed from the ocular surface in normal eyes. In *Lacrimal Gland, Tearfilm, and Dry Eye Syndromes 2* (eds D. A. Sullivan, D. Dartt and M. A. Meneray). Plenum Press, New York, pp. 675–681

Bergmanson, J. P. G., Doughty, M. J. and Blocker, Y. (1999) The acinar and ductal organisation of the tarsal accessory lacrimal gland of Wolfring in rabbit eyelid. *Exp. Eye Res.*, **68**, 411–421

Bernal, D. L. and Ubels, J. L. (1991) Quantitative evaluation of the corneal epithelial barrier: effect of artificial tears and preservatives. *Curr. Eye Res.*, **10**, 645–656

Beuerman, R. W. and Pedroza, L. (1996) Ultrastructure of the human cornea. *Microsc. Res. Tech.*, **33**, 320–335

Bron, A. J., Mengher, L. S. and Davey, C. C. (1985) The normal conjunctiva and its response to inflammation. *Trans. Ophthalmol. Soc. UK*, **104**, 424

Cameron, J. D., Waterfield, R. R., Steffes, M. W. and Furcht, L. T. (1989) Quantification of corneal organ culture migration: central and peripheral epithelium. *Invest. Ophthalmol. Vis. Sci.*, **30**, 2407–2413

Cavanagh, H. D., Ladage, P. M., Yamamoto, K., Li, L. *et al.* (2002) Effects of daily and overnight wear of a novel hyper-O_2 transmissible soft contact lens on bacterial binding and corneal epithelium: a 13-month clinical trial. *Ophthalmology*, **109**, 1957–1969

Chandler, J. W. (1996) Ocular surface immunology. In *Ocular Infection and Immunity* (eds J. S. Pepose, G. N. Holland and K. R. Wilhelmus). Mosby, St Louis

Chen, H. B., Yamabayashi, S., Ou, B. *et al.* (1995) Ultrastructural studies on the corneal superficial epithelium of rats by in vivo cryofixation with freeze substitution. *Ophthalmic Res.*, **27**, 286–295

Chen, H. B., Yamabayashi, S., Ou, B. *et al.* (1997) Structure and composition of rat precorneal tear film: a study by an in vivo cryofixation. *Invest. Ophthalmol. Vis. Sci.*, **38**, 381–387

Chodosh, J., Nordquist, R. and Kennedy, R. (1998) Anatomy of mammalian conjunctival lymphoepithelium. In *Lacrimal Gland, Tearfilm, and Dry Eye Syndromes 2* (eds D. A. Sullivan, D. Dartt and M. A. Meneray). Plenum Press, New York, pp. 557–563

Doane, M. (1980) Interactions of eyelids and tears in corneal wetting and the dynamics of the normal human eyeblink. *Am. J. Ophthalmol.*, **89**, 507–510

Doughty, M. (1997) Scanning electron microscopy study of the tarsal and orbital conjunctival surfaces compared to the peripheral corneal epithelium in pigmented rabbits. *Doc. Ophthalmol.*, **93**, 345–371

Doughty, M. and Panju, Z. (1995) Exploring the hidden surface of the underside of the eyelid. *Cont. Lens Spectrum*, **19**, 19–30

Ebato, B., Friend, J. and Thoft, R. A. (1988) Comparison of limbal and peripheral human corneal epithelium in tissue culture. *Invest. Ophthalmol. Vis. Sci.*, **29**, 1533–1537

Efron, N. (1997) Contact lens-induced papillary conjunctivitis. *Optician*, **213**(5583), 20–27

Estil, S. and Wilson, G. (2000) Apoptosis in shed human corneal cells. *Invest. Ophthalmol. Vis. Sci.*, **41**, 3360–3364

Fleiszig, S., Lee, E., Wu, C. *et al.* (1998) Cytotoxic strains of *Pseudomonas aeruginosa* can damage the intact corneal surface in vitro. *J. Cont. Lens Assoc. Ophthalmol.*, **24**, 41–47

Fogle, J. A., Yoza, B. K. and Neufeld, A. H. (1980) Diurnal rhythm of mitosis in rabbit corneal epithelium. *Albrecht V. Graefes Arch. Klin. Exp. Ophthalmol.*, **213**, 143–148

Gipson, I. (1994) Anatomy of the conjunctiva, cornea and limbus. In *The Cornea: Scientific Foundations and Clinical Practice* (eds G. Smolin and R. Thoft). Little Brown, Boston, pp. 3–24

Greiner, J. V., Leahy, C. D., Welter, D. A. *et al.* (1997) Histopathology of the ocular surface after eye rubbing. *Cornea*, **16**, 327–332

Haaskjold, E., Bjerknes, R. and Bjerknes, E. (1989a) Migration of cells in the rat corneal epithelium. *Acta Ophthalmol.*, **67**, 91–96

Haaskjold, E., Refsum, S. B. and Bjerknes, R. (1989b) Circadian variation in the mitotic rate of the rat corneal epithelium. *Virchows Archiv B. Cell. Pathol.*, **58**, 123–127

Haaskjold, E., Refsum, S. B. and Bjerknes, R. (1990) Circadian variations in the DNA synthesis of the rat corneal epithelium. *Virchows Archiv B. Cell. Pathol.*, **58**, 229–234

Hanna, C. and O'Brien, J. E. (1960) Cell production and migration in the epithelial layer of the cornea. *Arch. Ophthalmol.*, **64**, 88–91

Hingorani, M., Calder, V. L., Buckley, R. and Lightman, S. L. (1998) The role of conjunctival epithelial cells in chronic ocular allergic disease. *Exp. Eye Res.*, **67**, 491–500

Holden, B. A., Sweeney, D. F., Vannas, A. *et al.* (1985) Effects of long-term extended contact lens wear on the human cornea. *Invest. Ophthalmol. Vis. Sci.*, **26**, 1489–1501

Ichijima, H., Yokoi, N., Nishizawa, A. and Kinoshita, S. (1999) Fluorophotometric assessment of rabbit corneal epithelial barrier function after rigid contact lens wear. *Cornea*, **18**, 87–91

Imayasu, M., Petroll, W. M., Jester, J. V. *et al.* (1994) The relation between contact lens oxygen transmissibility and binding of *Pseudomonas aeruginosa* to the cornea after overnight wear. *Ophthalmology*, **101**, 371–388

Inatomi, T., Spurr-Michaud, S., Tisdale, A. S. and Gipson, I. K. (1995) Human corneal and conjunctival epithelia express MUC1 mucin. *Invest. Ophthalmol. Vis. Sci.*, **36**, 1818–1827

Inatomi, T., Spurr-Michaud, S., Tisdale, A. S. *et al.* (1996) Expression of secretory mucin genes by human conjunctival epithelia. *Invest. Ophthalmol. Vis. Sci.*, **37**, 1684–1692

Jester, J., Li, H.-F., Petroll, W. M. *et al.* (1998) Area and depth of surfactant-induced corneal injury correlates with cell death. *Invest. Ophthalmol. Vis. Sci.*, **39**, 922–936

Jumblatt, M. M., McKenzie, R. W. and Jumblatt, J. E. (1999) MUC5AC mucin is a component of the human precorneal tear film. *Invest. Ophthalmol. Vis. Sci.*, **40**, 43–49

Knop, E. and Brewitt, H. (1992) Conjunctival cytology in asymptomatic wearers of soft contact lenses. *Graefe's Arch. Clin. Exp. Ophthalmol.*, **230**, 340–347

Ladage, P. M. (2002) Corneal epithelial homeostasis during contact lens wear. PhD dissertation, College of Optometry, University of Houston, Houston, TX

Ladage, P. M., Yamamoto, K., Ren, D. H. *et al.* (2001a) Proliferation rate of rabbit corneal epithelium during overnight contact lens wear. *Invest. Ophthalmol. Vis. Sci.*, **42**, 2803–2812

Ladage, P. M., Yamamoto, K., Ren, D. H. *et al.* (2001b) Effects of rigid and soft contact lens daily wear on corneal epithelium, tear lactate dehydrogenase and bacterial binding to exfoliated epithelial cells. *Ophthalmology*, **108**, 1279–1288

Ladage, P. M., Yamamoto, K., Li, L. *et al.* (2002) Corneal epithelial homeostasis following daily and overnight contact lens wear. *Cont. Lens Ant. Eye*, **25**, 11–21

Ladage, P. M., Jester, J. V., Petroll, W. M. *et al.* (2003a) Vertical migration of epithelial basal cells towards the corneal surface during extended contact lens wear. *Invest. Ophthalmol. Vis. Sci.*, **44**, 1056–1063

Ladage, P. M., Ren, D. H., Jester, J. V. *et al.* (2003b) Eyelid closure, soft and silicone hydrogel contact lens wear: effects on the proliferation rate of the rabbit corneal epithelium. *Invest. Ophthalmol. Vis. Sci.*, **44**, 1843–1849

Latkovic, S. and Nilsson, S. (1997) The effect of high and low *Dk/L* soft contact lenses on the glycocalyx layer of the corneal epithelium and on the membrane associated receptors for lectins. *J. Cont. Lens Assoc. Ophthalmol.*, **23**, 185–191

Laurent, J. and Wilson, G. (1997) Size of cells collected from normal subjects using contact lens cytology. *Optom. Vis. Sci.*, **74**, 280–287

Lehrer, M. S., Sun, T.-T. and Lavker, R. (1998) A hierarchy of proliferative capacity exists within the transit amplifying (TA) cell population of the corneal epithelium. *Invest. Ophthalmol. Vis. Sci.*, **39**, s230

Li, L., Ren, D. H., Ladage, P. M. *et al.* (2002) Annexin V binding to rabbit corneal epithelial cells following overnight wear or eyelid closure. *CLAO J.*, **28**, 48–54

Liotet, S., Van Bijsterveld, O. P., Kogbe, O. and Laroche, L. (1987) A new hypothesis on tear film stability. *Ophthalmologica*, **195**, 119–124

Lohman, L. E., Rao, G. N., Tripathi, R. C. *et al.* (1982) In vivo specular microscopy of edematous human corneal epithelium with light and scanning electron microscopic correlation. *Ophthalmology*, **89**, 621–629

Mathers, W. D. and Lemp, M. A. (1992) Morphology and movement of corneal surface cells in humans. *Curr. Eye Res.*, **11**, 517–523

McNamara, N. A., Fusaro, R. E., Brand, R. J. *et al.* (1997) Measurement of corneal epithelial permeability to fluorescein: a repeatability study. *Invest. Ophthalmol. Vis. Sci.*, **38**, 1830–1839

McNamara, N. A., Polse, K. A. and Bonnano, J. A. (1998a) Fluorophotometry in contact lens research: the next step. *Optom. Vis. Sci.*, **75**, 316–322

McNamara, N. A., Polse, K. A., Fukunaga, S. A. *et al.* (1998b) Soft lens extended wear affects epithelial barrier function. *Ophthalmology*, **105**, 2330–2335

Nelson, J. D., Havener, V. R. and Cameron J. D. (1983) Cellulose acetate impressions of the ocular surface. *Arch. Ophthalmol.*, **101**, 1869–1872

Ren, H. and Wilson, G. (1994) The effect of ultraviolet-B irradiation on the cell shedding rate of the corneal epithelium. *Acta Ophthalmol.*, **72**, 447–452

Ren, H. and Wilson, G. (1996a) Apoptosis in the corneal epithelium. *Invest. Ophthalmol. Vis. Sci.*, **37**, 1017–1025

Ren, H. and Wilson, G. (1996b) The cell shedding rate of the corneal epithelium: a comparison of collection methods. *Curr. Eye Res.*, **15**, 1054–1059

Ren, H. and Wilson, G. (1997) The effect of a shear force on the cell shedding rate of the corneal epithelium. *Acta Ophthalmologica*, **75**, 383–387

Ren, D. H., Petroll, W. M., Jester, J. V. *et al.* (1997) The α, β, γ cell hypothesis for renewal of the corneal epithelial surface. In *Advances in Corneal Research: Selected Transactions of the World Cornea Congress on the Cornea* (ed J. H. Lass). Plenum Press, New York, pp. 463–464

Ren, D. H., Petroll, W. M., Jester, J. V. *et al.* (1999a) The relationship between contact lens oxygen permeability and binding of *Pseudomonas aeruginosa* to human corneal epithelial cells after overnight and extended wear. *J. Cont. Lens Assoc. Ophthalmol.*, **25**, 80–100

Ren, D. H., Petroll, W. M., Jester, J. V. *et al.* (1999b) Short-term hypoxia downregulates epithelial cell desquamation in vivo, but does not increase *Pseudomonas aeruginosa* adherence to exfoliated human corneal epithelial cells. *J. Cont. Lens Assoc. Ophthalmol.*, **25**, 73–79

Ren, D. H., Petroll, W. M., Jester, J. V. *et al.* (1999c) The effect of rigid gas permeable contact lens wear on proliferation of rabbit corneal and conjunctival epithelial cells. *CLAO J*, **25**, 136–141

Ren, D. H., Yamamoto, K., Ladage, P. M. *et al.* (2002) Adaptive effects of 30-night wear of hyper-O_2 transmissible contact lenses on bacterial and corneal epithelium: a 1-year clinical trial. *Ophthalmology*, **109**, 27–40

Tseng, S. C., Hirst, L. W., Maumenee, A. E. *et al.* (1984) Possible mechanisms for the loss of goblet cells in mucin-deficient disorders. *Ophthalmology*, **91**, 545–552

Tsubota, K., Hata, S., Toda, I. *et al.* (1996) Increase in corneal epithelial cell size with extended wear soft contact lenses depends on continuous wearing time. *Br. J. Ophthalmol.*, **80**, 144–147

Ubels, J. (1998) Conjunctival permeability and ultrastructure. In *Lacrimal Gland, Tearfilm, and Dry Eye Syndromes 2* (eds D. A. Sullivan, D. Dartt and M. A. Meneray). Plenum Press, New York, pp. 723–735

Versura, P., Profazio, V., Cellini, M. and Torreggiani, A. (1999) Eye discomfort and air pollution. *Ophthalmologica*, **213**, 103–109

Wang, Y., Chen, M. and Wolosin, J. M. (1993) ZO-1 in corneal epithelium: stratal distribution and synthesis induction by outer cell removal. *Exp. Eye Res.*, **57**, 283–292

Watanabe, H., Fabricant, M., Tisdale, A. S. *et al.* (1995) Human corneal and conjunctival epithelia produce a mucin-like glycoprotein for the apical surface. *Invest. Ophthalmol. Vis. Sci.* **36**, 337–344

Wei, Z.-G., Wu, R.-L., Lavker, R. M. and Sun, T.-T. (1993) In vitro growth and differentiation of rabbit bulbar fornix, and palpebral conjunctival epithelia. *Invest. Ophthalmol. Vis. Sci.*, **34**, 1814–1828

Wei, Z.-G., Cotsarelis, G., Sun, T.-T. and Lavker, R. M. (1995) Label-retaining cells are preferentially located in fornical epithelium: implications on conjunctival epithelial homeostasis. *Invest. Ophthalmol. Vis. Sci.*, **36**, 236–246

Wei, Z.-G., Sun, T.-T. and Lavker, R. M. (1996) Rabbit conjunctival and corneal epithelial cells belong to two separate lineages. *Invest. Ophthalmol. Vis. Sci.*, **37**, 523–533

Wilson, G. (1994) The effect of hypoxia on the shedding rate of the corneal epithelium. *Curr. Eye Res.*, **13**, 409–413

Wilson, G. (1996) The effect of osmolality on the shedding rate of the corneal epithelium. *Cornea*, **15**, 229–334

Wilson, G. and Laurent, J. (1998) The size of corneal epithelial cells collected by contact lens cytology from dry eyes. In *Lacrimal Gland, Tearfilm, and Dry Eye Syndromes 2* (eds D. A. Sullivan, D. Dartt and M. A. Meneray). Plenum Press, New York, pp. 675–681

Wilson, G. and Primo, E. (1997) The effect of sequential contact lens cytology on the corneal epithelium. *Invest. Ophthalmol. Vis. Sci.*, **38**, s863

Wilson, G., Schwallie, J. D. and Bauman, R. E. (1998) Comparison by contact lens cytology and clinical tests of three contact lens types. *Optom. Vis. Sci.*, **75**, 323–329

Wolff, E. (1976) *Anatomy of the Eye and Orbit*. W. B. Saunders, Philadelphia

Wolosin, J. M. and Chen, M. (1993) Ontogeny of corneal epithelial tight junctions: stratal locale of biosynthetic activities. *Invest. Ophthalmol. Vis. Sci.*, **34**, 2655–2664

Yamamoto, K., Ladage, P. M., Li, L. *et al.* (2001a) Bcl-2 expression in the human cornea. *Exp. Eye Res.*, **73**, 247–255

Yamamoto, K., Ladage, P. M., Li, L. *et al.* (2001b) Effects of low and hyper *Dk* rigid gas permeable contact lenses in Bcl-2 expression and apoptosis in the rabbit corneal epithelium. *CLAO J*, **27**, 137–143

Yamamoto, K., Ladage, P. M., Li, L. *et al.* (2001c) Epitope variability of Bcl-2 immunolocalization in the human corneal epithelium. *CLAO J*, **27**, 221–224

Yamamoto, K., Ladage, P. M., Li, L. *et al.* (2002) The effect of eyelid closure and overnight contact lens wear on viability of surface epithelial cells in rabbit cornea. *Cornea*, **21**, 85–90

You, L., Kruse, F. E., Pohl, J. and Volcker, H. E. (1999) Bone morphogenetic proteins and growth and differentiation factors in the human cornea. *Invest. Ophthalmol. Vis, Sci.*, **40**, 296–311

Zaidi, T. S., Fleiszig, S. M., Preston, M. J. *et al.* (1996) Lipopolysaccharide outer core is a ligand for corneal cell binding and ingestion of *Pseudomonas aeruginosa*. *Invest. Ophthalmol. Vis. Sci.*, **37**(6), 976–986

Chapter 3

Tear mixing under soft contact lenses

Kimberly L. Miller, Meng C. Lin, Clayton J. Radke and
Kenneth A. Polse

INTRODUCTION

Disposable soft contact lens (SCL) extended wear (EW) has previously been associated with ocular complications, many caused by corneal hypoxia (Lebow, 1980; Mertz and Holden, 1981; Holden *et al.*, 1985; Schein *et al.*, 1989; Sankaridurg *et al.*, 1999). The recent development of silicone hydrogel SCLs with high oxygen transmissibility (Dk/t) has all but eliminated contact lens-induced corneal hypoxia, along with the physiological complications associated with low oxygen tension (e.g. corneal swelling, epithelial microcysts and corneal acidosis; Humphreys *et al.*, 1980; Kenyon *et al.*, 1986; Lemp and Gold, 1986; Polse *et al.*, 1990; Tsubota *et al.*, 1996). Nevertheless, clinicians continue to observe that some patients wearing silicone hydrogel SCLs develop adverse ocular responses such as superior epithelial arcuate lesions (SEALs), superficial punctate keratitis, contact lens-induced peripheral ulcers (CLPU), corneal infiltrates, contact lens-induced acute red eye (CLARE), microbial keratitis, contact lens-induced papillary conjunctivitis (CLPC) and corneal erosions (Holden *et al.*, 2001; Dumbleton, 2002; Sweeney *et al.*, 2002). Apparently many of these events occur with a frequency similar to that reported with standard low oxygen-permeable lenses worn for EW (Sankaridurg *et al.*, 1999; Fonn *et al.*, 2002).

The aetiology of the adverse clinical events associated with silicone hydrogel SCL wear is not completely understood, but most clinicians and investigators believe that corneal hypoxia is not the underlying mechanism. More likely these complications are related to lens performance factors involving lens/lid pressure, lens movement, lens surface properties, post-lens tear film (PoLTF) and the rate of tear exchange under the lens. Inflammatory cells, metabolic by-products and debris that accumulate under the lens and are not removed efficiently may lead to adverse responses of both biochemical and mechanical origin. This chapter focuses on assessment of and improvement in tear mixing under hydroxyethyl methacrylate (HEMA) and silicone hydrogel SCLs.

In the normal eye, without the presence of a contact lens, blinking and tear drainage facilitate clearance of bacteria and other potentially harmful pathogens.

Further, proteins in the tear film aggregate and kill bacteria, glycocalyx on the epithelial cell surface repels bacteria, ocular mucus binds bacteria to inhibit adherence, and surface epithelial cells which internalize bacteria are exfoliated and removed from the eye on a regular basis. All these functions of the tear and corneal epithelium contribute to the innate defence of the eye. Since fresh tears filled with electrolytes and nutrients are essential to maintain the extracellular environment for the health of the corneal epithelial cells (Thoft and Friend, 1975; O'Leary et al., 1985), changes in composition of the tear film and alterations in corneal epithelial physiology due to lack of tear exchange during contact lens wear may leave the eye unprotected.

Studies have shown that when contact lenses are worn normal tear drainage is impeded and the glycocalyx is depleted, exposing receptors for bacteria and increasing their adherence to the cornea (Latkovic and Nilsson, 1997). Moreover, bacteria under an SCL enter surface epithelial cells and remain in contact with the ocular surface for longer than normal periods of time due to a decreased shedding rate of the epithelial cells (Tsubota et al., 1996; Ren et al., 2002). In addition, studies by Fleiszig et al. (1996, 1998) show that stagnation of cytotoxic bacteria adjacent to the corneal surface contributes to the pathogenesis of infection associated with the use of SCLs. When there is sufficient contact time, these pathogens can damage the cornea by interacting with cells that are not polarized properly. The stagnant tear film in the closed eye condition is rich in inflammatory cells (Sack et al., 2000). Thus, slow removal of these cells after eye opening may lead to adverse clinical events such as infiltrative keratitis, red eye and infection. In summary, efficient replenishment and exchange with fresh tears are important to maintain the homeostasis of the PoLTF and the ocular-surface physiology.

Mechanically driven adverse responses also highlight the importance of PoLTF flushing to safe SCL EW. Recent studies that measured the permeability of the epithelium (P_{dc}) to sodium fluorescein have found that overnight wear with both high- and low-Dk/t lenses causes significant changes in epithelial barrier function (McNamara et al., 1998; Lin et al., 2002a). Although the changes in P_{dc} with low-Dk/t materials were greater compared with silicone hydrogel SCL, it appears that SHSL wear (i.e. normoxia) during eye closure can alter epithelial status, suggesting that these alterations are, in part, due to mechanical irritation. In these studies, subjects reported to the laboratory with only one eye patched and, interestingly, the unpatched eye showed greater increases in P_{dc} compared to the fellow (patched) eye (Lin et al., 2002a). One possible explan-ation is that lens movement for the unpatched eye initiated after awakening causes the retained debris, sandwiched between the lens and cornea, to rub against the epithelium and exacerbate the mechanical effect of a soft lens on the epithelial surface. If the trapped debris is removed quickly after eye opening, mechanical abrasion to the epithelial cells is minimized. Compared to soft lenses, rigid gas-permeable (RGP) lenses have very fast tear exchange rates, and trapped debris is seldom observed after eye opening. It is likely that the rapid tear mixing rate of RGP lenses produces less mechanical insult to the epithelium and helps explain the low rate of corneal complications accompanying RGP EW (Lin et al., 2002b).

An association between mechanical adverse responses and inefficient tear mixing can be reasoned as follows. During sleep there is a build-up of debris and inflammatory cells under the contact lens. However, because the lens is stationary, the epithelium is sequestered from the mechanical effects of lens movement and rubbing of the debris against the epithelium. Upon eye opening, the debris in the PoLTF is not quickly removed because of the inefficient tear mixing; when normal blinking resumes the debris sandwiched between the lens and cornea is mechanically agitated against the epithelium with each movement of the lens. Ultimately, for some contact lens wearers, this repeated mechanical agitation alters epithelial cell integrity and provides a pathway for abnormal physiological responses such as inflammation, CLPU, CLARE and SEALs.

Given the likely connection between inefficient tear mixing and adverse response to extended and closed-eye lens wear, we argue that timely removal of debris is a prudent requirement for safe EW. To develop lenses with improved tear mixing we must understand the fundamental physical and physiological factors that affect tear exchange. Using engineering science design principles, we construct a mathematical mixing model and test it by measuring fluorescein isothiocyanate (FITC)-dextran flushing from the PoLTF of currently available SCLs. The resulting analysis of clinical tear mixing data can be used to refine the mixing model further. Thus the interactive process between empirical data analysis and refinement of the mixing model assists in the development of new lens designs to enhance tear mixing.

In this chapter we report our progress and the progress of others in (1) describing lens motion during blinking, (2) developing a tear mixing model, (3) estimating tear exchange rates for some currently available hydrogel and silicone hydrogel SCLs, and (4) identifying some ocular and lens parameters that affect tear exchange and exploring strategies for new lens designs to enhance tear mixing. Because lens motion is critical to understanding mixing in the PoLTF, we begin with this topic.

LENS MOTION

FLUSHING OF THE PoLTF

Experiments on FITC-dextran intensity decay from behind SCLs, described fully below, confirm that the PoLTF can indeed be flushed. By way of example, Figure 3.1 shows typical experimental decay histories (symbols) of the relative intensity or relative average dye concentration under two SCLs (i.e. etafilcon A and lotrafilcon A(exp)) and near the centre of the cornea, C/C_o, as function of time, t, in minutes on a semi-logarithmic scale. After a few minutes of initial lens wear, the fit straight lines to the measured data in Figure 3.1 indicate that the FITC-dextran concentration in the PoLTF obeys an exponential decay, i.e. $C/C_o = \exp(-t/T)$, where T is a characteristic decay time, which is given by the negative slope of the fit line. Typical characteristic decay times are around 10 minutes, meaning that 95 per cent of the dye is flushed within $3T$ or 30 minutes. However, because a blink directly flushes only the pre-lens tear film (PrLTF), the mechanism for dye (or other chemical species) removal from the PoLTF is not obvious.

The first thought might be that gravity flushes the PoLTF. To assess the importance of the gravity flow we write the characteristic velocity for vertical drainage from a narrow slit as $\rho g h^2/3\mu$ (Bird *et al.*, 1960), where ρ and μ are the density and Newtonian viscosity of tear respectively, g is the acceleration due to gravity, and h is the PoLTF thickness (PLTT). Using the known physical properties of tear and a PLTT of $10\,\mu m$, the characteristic gravity flushing velocity is $10^{-4}\,cm/s$. For comparison, typical lid velocities that drive lens motion are $5\,cm/s$ (Doane, 1980, 1981, 1984). Accordingly, gravity drainage is completely overwhelmed by lens movement (Creech *et al.*, 2001).

A second mechanism for removing species from the PoLTF is molecular diffusion. However, the characteristic time for diffusion is L^2/D, where L is the radius of the lens and D is the molecular diffusivity of FITC-dextran. For a $14\,mm$ diameter lens and with $D = 7.5(10^{-7})\,cm^2/s$ (Guiot *et al.*, 2000), the time for diffusion removal of the fluorescent dye is 180 hours. Compared to the characteristic measured times, T, in Figure 3.1 of 10 minutes, diffusion is much too slow to provide any contribution to the observed dye removal. Our conclusion is that another mechanism is responsible for flushing of the PoLTF and that lens motion

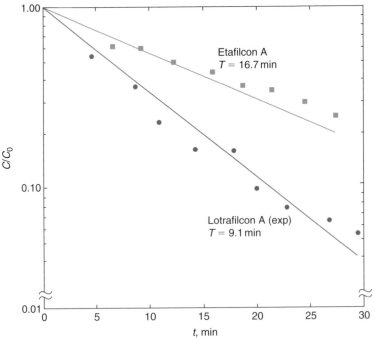

Figure 3.1 Typical fluorescence decay of FITC-dextran from the PoLTF of an etafilcon A and a lotrofilcon A(exp) lens. Relative dye concentration, C/C_o, equivalent to the relative fluorescence intensity is shown (closed symbols) as a function of time, t, on a semi-logarithmic scale. Straight line fits indicate exponential decay after about a 5-minute delay. Efficiency of dye flushing is gauged by the characteristic exponential decay time, T, which is around 10 minutes for these particular lenses and subjects. After Creech *et al.* (2001)

during blinking must surely be important. Therefore, before discussing the proposed mixing model, we review and augment what is known about lid and lens motion as related to PoLTF flushing.

TYPES OF LENS MOTION

Movement of an SCL on the eye during and just after a blink is crucial to vision correction, lens comfort and efficient cleansing of the PoLTF. It is therefore important to discuss how an SCL responds to the motion of the lids during blinking. On the eye, an SCL is subject to the forces applied by the eyelids that cause it to move and deform, as pictured in Figure 3.2 (Chauhan and Radke, 2001a). Three basic types of lens movement are documented: (1) up–down or vertical motion, (2) in–out or transverse motion, and (3) temporal–nasal or sideways motion (not shown). Each of these motions is described below in the context

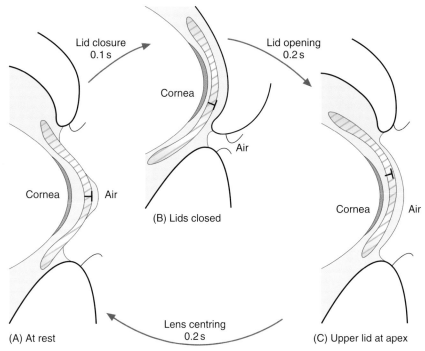

Figure 3.2   Schematic of a soft contact lens covered eye in cross-section during a blink cycle (not to scale). Eyelids are outlined with thick black lines, the contact lens is shown in cross-hatching and the PrLTFs and PoLTFs that envelop the lens are shown as lightly dotted. Large arrows prescribe the blink sequence starting at the top left and proceeding clockwise. To track its motion the lens is shown as marked in the centre with a cross: (A) contact lens at rest during the interblink period after centring. Note that the PrLTF is shown as ruptured; (B) contact lens descending during upper lid closure; (C) contact lens ascending during upper lid opening. During this period, a fresh PrLTF is deposited on the lens. After Chauhan and Radke (2001a), with permission

of Figure 3.2, which demonstrates three sequential lens configurations occurring during a blink. This physical picture of the various lens configurations in a blink is based on qualitative observations from video camera recording done in our laboratory and in literature documentation (Doane, 1980, 1981, 1984). In the figure, arrows delineate the blink cycle. Eyelids are outlined with thick black lines, the contact lens is shown in cross-hatch and the PrLTFs and PoLTFs are lightly dotted. The cornea is shown in grey with the sclera extending beyond. To track its motion, the lens in Figure 3.2 is shown marked in the centre with a cross. Observe that after completion of a blink in Figure 3.2C the lens is covered by a PrLTF and separated from the cornea by a PoLTF, completely enveloping the lens in tear. Thus if the PrLTF remains intact until the next blink event, lens wettability plays little or no role in lens motion during blinking.

Basically, during vertical excursion, the lens is first dragged towards the inferior lid by the downward motion of the upper eyelid. Soon thereafter the lens is then pulled up during the opening phase of the blink, now by the upward motion of the upper lid. When the blink is complete and the upper lid remains stationary, the lens centres back to its original location over the cornea. The entire blink process occurs within tenths of seconds, and then repeats after a 4- to 5-second interblink of interval.

UP–DOWN (VERTICAL) MOTION

First, Figure 3.2A shows a centred contact lens during the interblink period. The PrLTF is depicted as partially broken because we find that tear film rupture before the next blink is common on SCLs. In Figure 3.2B the downward motion of the upper eyelid drags the lens downwards. It is primarily the leading edge of the upper lid near the grey line (i.e. the line of Marx) that propels the lens. Direct or molecular attachment of the upper lid to the lens during this process is not expected. More likely, a thin film of lubricating tear and mucin separates the superior marginal palpebral conjunctiva from the lens anterior surface. The thickness of this film is not known but an estimate of 1 μm is reasonable (Chauhan and Radke, 2001a). As the lid traverses downward, this thin tear film is dragged downward and, in turn, drags the lens with it by transmitting the lid shear force. At the leading edge of the closing upper lid, some of the PrLTF covering the anterior lens surface provides a new thin lubricating tear film between the upper lid and the lens, and the remainder is pushed ahead. If the lens becomes non-wetting due to repeated contamination, for example with continued lipid build-up or with airborne oily debris, then rupture of the PrLTF can be extensive and much of the anterior surface of the lens is in contact with air. Subsequently, during the downward blink, the upper lid must slide over dry patches that have no thin lubricating tear layer. Here dry friction may occur, and physical irritation is possible. This is one explanation for the so-called 'lid wiper' phenomenon where, for dry-eye subjects, staining of the upper lid marginal epithelium occurs (Korb et al., 2002). Because of the wiper mechanics of the upper lid, the shear force applied by the upper lid is not uniform over the tarsal area, but rather is focused along a narrow band at the very edge of the lid. Thus, during blinking, the upper lid behaves similarly to a squeegee.

As pictured in Figure 3.2, there is also a thin film of tear sandwiched between the lower lid palpebral conjunctiva and the anterior lens surface. This film is more uniform in thickness and offers a resistive shear force as the lens is driven into the lower fornix. There are two other resistive forces to downward lens motion. First, the PoLTF resists being dragged downward by the lens and, in turn, exerts a shear force on the cornea and sclera similar to that when the lens is not present. Secondly, since the sclera is flatter than either the cornea or the lens, the downward motion of the lens causes an increase of stored elastic energy due to the stretching and bending of the lens as it rides over the sclera. The resulting elastic force acting on the lens is directed upwards, retarding lid closure. The gravitational force acting on the lens is negligible in comparison to the drag and elastic forces (Funkenbusch and Benson, 1999; Chauhan and Radke, 2001a).

During upward motion of the upper eyelid, the same processes mentioned above occur but in the opposite direction. The thin lubricating tear film separating the upper lid margin and the lens now drags the lens upward with viscous drag from the PoLTF and from the lubricating tear between the inferior palpebral conjunctiva and the lens, again retarding lens movement. As depicted in Figure 3.2C, the lens is progressively unbent from the inferior sclera and bent and stretched over the superior sclera. Here the net elastic force changes sign, eventually acting downward when the lens reaches its apex. Once at its apex when the upper lid is effectively motionless, the lens centres back down to its rest position in Figure 3.2A. Centring is primarily due to the elastic deformation energy stored in the lens, as gravity contributes little to lens motion (Funkenbusch and Benson, 1999; Chauhan and Radke, 2001a).

Based on the above lens vertical motion scenario, Chauhan and Radke (2001a) predict quantitatively the up–down motion of an SCL. For the elastic deformation energy, Chauhan and Radke adopt the simplified expression derived by Taylor and Wilson (1996) for elastic bending. Figure 3.3 displays the resulting predicted vertical motion of two lenses of differing elastic modulus (solid lines), along with the corresponding upper lid motion (dashed line), taken from the studies of Doane (1981, 1984). Lid motion is gauged from the tip, whereas lens motion is measured relative to the centre of the cornea. Note that the lens moves upward slightly before the upper lid reverses its downward direction and that the lens rides downward before the lid stops its upward travel. Both of these effects arise because of lens elasticity that works toward centring the lens. Also note that the lens vertical motion is not symmetric about the rest position. There is a decidedly larger downward excursion than upwards. The most important conclusion from Figure 3.3 for PoLTF mixing is that lens vertical travel is significantly larger than that normally measured. This is because, in a typical vertical motion measurement, a mark on the lens is tracked and the mark is buried under the upper lid for much of the lens motion (see Figure 3.2). Only the very last centring motion of the mark from the maximum to rest position is observed experimentally, as labelled by Δ in Figure 3.3. Accordingly, actual lens vertical travel can be two or three times larger than that commonly accepted (Chauhan and Radke, 2001a).

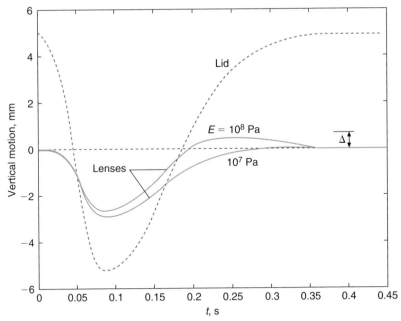

Figure 3.3 Experimental travel history of the upper lid (dashed line; Doane, 1980, 1981, 1984) and calculated vertical motion of two lenses with moduli $E = 10^7$ and 10^8 Pa (solid lines; Chauhan and Radke, 2001a). Centre mark vertical lens detected motion is labelled as Δ. Parameters in the theory are: lens diameter $2L = 14$ mm, lens thickness $b = 100\,\mu$m, lens base curve radius (BCR) $= 7.9$ mm, scleral radius $= 12$ mm, palpebral aperture size (PAS) $= 12$ mm, thickness of PrLTFs and PoLTFs $= 1\,\mu$m and tear viscosity $\mu = 1.5$ mPas. After Chauhan and Radke (2001a), with permission

Clinical observations

In a recent study on tear mixing discussed later, Lin *et al.* (2002c) measured the vertical motion of 58 subjects wearing 14 mm diameter polymacon lenses using the centre mark method of Figure 3.2. Two different base curve radii (BCR) were investigated: 7.9 mm (steep) and 8.7 mm (flat). These authors confirm the expected result that lens vertical motion is larger (0.7 ± 0.1 mm) for the flat lenses compared to the vertical motion of the steeper lenses (0.4 ± 0.1 mm). The modelling effort of Chauhan and Radke (2001a) in Figure 3.3 does not correctly reflect the role of BCR in vertical lens motion primarily because the stretching elastic energy of the lens is not accounted for (Funkenbusch and Benson, 1999) and also because the lens bending energy expression of Taylor and Wilson is oversimplified.

Birth of the PrLTF

As the upper lid translates upward during the eye-opening portion of each blink in Figure 3.2C, a new PrLTF is created on the lens exterior. Tear from the translating upper lid meniscus is deposited on to the lens anterior surface in a coating process. Liquid in the upper lid meniscus is under a suction force due to its curvature, tending to pull liquid into the tear lake. At the same time, shear forces from the contact lens drag liquid out of the superior tear lake to coat the lens anterior surface. A balance between these two forces specifies the thickness, h_o, of the PrLTF over the contact lens (Wong $et\ al.$, 1996):

$$\frac{h_o}{R} = 2.12\left(\frac{\mu U}{\sigma}\right) \qquad (1)$$

where R is the mean radius of curvature of the tear in the lid meniscus, μ is the tear viscosity, σ is the tear surface tension, and U is the opening speed of the upper lid. Since the upper lid moves slowly at first, speeds up, and then slows down during upward motion (Doane, 1980, 1981, 1984; Figure 3.3), the deposited PrLTF is thicker near the centre of the cornea and thinner near the lid margins. Using expected values for the tear properties and the meniscus curvature, along with the measured lid velocities of Doane (1981, 1984), Wong $et\ al.$ (1996) demonstrate that Equation (1) provides reasonable estimates of the PrLTF thickness of around 10 μm. Since the volume of tear in the lid meniscus increases linearly with R^2, another interpretation of Equation (1) is that subjects with larger tear volumes exhibit thicker PrLTF.

Creech $et\ al.$ (1998) measured the meniscus curvature of the inferior lid at the cornea meridian for a number of human subjects, both with and without SCL wear. Given typical values for the tear properties of tension and viscosity and for the upper lid velocity, the PrLTF thickness at the centre of the cornea was established using Equation (1). PrLTF thicknesses over SCLs ranged from 3 to 15 μm (Creech $et\ al.$, 1998). Actual PrLTF thickness is likely to be somewhat smaller because the velocity appearing in Equation (1) is the relative value of the upper lid and the lens, a factor not taken into account by Creech $et\ al.$ (1998). Fascinatingly, the precorneal film thickness (over the nascent cornea without a contact lens in place) was always larger than that over contact lenses for every subject, ranging from 5 to 25 μm (Creech $et\ al.$, 1998). The meaning, apparently, is either that during SCL wear tear production is not as large as that without lens wear, or that the produced tears are unable to reach the tear lake.

Once the PrLTF is established and the lens centres into its rest position, the lid menisci remain under a suction curvature, and tend to draw in liquid from the bulk of the tear film. Because the lid and lens are now essentially static, there is no longer an offsetting drag force from a moving lens surface and tear flows into the 'thirsty' lower and upper menisci (McDonald and Brubaker, 1971). However, the PrLTF is thin and resists flowing as a whole. The result is deep, local thinning directly adjacent to the menisci (Wong $et\ al.$, 1996; Miller $et\ al.$ 2002) to form the so-called 'black lines' first reported by McDonald and Brubaker (1971). These very thin horizontal strips form quickly once lid motion ceases, in less than hundredths of a second (Miller $et\ al.$, 2002), and prevent drainage from or flow into the initially deposited PrLTF. Basically the PrLTF is trapped or 'perched' on the lens (or on the cornea with no lens wear) during the interblink period (Fatt, 1991; Miller $et\ al.$, 2002).

Shortly after lens centring, a curtain of molecularly thin, oily lipid spreads upwards from the meibomian glands in the inferior lid and over the deposited tear film (McDonald, 1969). When viewed under white light, this superficial oily layer is thin enough to give rise to colourful interference patterns that are used as one gauge of dry-eye syndrome (Doane, 1994; Korb and Greiner, 1994). Surface tension gradients, caused by composition or thickness differences in the lipid layer, drive the curtain upwards carrying some tear film along (Berger and Corsin, 1974).

Visualization of the interblink PrLTF under fluorescein instillation reveals the appearance of random black spots or streaks that are ascribed to local rupture of the film, as illustrated in Figure 3.2A. Although the exact mechanism of PrLTF rupture remains in doubt (Cho, 1991), thin deposited tear films (Sharma and Ruckenstein, 1990; Creech et al., 1998) and strongly non-wetting lenses (i.e. those with relatively large water-receding contact angles; Sharma and Ruckenstein, 1990) clearly exacerbate tear break-up. Dry spots on the lens during the interblink are particularly vulnerable to hydrophobic contamination from the air and from the superficial lipid layer, leading to a vicious cycle of increasing contamination and further and more extensive break-up in subsequent blinks. The significance of PrLTF rupture for lid and lens motion is the dry friction and possible upper lid irritation (mentioned above) that may occur during lid closure. However, significant dry friction is not anticipated unless break-up of the PrLTF is extensive. For sparse, isolated black spots, the extending upper lid pushes tear fluid ahead, likely covering the dry patches.

IN–OUT (TRANSVERSE) MOTION

The palpebral marginal region of the upper eyelid also drives the in–out motion or pumping of the lens. Immediately after placement on the eye, the lens is relatively stress-free, and the PoLTF is quite thick, around 0.1 mm or more. During the blink pictured in Figure 3.2B and C, the squeegee action of the upper eyelid applies a normal force to the intervening, incompressible PrLTF that, in turn, pushes the lens closer to the cornea. Some of the PoLTF is squeezed out, and the lens is bent and stretched, increasing its elastic energy. During the interblink, when the upper eyelid force is removed, the elastic energy stored in the lens, due to its deformation, is released, causing it to recoil and move away from the cornea. This also pulls liquid into the PoLTF from the tear lakes in the fornix vaults and possibly from surrounding tear on the sclera. Initially, when the PoLTF thickness is large, the inward motion of the lens during the blink is more than the outward motion during the interblink; this causes the lens to translate closer to the cornea, giving rise to the well-known phenomenon of lens settling. Eventually there may be a balance of the inward motion during the blink and the outward motion during the interblink. If so, the lens subsequently exhibits periodic steady-state motion in the in–out (and up–down) direction. This behaviour is the commonly accepted scenario of lens settling to a periodic steady state and sets the eventual time-averaged PLTT. However, a balance between inward and outward motion may not necessarily be achieved, in which case the lens continues to settle slowly, but endlessly. If this happens, thin film interactions between the mucin-covered corneal and scleral surfaces and the posterior lens surface determine whether the PoLTF ruptures, and the lens actually touches the cornea, possibly adhering.

Occurrence of SEALs suggests that the lens can mechanically abrade the cornea and lead to lesions (O'Hare *et al.*, 2000) which possibly increase the chances of bacterial infection. Thus, it is important to determine whether the lens eventually executes a time periodic motion with a stable PLTT profile or whether the lens continues to settle until the PLTT becomes small enough to allow direct physical adherence of the lens with the cornea or sclera.

To answer this question Chauhan and Radke (2002) modelled the lens as a deformable elastic shell and the cornea as a flat non-deformable body. The tear fluid was assumed to be Newtonian, and the lens was characterized by an elastic modulus and a Poisson ratio. Lubrication hydrodynamic equations under creeping flow were implemented to solve the fluid flow problem, while the thin shell approximation was applied to the solid lens. Figure 3.4 reports, on log-log scales, a calculated lens settling history of the PLTT, h, in micrometres at the lens centre and at the lens periphery as a function of time in hours. A 14 mm diameter lens of uniform thickness $b = 100\,\mu m$, an elastic modulus $E = 1$ MPa and a non-uniform applied pressure, p_o, were chosen in the calculation (Chauhan and Radke, 2002). The lens settles starting from a PLTT of 100 μm over a time-scale of 1000 hours with 5-second interblink times under the influence of a 100 Pa axisymmetric driving force that diminishes quadratically from the lens centre and that is applied

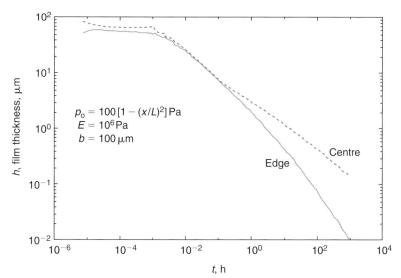

Figure 3.4   Calculated lens settling history on a log–log scale. PLTT, h, versus time, t, is shown at the lens centre and periphery. Each blink comprises a 5-second interval. Lens properties include: $E = 1$ MPa and $b = 100\,\mu m$, while the tear viscosity is $\mu = 1.5\,mPas$. The applied lid pressure, p_o, is quadratically distributed, as listed where x is the radial distance from the lens centre and L is the lens radius. After Chauhan and Radke (2002), with permission

only during the 0.1-second blink period. Fascinatingly, the elastohydrodynamic lens settling model of Chauhan and Radke (2002) predicts no periodic steady state, but rather a continual recession towards the corneal surface, especially near the lens edge. Such continued settling behaviour, especially near the lens periphery, provides an explanation for the cited occurrences of SEALs and, in some cases, even lens adherence. Very thin local thicknesses at the lens edge clearly impede tear replenishment and may not allow the PoLTF to have the same composition as that of the PrLTF, essentially compartmentalizing the overall tear film. Effective tear mixing in the PoLTF then becomes a major challenge for both the biochemical and physical health of the cornea.

Clinical observations

Currently, a technique to measure directly the amount of transverse lens motion is not available. However, using optical pachometry, Lin *et al.* (1999) showed that it is possible to estimate the thickness of the central PoLTF under a soft lens. Thus, to verify the temporal dynamics of the PoLTF, Polse *et al.* (2002) monitored changes in the central PLTT for an etafilcon A (14 mm diameter, BCR = 8.8 mm) commercial lens and an experimental lotrafilcon A(exp) lens (14 mm diameter, BCR = 8.6 mm) over a 7-hour wearing period. Figure 3.5 illustrates these changes by closed symbols that represent the average of 11 subjects, with error bars reflecting the standard error. Lines in this figure simply connect the data points. For the lotrafilcon A(exp) lens, starting from around 10 μm, the central PLTT slowly diminished down to less than 4 μm. For the etafilcon A lens after 30 minutes of wear, the average PLTT was about 10–12 μm. Over the course of the 7-hour

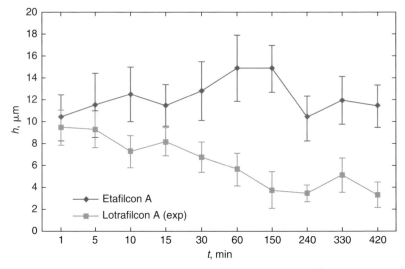

Figure 3.5   The central PLTT, *h*, as a function of time, *t*, for etafilcon A (closed diamonds) and lotrafilcon A(exp) (closed squares) lenses in an 11-subject study. Lines connect the data points, and vertical bars denote the standard error. After Polse *et al.* (2002)

wearing period, the PLTT apparently stabilized at about 12 μm. The PLTT measurements in Figure 3.5 suggest that the PoLTF is stable during open-eye lens wear. This conclusion is not necessarily inconsistent with the continued settling prediction in Figure 3.4 because of the very long wear times reported in that calculation (up to 1000 hours). Also, the theory underlying Figure 3.4 is highly simplified and does not account for simultaneous up–down lens motion or for the actual lid wiper forces driving settling. Next, there may be tear supply to the PoLTF from the aqueous humour through the cornea (Fatt and Weisman, 1992). Finally, since there is a pressure difference established between the anterior and posterior sides of the lens during the blink cycle, water can enter the PoLTF through the lens (Nicolson *et al.*, 1999). In the dispersive mixing model (DMM) described below, we assume that the SCL is impervious and moves periodically in both the up–down and in–out directions with amplitudes of Δ and Δ', respectively, and with a stable and uniform PLTT.

Precisely what determines the PLTT (and the motion amplitudes Δ and Δ') for various lens designs on different eyes is not known. For this reason, and because of the importance of the PLTT to tear mixing, Lin *et al.* (2002d) measured this quantity using optical pachometry for four different SCLs. Table 3.1 displays these results in column 4 for the average central PLTTs after 30 minutes of settling. Also shown are the subject sample sizes, n, along with the lens modulus (i.e. E) and the BCR in millimetres. The average PLTT values range from 11 to 16 μm in thickness. Such values are similar to the thickness of the pre-corneal tear film (e.g. with no lens; Danjo *et al.*, 1994; Creech *et al.*, 1998). This finding suggests that soft lenses basically conform to the shape of the cornea. However, a PLTT value of 11 μm beneath etafilcon A lenses is thicker than that reported by Nichols and King-Smith (2000), who found an average PLTT of 2 μm using interferometry and by Wang *et al.* (2003), who found an average PLTT of 5 μm using optical coherence tomography. Disagreements in the PLTT measurements may be due to differences in instrumentation, location of measurements (i.e. as shown below, the PLTT is not uniform across the cornea), amount of wearing time, calibration techniques, or subject sample size. Further investigation is needed before precise measurements of the PLTT are known. We stress, however, that the relative changes in PLTT reported in Table 3.1 are reliable.

Table 3.1   Central PLTT variations with contact lens BCR and ethnicity

Lens	BCR (mm)	Modulus of rigidity (MPa)	Central PLTT			n
			Avg. (μm)	Asian (μm)	Non–Asian (μm)	
Etafilcon A	8.8	0.28	11	11	12	23
Polymacon	7.9	0.81	16	10	20	38
	8.7	0.81	12	9	17	38
Lotrafilcon A(exp)	8.6	1.20	14	12	18	11

$n =$ number of subjects.

Since eyelid anatomical characteristics that may influence the PLTT are different between Asian and non-Asian eyes, most notably the palpebral aperture size (PAS) and lid tension, Lin *et al.* (2002d) stratify the data in Table 3.1 by Asian and non-Asian eyes in columns 5 and 6. Foremost, upon stratification by ethnicity, the PLTTs in non-Asian eyes are substantially thicker for all lenses except for the low-modulus etafilcon A lens. Accordingly, PLTT values obtained using the same lens design and material are greater on eyes with larger PAS compared to smaller PAS. Next, BCR in column 2 has a significant effect for the non-Asian eye, whereby a smaller radius (i.e. a steeper lens) has a larger PLTT. This finding is physically reasonable because of the larger sagittal depth of the steeper lens. Finally, different moduli lenses with the same BCR (i.e. etafilcon A and lotrafilcon A(exp)) on non-Asian eyes exhibit thicker PLTT with the larger-elasticity lens. Apparently, lens recoil is larger with a higher-modulus lens leading to a thicker PoLTF (Chauhan and Radke, 2002). However, more data are necessary to establish this conclusion firmly.

Confounding results are seen for the Asian eye in that the PLTT is not sensitive to either lens modulus or BCR (Lin *et al.*, 2002d). It is possible that the small vertical palpebral apertures and tighter lids found in Asian eyes create a strongly localized lid wiper pressure on the lens and make the central PLTT value less susceptible to changes in BCR or modulus compared to the larger PAS found in non-Asian eyes. Such effects are currently beyond our modelling capabilities. We do learn, however, that the physical mechanisms determining the central PLTT are multifaceted and complicated.

Although measurement and understanding of the central PLTT are extremely helpful, even more relevant to mixing in the PoLTF is the distribution of tear thickness. Figure 3.4 reveals that the PLTT distribution under an SCL need not be uniform in that the lens edge settles more quickly than the lens centre. Data for the PLTT distribution under an SCL are not available but are highly valuable because tear mixing depends on the thickness of the PoLTF under the entire lens. Miller *et al.* (2003) suggested a strategy for estimating the PLTT distribution across the horizontal meridian of a soft lens by using a fluorogram and the central PLTT determined from optical pachometry. The technique involves first photographing a Fluorosoft-stained PoLTF under a lotrafilcon A(exp) lens (14 mm diameter and BCR = 8.9 mm), as illustrated in Figure 3.6A. From the photograph, a schematic of the dye distribution under the lens is constructed by visual inspection of the light and dark bands in the photomicrograph (Figure 3.6B). Dark areas in Figure 3.6A and B indicate minimal fluorescence corresponding to regions of thin PoLTF, and brighter areas indicate a locally thicker PoLTF. The schematic in Figure 3.6B shows the brightest (or thickest) ring of the tear film located at 4.5 mm from the lens centre, flanked by approximately 1 mm wide thin regions at 3.8 and 5.2 mm from the lens centre.

Using a 5 subject average central optical pachometry measurement of PLTT = 5 μm as a reference, Miller *et al.* (2003) estimated the PLTT distribution under a lotrafilcon A(exp) lens after 10 minutes of settling. The distribution is reported in Figure 3.6C by the variation of h as a function of the distance from

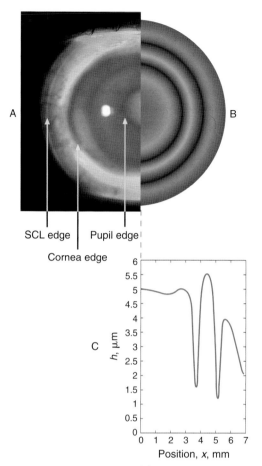

SCL edge | Pupil edge

Cornea edge

Figure 3.6   Thickness profile in the PoLTF: (A) composite photomicrograph after 30 minutes of settling; (B) schematic of observed fluorescein pattern in A; (C) estimated thickness profile, $h(x)$, where x is the radial position from the lens centre. From Miller *et al.* (2003), with permission

the lens centre $(x = 0)$ to the edge of the lens $(x = 6.9\,\text{mm})$. Since central PLTT values for lotrafilcon A(exp) lenses as thin as $2\,\mu\text{m}$ are detectable after 7 hours of settling (see Figure 3.5), Miller *et al.* (2003) set the thinnest or black regions of the fluorogram in Figure 3.6A and B as less than about $2\,\mu\text{m}$. Thus, based on the Fluorosoft patterns in Figure 3.6A and B, the PoLTF thickness distribution can be estimated, as graphed in Figure 3.6C. These estimates accentuate the non-uniform distribution of the PoLTF. However, improved strategies for obtaining tear thickness distributions and for modelling this behaviour must be developed if this information is to have useful clinical application. Figure 3.6 does highlight the difficult task of lens design for improved motion, tear mixing and comfort.

HORIZONTAL (SIDE-TO-SIDE) MOTION

In addition to the anterior–posterior and inferior–superior motion, SCLs exhibit side-to-side (i.e. lateral) and rotational motions. Just before the upper lid closes in Figure 3.2B, the lower lid translates nasally and then returns, thereby expressing tear in the lid menisci toward the puncta (Doane, 1984) and imparting a small horizontal motion to the upper lid (Lemp and Weiler, 1983; Doane, 1984). This repeated gull-wing-like motion, in principle, induces sideways and rotational motions in the SCL. Videophotographic measurements with marked and well-fitted lenses, however, demonstrate repeated side-to-side movement, but no persistent rotation (M. C. Lin, unpublished research, 2002). As part of the 58-subject study mentioned earlier with centre-marked polymacon lenses, Lin (2002) measured horizontal excursions of 0.11 ± 0.01 mm for the steep lens (BCR = 7.9 mm) and 0.15 ± 0.01 mm for the flat lens (BCR = 8.7 mm). Again, the flatter lens moves more, as is true for vertical motion. Nevertheless, the magnitude of the sideways and rotational movements is small relative to the vertical lens motion. Clearly, the most important lens motions pertinent to tear mixing are those in the in–out and up–down directions.

PoLTF flushing

Lens motion alone does not permit flushing of the PoLTF, except near the edges of the lens. The reasoning is as follows. Imagine coloured dye initially extending throughout the PoLTF. Upon the first downward portion of a blink some dye is squeezed out of the PoLTF near the periphery and into the surrounding tear lake, where it is mixed well into a colourless solution. Then, during the upward portion of the blink colourless liquid is drawn back into the PoLTF equal to the amount of dyed tear initially squeezed out. Now, in following blinks, colourless liquid is squeezed out and drawn in with no mixing penetration into the centre of the PoLTF. Consequently, lens motion alone cannot flush the PoLTF. Mixing occurs only at the edge of the lens and then only on the first blink. Some other mechanism must be the origin of the flushing action documented experimentally in Figure 3.1.

THE PHYSICS OF TEAR MIXING

MECHANISM

The physical forces controlling PoLTF mixing can be explained using a DMM based upon lid-induced vertical (up–down) and transverse (in–out) motion of the contact lens (Creech *et al.*, 2001). These two lens motions control the mass transfer of tear components in the PoLTF. The DMM can be explained by following the path of a small depot or pulse of dye initially with uniform concentration under a lens, as illustrated in Figure 3.7. In this figure the right half of the PoLTF is shown in a horizontal orientation over a blink cycle. Light grey denotes the SCL, dark grey corresponds to the cornea, intermediate levels of grey indicate the dye

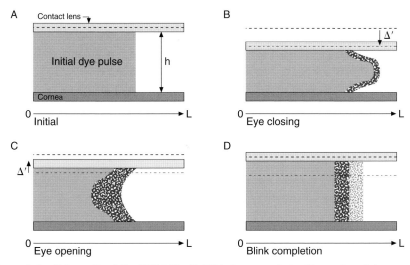

Figure 3.7 Schematic of the DMM. The PoLTF is impregnated with a pulse of dye, shown in intermediate grey colour. Dark grey denotes the cornea and light grey corresponds to the SCL. Each frame pictures how the pulse of dye spreads due to the pumping action of the lens with amplitude Δ′. Note that the dye disperses due to fluid stretching by the combined action of squeeze flow and molecular diffusion in the transverse direction, normal to the PoLTF. This drawing is not to scale

concentration; the amplitude of the transverse or in–out motion is shown as Δ′. This sketch accentuates the PoLTF and is not to scale.

When the lens is stationary, the only pathway for the dye depot to escape is by molecular diffusion. As noted above, however, time-scales for molecular diffusion parallel to the lens are very long, particularly for the larger molecules found in the tear film. However, the lens is not stationary, and under lid blink action the lens moves in-and-out and up-and-down. This causes the pulse of dye to lengthen according to the lens motion into a combined Couette[1] and squeeze velocity profile, as illustrated in Figure 3.7 for the squeeze profile only. In the stretched position of the eye closing phase of Figure 3.7B, the edges of the dye depot blur due to both transverse diffusion (normal to the PoLTF) and radial diffusion (parallel to the PoLTF). However, transverse diffusion occurs on a much shorter time-scale than diffusion along the lens because of the much shorter distance scale (i.e. the thickness of the PoLTF is 10 μm whereas the lens radius is 7 mm). This means that after many blinks the transverse-diffusion contribution dominates the mixing process. During the eye-opening portion of a blink, the dye pulse returns to its initial position but, as pictured in Figure 3.7C, transverse diffusion continues to cause blurring near the dye edge. At the end of each blink in Figure 3.7D, the lid force is released; the lens returns to its original position, but the dye now smears further towards the edge of the contact lens. As the blurring process

---

[1] The word Couette refers to rectilinear flow in a narrow gap between two parallel, semi-infinite flat plates sliding with respect to each other.

repeats during continued blinking, the shape of the dye concentration profile eventually takes on a Gaussian distribution, as if radial diffusion were responsible for the redistribution (or dispersion) of the dye. However, the mechanism is not one of molecular diffusion but rather of a mechanically driven mixing (i.e. due to the periodic lens motion). Combination of repeated lens motion and transverse molecular diffusion leads to mechanical removal of the dye from under the lens and is referred to as dispersive mixing (Creech *et al.*, 2001). Without lens motion, mixing in the PoLTF is reduced to molecular diffusion along the lens, which, again, occurs much too slowly to explain the 10-minute characteristic mixing times found experimentally in Figure 3.1 for FITC-dextran.

DISPERSIVE MIXING MODEL

Based on the mechanical mixing physics described in Figure 3.7, Creech *et al.* (2001) derived a DMM to quantify the measured FITC-dextran decay data in Figure 3.1 and to provide new design strategies for improving flushing of the PoLTF. Using periodically steady squeeze and Couette velocity profiles, of amplitudes Δ and Δ', to reflect the in–out and up–down lens motions respectively, Creech *et al.* (2001) established that dispersive mixing obeys Fick's second law for diffusion but with an effective diffusion or dispersion coefficient, and that the transverse average dye concentration decays exponentially at later times, consistent with Figure 3.1. Species dispersivities, D^*, in the PoLTF are three orders of magnitude larger than their corresponding molecular diffusion coefficients, D (Creech *et al.*, 2001). Hence, the characteristic time for FITC-dextran removal from the PoLTF becomes $T = L^2/D^*$, or about 10 minutes, a number quite in accord with the typical experimental FITC-dextran flushing times in Figure 3.1.

Creech *et al.* (2001) also derive a mathematical formula to predict D^* from lens and tear properties:

$$\frac{D^*}{D} = f\left(\frac{\omega h^2}{D}, \frac{\Delta}{h}, \frac{\Delta'}{h}\right) \tag{2}$$

where f denotes a known function (Creech *et al.*, 2001), h is the (uniform) PLTT, and ω is the blink frequency in radians. In general, increasing either the vertical amplitude, Δ, or the transverse amplitude, Δ', increases the dispersion coefficient and hence improves flushing from the PoLTF. Thus, we again learn that lens motion and the PLTT are crucial components of tear mixing. Consequently, information about these two components is critical to developing lens design strategies to optimize tear mixing. We also stress from Equation (2) that mixing times in the PoLTF are not universal. That is, bacteria do not have the same flushing times as FITC-dextran because these two species have quite different molecular diffusion coefficients. Intuitively, we expect that bacteria with larger diffusion coefficients than FITC-dextran take longer to flush from the PoLTF. However, this presupposition depends on the particular value of the parameter $\omega h^2/D$ pertinent to the PoLTF. Armed with the DMM, we now consider the roles of various lens properties and lid anatomy on flushing of the PoLTF.

TEAR MIXING MEASUREMENTS

METHODS

Tear mixing under an SCL has been estimated by measuring the time required for a tracer material (e.g. dye, microspheres, red blood cells) to be removed from under the contact lens (Guillon and McGrogan, 1997; McGrogan et al., 1997). Most tear-mixing estimates have been made using a fluorometer, which can measure the change in fluorescence under a contact lens over a specified wearing period. Either high-molecular-weight sodium fluorescein (Fluorosoft, MW = 600 Da) or a dye formulated as a fluorescein-tagged dextran (FITC-dextran, Smith Chemical; available over a molecular weight range from 1 to 12 kDa) is used in the fluorometric measurement. Fluorosoft is absorbed by lenses with water content greater than about 50 per cent. Therefore, most measurements are done here using FITC-dextran (MW = 9–12 kDa) to avoid underestimates of tear mixing that might occur with lens or ocular absorption of the tracer dye.

INSTRUMENTATION

Two fluorometric methods are currently used to estimate tear mixing. One technique uses a modified slit-lamp with light focused on the PoLTF as changes in fluorescence intensity (FI) are monitored. This technique has the advantage of placing the excitation light directly on the target area (e.g. tear film; Bergman et al., 1970; Polse, 1979). An alternative IV fluorometric technique uses a scanning fluorometer (Ocumetrics Inc., Mountain View, CA) that drives the excitation light from the PrLTF to the cornea using a computer-driven stepper motor. The instrument makes a series of FI readings and provides FI data centred around the peak FITC-dextran fluorescence under the SCL (McNamara et al., 1999). This instrument is very sensitive to low levels of fluorescent dye. Unfortunately, since the placement of the light cannot be controlled precisely, the tear-mixing estimate assumes that there is no fluorescence on the anterior lens surface. This assumption is valid for lenses with slow tear-mixing rates. However, if there is efficient tear mixing (e.g. with RGP lenses), the measurement is invalid because it is not possible to separate intensity decay from the PrLTF and PoLTF when the decays occur on the same time-scales. The result is an overestimate of the amount of tear mixing in the PoLTF. Details of each instrument are covered extensively in other publications (Polse, 1979; Kok et al., 1992; McNamara et al., 1999; Paugh et al., 2001).

MEASUREMENT PROCEDURES

The procedure for estimating tear mixing is as follows: baseline (B_o) autofluorescence readings (cornea + lens) are obtained with the lens on the eye. The lens is then removed, a small amount (e.g. 1 μl) of FITC-dextran solution is placed on the posterior lens surface, and then the lens is reinserted directly on to the cornea. Next, the FI is monitored for 30 minutes. Subjects are either allowed to blink at their normal rate or asked to blink at a rate of 15 blinks/minute (average blink rate) cadenced using a metronome. The rate of dye depletion is determined by fitting an exponential decay model to the FI values obtained over the 30-minute observation period (McNamara *et al.*, 1999), as illustrated in Figure 3.1. The straight lines seen in the semi-logarithmic graph of Figure 3.1 confirm exponential decay. After approximately 30 minutes there is little or no detectable change in FITC-dextran intensity.

The exponential decay rate is expressed as a time constant, T, defined as the time required to deplete 63 per cent of dye from under the lens. For the computation, we eliminate the first 5 minutes of data because reflex tearing may occur as the lens is initially inserted and because the DMM applies at a later time. The efficiency of tear mixing is expressed as the time required to deplete 95 per cent of the dye from under the lens or $3T$, which we denote as T_{95}. Other investigators have expressed tear exchange as a change in percentage volume per blink (tear replenishment rate (TRR); Polse, 1979) or as the time needed to eliminate the dye from under the lens (ER). We choose T_{95} as the measure of PoLTF flushing because it has a physically transparent meaning, and it is directly related to the DMM. Also, T_{95} is obtained immediately from the FI decay data without further data manipulation. Conversion among all three measures of PoLTF flushing is straightforward (Miller, 2002).

VALIDATION

It is possible that the clinical estimates of tear mixing with fluorescent dye are not due to dispersion-assisted mixing, but rather to the settling of the lens after insertion. For example, the settling action of the lens might expel fluorescence stained tears without changing the dye concentration in the PoLTF. As the tear film thins, there are fewer photons emitted, giving rise to a smaller fluorescence signal that can be misinterpreted as fluorescence decay. To determine whether dye actually 'mixes' (i.e. moves from under the lens to outside the lens boundary), the movement of a small amount of dye placed outside the lens can be followed by careful slit-lamp observation. If dye does not appear under the lens, the change in FI measured during lens wear is likely due to the settling of the lens and not to dispersive tear mixing and vice versa.

Miller (2002) traced the movement of dye by placing 5 µl of FITC-dextran solution (4.4 kDa) on to the temporal bulbar conjunctiva and visually observing the time course of the dye through a slit-lamp at the 6 o'clock position over a 240-minute wearing period as it transported from outside to under the lens. Results are summarized in Figure 3.8, which gives the time for appearance under the lens (y-axis) at 10, 30 and 240 minutes of wear time (x-axis) at the peripheral (closed squares) and centre positions (open squares) for lotrafilcon A(exp) lenses (14 mm diameter, BCR = 8.9 mm). The plot displays the mean time for the appearance of the dye on four subjects. Error bars represent one standard deviation above and below the mean of each measurement and lines connect the data points. For all four subjects, the dye travelled from outside to under the lens.

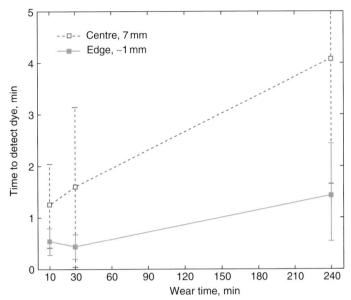

Figure 3.8   Time to detect visually FITC-dextran under lotrafilcon A(exp) lenses after instillation on the temporal conjunctiva for four subjects as a function of wear time. Observations are made at the 6 o'clock position for two locations under the lens: 1 mm from the lens edge (closed squares) and 7 mm from the edge at the lens centre (open squares). Lines connect data points

Note that it takes considerably longer for the dye to reach the centre compared to the edge of the lens. Also, the longer the lens is on the eye, the greater is the time for the appearance of dye at both the edge and central positions. This is because the lens settles over long time periods (see Figures 3.4 and 3.5) and because dispersive mixing slows for smaller PLTT, as discussed below. Since dispersion-assisted mixing is independent of the direction of dye travel, both of these observations are in harmony with the proposed DMM. We conclude that the changes in dye intensity measured during fluorometry of the PoLTF (see Figure 3.1) are likely due to dispersive mixing and not simply to lens settling. Figure 3.5 further reinforces dispersive-assisted mixing as the operative PoLTF flushing mechanism, since there is very little settling of the lotrafilcon A(exp) lens between 5 and 30 minutes, the time-scale of the FI measurements.

CLINICAL TEAR MIXING RESULTS

PREVIOUS MIXING ESTIMATES

Several reports are available on the mixing efficiency under hydrogel and silicone hydrogel SCLs. Early studies were performed with low water content (e.g. 38 per cent) HEMA materials. FI data were obtained with a slit-lamp fluorometer, and tear mixing was expressed as a TRR, the percentage volume of tear replaced per

Table 3.2   Tear-mixing rates for selected HEMA and silicone hydrogel lenses

Research group	Dye	Instrument	Lens type	TRR (%/blink)	T_{95} (min)	n
Polse (1979)	Fluorosoft	Slit-lamp fluorometer	Polymacon	0.27	73.1	1
			Tetrafilcon	0.39	50.8	1
			Bufilcon A	0.38	52.6	1
McNamara et al. (1999)	FITC-dextran	Scanning fluorometer	Isofilcon (13 mm diam.)	1.34	14.9	22
Paugh et al. (2001)	FITC-dextran	Slit-lamp fluorometer	Lotraficon A (prototype)	0.95	21.1	7
			Etafilcon A	0.59	34.0	11
			Polymacon	0.90	22.2	49
Miller (2002)	FITC-dextran	Scanning fluorometer	Etafilcon A	0.66	30.2	23
			Ocufilcon D	0.64	31.1	22
			Lotrafilcon A(exp)	0.87	22.9	21

n = number of subjects.

blink. TRR values ranged from 0.9 to 2.2 per cent (Polse, 1979). Quantifying tear mixing as a TRR is not strictly correct since a volume of tear is not actually removed with each blink. A more accurate description of tear exchange is given by the T_{95} value. Conversion of the 2.2–0.9 per cent TRR values corresponds to T_{95} values of 9–22 minutes. More recently, several tear-mixing estimates on both hydrogel and silicone hydrogel SCLs have been made using highly sensitive fluorometers. Table 3.2 summarizes the tear-mixing estimates from these studies and shows that, in general, tear-mixing rates in the PoLTF are low (i.e. 20–30 minutes).

EFFECT OF LENS DIAMETER

The effects of lens diameter have been studied over a range from 12.0 to 13.5 mm for 23 subjects wearing lathe-cut isofilcon lenses (McNamara et al., 1999). Figure 3.9 displays these results as T_{95} both as a function of the lens diameter squared (bottom abscissa) and as lens diameter (top abscissa). The reason for plotting the square of the lens diameter is that the characteristic time for dispersive mixing scales is calculated as L^2/D^*. Closed squares reflect the experimental mean mixing times with standard deviations corresponding to about the size of the data points. Tear mixing improves slightly (i.e. T_{95} diminishes) as the diameter decreases from 13.5 to 12.0 mm. Solid lines in this figure reveal the DMM predictions (i.e. from Equation (2) using the physical parameters listed). Since the amplitude of lens transverse motion is not known, Creech et al. (2001) estimated it from known results for squeeze flow and the normal lid force. Unfortunately pachometry

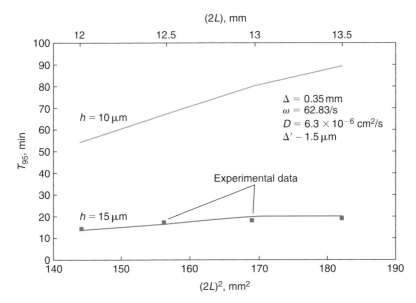

Figure 3.9   Comparison of the DMM (solid lines) to experimental T_{95} values for FITC-dextran flushing under isofilcon lenses worn by 23 subjects (solid squares). The effect of lens diameter is studied. Parameters used in the DMM are listed in the figure. An average PLTT of around 15 μm fits the dye mixing data adequately. From Creech *et al.* (2001), with permission

estimates of the PLTT were not available. Hence, Figure 3.9 adopts two reasonable values: 10 and 15 μm. A 15 μm value for h provides a good fit of the DMM to the experimental data, indicating that the proposed mixing theory provides a useful tool for guiding designs of improved flushing of the PoLTF.

Although these findings are in accord with the DMM, the amount of change with lens diameter is modest. We caution that when the lens diameter was changed, the BCR was simultaneously altered to achieve an acceptable lens fit. The simultaneous change of lens diameter and BCR is the likely reason why the up–down lens motion is about the same for all four different diameter lenses studied in Figure 3.9. So we cannot conclude that smaller-diameter lenses necessarily improve tear exchange. In any case, from a clinical perspective, diameters less than 12.5 or greater than 14 mm are not prescriptable because of comfort and physiological restraints and, therefore, major improvements in tear flushing solely by reducing lens diameter are unlikely to be effective.

EFFECT OF LENS PLTT

The DMM predicts that T_{95} decreases with increasing PLTT (Creech *et al.*, 2001). As noted in the discussion of lens motion, complicated lid and lens mechanics set the PLTT; thus the PLTT is influenced by many factors including lens BCR, lens modulus, vertical PAS, central corneal curvatures and ethnic background (Asians versus non-Asians), among others. Although we find that BCR, lens modulus,

Table 3.3   Effects of BCR and vertical movement on 58 subjects wearing polymacon lenses

	BCR = 8.7 mm	BCR = 7.9 mm	
	Mean ± SE	Mean ± SE	p-Values
Vertical movement (mm)	0.7 ± 0.1	0.4 ± 0.1	0.001
Horizontal movement (mm)	0.17 ± 0.01	0.11 ± 0.01	0.001
T_{95} (min)	23 ± 1	24 ± 1	0.643

vertical PAS, and ethnic background all influence the PLTT (see Table 3.1), there are few clinical data to establish this. Lin *et al.* (2002c) recently completed preliminary studies using lathe-cut polymacon lenses. They find that tear mixing is more efficient as the PAS increases. Similarly, Brennan *et al.* (2001) recently correlated a qualitative measure of PLTT to fluorometric estimates of tear mixing and found that thinner PLTT values are associated with poor tear mixing. Thus it is theorized that eyes with large PAS tend to have thicker PLTT and, hence, more efficient tear mixing. These preliminary clinical observations are in agreement with the predictions of the DMM, which state that the tear mixing rate increases with the PLTT (see also Figure 3.9). Nevertheless, more work is needed to understand the PLTT–T_{95} relationship.

EFFECT OF LENS VERTICAL MOVEMENT

Recently, Lin *et al.* (2002c) explored the relationships between lid anatomy, lens design and performance by measuring aperture size, vertical and horizontal movement, and tear mixing on a series of 58 Asian and non-Asian subjects wearing polymacon lenses. Table 3.3 summarizes the results of these studies and shows that flatter lenses move more than steeper lenses in both the vertical and horizontal directions, as noted earlier. However, tear mixing was not significantly different between the two lens groups with $T_{95} \cong 25$ minutes for each. These clinical results suggest that changes in vertical or horizontal lens movements in the range that provide acceptable comfort do not have a significant impact on tear mixing. Miller (2002) used the DMM to estimate the change in T_{95} as a function of vertical movement when all other parameters are held constant. Figure 3.10 shows the calculated change in tear mixing, in minutes as a function of vertical lens movement, ΔT_{95}, using a lens with a 14 mm diameter, a uniform PLTT of 10 µm, and a transverse motion of 3 µm. Under these conditions, an increase in lens travel from 0.25 to 0.75 mm results in a reduction in T_{95} of only 1 minute. Even over the entire range of lens travel (i.e. 1.5 mm), the DMM predicts that T_{95} changes by only 4 minutes. Although we cannot be certain that the constants used in the modelling effort are entirely correct, they are reasonable. In addition, vertical lens travel is not correctly estimated using the centre mark method, and the DMM considers a symmetric vertical motion that is not expected to be correct (see Figure 3.3). Nevertheless, based on our current T_{95} data and on concern

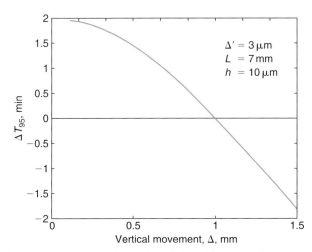

Figure 3.10   The change in PoLTF mixing time, ΔT_{95}, with vertical lens movement, Δ, from the DMM. Lens transverse motion, Δ', is held constant at 3 μm. Remaining parameters in the DMM are listed in the figure. The reference T_{95} is for a vertical lens displacement of 1 mm

over lens comfort, we surmise that strategies aimed at increasing vertical lens movement alone may not be a clinically effective way to enhance tear mixing.

EFFECT OF LENS TRANSVERSE MOVEMENT

The DMM shows that increased transverse lens motion (anterior–posterior lens motion) enhances tear exchange. Since we do not anticipate in–out motion of the lens to affect comfort, it is useful to explore strategies to increase transverse motion. Chauhan and Radke (2001b) employ a lubrication hydrodynamic model to show that, by inserting multiple fenestrations or channels into the lens, fluid resistance in the PoLTF against transverse motion is reduced. Fenestrations allow the PoLTF to escape through the holes, rather than only through the lens periphery, while channels permit alternative escape routes to the lens periphery. We reiterate that simply permitting additional escape routes for the PoLTF does not improve overall flushing of unwanted species, since only the edge regions are influenced (Miller *et al.*, 2003). The argument is identical to that made earlier for the repeated squeezing in and out of clear fluid near the lens periphery. Rather, fenestrations or channels reduce the flow resistance for lens pumping, subsequently increasing Δ' in Equation (2). Said in another way, reduction of the hydro-dynamic resistance to fluid flow allows for increased transverse motion and a concomitant increase in dispersive tear mixing (Chauhan and Radke, 2001b; Miller *et al.*, 2003).

Very recently, Miller *et al.* (2003) completed preliminary work to explore the effects of multiple fenestrations on tear mixing with experimental lotrafilcon A(exp) lenses in which an array of 40 fenestrations of 50 μm diameter each is placed in two concentric, circular rows near the lens periphery. These researchers compared the tear mixing behind the fenestrated lenses to lenses of the same lens design except for the holes. Figure 3.11 illustrates the clinical effects of fenestrations for 20 subjects wearing both the fenestrated (F) and standard, unfenestrated (S-uF) lenses. A line connects the T_{95} value for each of the two lens types. The majority of subjects (16/20) had lower T_{95} rates for the F lenses. The average T_{95} for the 20 subjects (mean $\pm$ SE) was 22.6 $\pm$ 1.0 minute and 18.3 $\pm$ 1.0 minute for the S-uF and F lens, respectively. This difference corresponds to a 23 per cent improvement in tear mixing efficiency and is statistically significant (paired $t = 4.86$, $p < 0.005$). Although such changes in T_{95} probably do not provide the optimal tear-mixing rates that are needed for safe EW, the data do suggest that strategies aimed at increasing transverse lens motion should be considered along with other approaches to improve tear exchange. For example, Miller *et al.* (2003) argue that precise placement of the fenestrations can have a significant influence on improving tear-mixing efficiency.

The theoretical study of Chauhan and Radke (2001b) suggests that channels are even more effective than fenestrations in improving flushing from the PoLTF. As with fenestrations, the predicted mechanism is increasing the transverse motion, thereby making the dispersion coefficient larger and lowering the mixing time, T_{95}. Since channels provide escape paths all along their length, they are more effective than fenestrations that act somewhat as point escapes. Miller (2002) recently studied, both theoretically and clinically, the behaviour of channelled ocufilcon D lenses (14.2 mm diameter, 8.6 mm BCR) with rectangular channels in the posterior side. Channels were equally spaced, numbered between

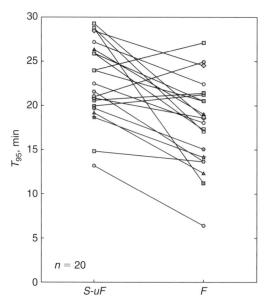

Figure 3.11 T_{95} clinical results for 20 subjects wearing otherwise identical lotrafilcon A(exp) lenses with fenestrations (F) or standard with no fenestrations (S-uF). Lines connect the data points for each subject. From Miller *et al.* (2003), with permission

10 and 40, and extended radially outward from the optic zone to a distance of 4 mm. All channels were 20 μm deep and 0.24 mm wide. The initial clinical result of placing the channelled lenses on five subjects was a universal and rapid settling to an uncomfortable state of almost no vertical movement. Otherwise identical lenses with no channels exhibited a range of vertical motion from 0.25 to 0.75 mm and produced no discomfort. Incorporation of channels permitted such rapid egress of the PoLTF that almost complete settling occurred within several blinks. Thus, the channels accomplished the goal of easier egress (and ingress) of tear from underneath the lens. Although the particular studied channelled lenses are not viable clinically, their efficient pumping action provides clues for improving channel designs with both lower resistance to tear flow under the lens and with a stable PoLTF.

EFFECT OF LENS MODULUS

Tear-mixing measurements with four different modulus lenses ranging from 0.28 to 1.2 MPa of essentially the same diameter and BCR indicate that the higher the modulus, the more efficient is the tear exchange (Miller, 2002). Table 3.4 lists average T_{95} values for the four studied soft lenses, along with the lens initial water content and the subject sample sizes. No differences in the comfort ratings of the lenses were observed (Miller, 2002).

The proposed explanation is that modulus plays an indirect role of increasing the in–out motion of the lens (Miller, 2002). Although the vertical motion of the four lenses was not recorded, it is improbable that there are large differences in up–down movement of these lenses. Further, as noted in Figure 3.10, vertical motion does not appear to play a major role in tear mixing. However, transverse motion can potentially affect tear mixing more dramatically. Figure 3.12 is a companion graph to Figure 3.10 and reports the calculated change in mixing times, ΔT_{95}, as a function of transverse motion, Δ', compared to a reference lens 14 mm in diameter with a uniform PLTT of 10 μm and with a vertical motion amplitude of 1 mm (Miller, 2002). Small changes in transverse motion are seen to alter T_{95} substantially. Thus Miller (2002) argues that the improved mixing times reported in Table 3.4 for the higher-modulus lenses are due to increased transverse motion leading to improved PoLTF flushing per the DMM. Since no

Table 3.4 Changes in tear exchange with lenses of various moduli of rigidity

Material	Diam. (mm)	BCR (mm)	H₂O content	Modulus of rigidity (MPa)	n	T_{95} (min)
Etafilcon A	14.0	8.7	58%	0.28	22	30.2 ± 1.5
Ocufilcon D	14.2	8.6	55%	0.52	22	31.1 ± 1.6
Polymacon	14.0	8.7	38%	0.81	49	22.2 ± 1.1
Lotrafilcon A(exp)	13.8	8.6	24%	1.20	21	22.9 ± 1.6

n = number of subjects.

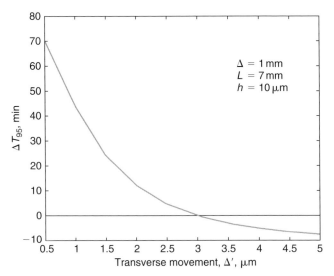

Figure 3.12   The change in PoLTF mixing time, ΔT_{95}, with transverse lens movement, Δ', from the DMM. Lens vertical motion, Δ, is held constant at 1 mm. Remaining parameters in the DMM are listed on the figure. The reference T_{95} is for a transverse lens displacement of 3 μm

direct measures of Δ' are available and since the current modelling efforts to predict lens motion are rudimentary (Chauhan and Radke, 2001a, 2002), confirmation of this reasoning is lacking. Further, the PLTT distribution under the ocufilcon D, etafilcon A and polymacon lenses differs from that of the lotrafilcon A(exp) lens (see Figure 3.6; Miller, 2002). Additional and more detailed examination of the tear film thickness profiles under SCLs is needed to understand the mechanism(s) of tear exchange.

SUMMARY

Efficient tear mixing and timely removal of cellular debris, bacteria or unwanted chemical species that accumulate between the lens and cornea during extended and especially during closed-eye contact lens wear appear necessary for safe lens wear. The tear flushing rate can be estimated using fluorometry to measure the exponential concentration decay of a high-molecular-weight dye (i.e. FITC-dextran) from under the lens. Mixing efficiency is expressed as T_{95}, the time required for 95 per cent of the dye to be removed from under the lens. Several clinical studies demonstrate that the tear exchange process with current soft lenses is slow (e.g. $T_{95} = 20$–30 minutes), and if the occurrence of mechanically induced complications associated with overnight wear is to be significantly reduced, more efficient tear mixing is required. We emphasize that time constants for FITC-dextran removal from the PoLTF most likely underestimate those of larger contaminants in the PoLTF, such as bacteria or debris, that exhibit larger molecular diffusion coefficients. Consequently, the optimal T_{95} is not known. Provisionally, we suggest that time constants for FITC-dextran removal similar to those observed with rigid lenses (e.g. ~5–7 minutes) might significantly lower the frequency of several types of adverse clinical events associated with closed-eye lens wear.

Mixing of chemical species in the PoLTF is driven primarily by lid motion during blinking. Little or no radial molecular diffusion directly transports material from the PoLTF because the rate of this process is much too slow. Rather, lid motion drives movement of the contact lens that, in turn, leads to a mechanical stretching of fluid elements in the PoLTF. This flow stretching, in concert with transverse molecular diffusion, leads to a dispersion-assisted species mixing process that behaves identically to molecular diffusion, but with an effective dispersion coefficient, D^*. In the PoLTF, D^* is thousands of times larger than the molecular diffusion coefficient, D. Four types of lens motion potentially contribute to dispersive mixing in the PoLTF: up–down or vertical motion, in–out or transverse motion, side–side or lateral motion, and rotational motion. Efforts to understand and quantify lens motion are crucial not only for better PoLTF flushing but also for improved lens design. In particular, exactly how a lens settles into a time periodic state with a stable PoLTF, or whether a stable periodic motion is even established, remains an open issue. Of the documented lens motions, vertical and transverse movements appear to be the most important to tear mixing.

Based on periodic vertical and transverse lens motion and well-established hydrodynamic principles, we developed a DMM to quantify tear mixing and to guide lens design for improved flushing from the PoLTF. The model shows that tear exchange under a contact lens is a complex process depending on many lens and ocular factors. Although it is possible to modify some of the factors that might improve tear mixing (e.g. PLTT, lens design, modulus), other factors cannot be changed (e.g. lid tension, PAS, corneal shape). In essence, the DMM predicts that increased amplitudes of vertical and transverse motion, Δ and Δ', respectively, reduce T_{95}. Ultimately, the appropriate selection of lens mater-ials and designs is critical to the improvement of tear mixing. To develop optimal lenses we adopt a strategy of obtaining clinical data which are then used to refine and improve the DMM. Our current findings include the following.

The DMM predicts and clinical data confirm that increased PLTT improves PoLTF flushing. This is because, for a given applied lid force, the transverse movement of the lens is larger. Average central PLTT values, obtained here by optical pachometry, are around $10\,\mu m$. However, this value is significantly influenced by PAS and lid tension, such that smaller PAS and tighter lids (e.g. Asian eyes) have significantly thinner PLTT compared to larger PAS and looser lids (non-Asian eyes). A caveat is that central PLTTs are insufficient to characterize the entire PLTT profile under the SCL. Thin regions of the PoLTF can have a dominant negative effect on tear mixing by lowering transverse and vertical lens movement. There is currently a paucity of information on the PoLTF thickness profile and how it changes with lens design and ocular anatomy.

Larger lens BCR (i.e. flatter lenses) improve both vertical and horizontal lens motions. Surprisingly, we find that the increased motion does not necessarily translate into lowering of T_{95} and into better tear mixing. Calculations using the DMM suggest that T_{95} is not highly sensitive to increases in vertical motion, but rather is more sensitive to improvement in transverse lens motion (see Figures 3.10 and 3.12). Further, comfort constraints limit the amount of vertical lens motion that can be tolerated. We caution, however, that this conclusion is reached only for FITC-dextran flushing and not for bacteria or debris flushing, which may behave somewhat differently because of the larger molecular diffusion coefficients for such species. Lenses with smaller BCR (i.e. steeper lenses) exhibit larger central PLTTs. Investigation of this effect alone on tear mixing is masked by simultan-eous changes in vertical and lateral lens motion.

A higher lens modulus improves the efficiency of mixing in the PoLTF. Our explanation is that higher moduli permit more recoil during the interblink, thereby increasing the lens in–out motion. However, we have no confirmation of this proposal since currently no direct means are available for measuring the transverse lens motion.

According to the DMM, lessening the lens diameter enhances mixing efficiency. The predicted effect is two-fold. First, the path length for species flushing is reduced for smaller lenses; second, smaller-diameter lenses travel more in both the vertical and transverse directions because of lower hydrodynamic resistance. Clinical measurements show a minor improvement in tear mixing with smaller lens diameters. However, our studied lenses also had different BCR to maintain good fits, so the effect of lens diameter was not isolated.

Finally, the DMM suggests that holes or channels enhance tear mixing. The effect is not that of providing escape routes for the unwanted species but rather that of increasing transverse lens movement. For lotrafilcon A(exp) lenses, we find a 23 per cent improvement in FITC-dextran mixing efficiency with 50 μm holes placed in two concentric, circular rows of 20 holes each. Model predictions indicate that more careful placement of the holes increases the mixing efficiency more substantially. The DMM also predicts that channels improve tear-mixing efficiency even more than fenestrations by providing reduced flow resistance for improved tear pumping. Clinical evaluation of this prediction needs to be performed.

In conclusion, we argue that engineering analysis is extremely helpful to develop new lens prototypes that can be tested in the clinical laboratory. Data from these measurements can be used to refine the model further. Hopefully this process results ultimately in optimized lens prototypes that exhibit significantly enhanced tear mixing. Once such lenses are available, it is important to evaluate the hypothesis that inefficient tear mixing associated with closed-eye lens wear can lead to adverse clinical events.

REFERENCES

Berger, R. E. and Corsin, S. (1974) A surface tension gradient mechanism for driving the pre-corneal tear film after a blink. *J. Biomechanics*, 7, 225–238

Bergman W., Maurice, D. M. and Ruben, M. (1970) Effect of channelling on hydrostatic pressure behind a haptic lens. *Br. J. Ophthalmol.*, **54**, 484–485

Bird, R. B., Stewart, W. E. and Lightfoot, E. N. (1960) *Transport Phenomena*. Wiley: New York, p. 40

Brennan N., Jaworski A., Shuley, V. *et al.* (2001) Studies of the post-lens tear film. *Optom. Vis. Sci.*, **78**(12s), 51

Chauhan, A. and Radke, C. J. (2001a) Modeling the vertical motion of a soft contact lens. *Curr. Eye Res.*, **22**, 102–108

Chauhan, A. and Radke, C. J. (2001b) The role of fenestrations and channels on the transverse motion of a soft contact lens. *Optom. Vis. Sci.*, **78**, 732–743

Chauhan, A. and Radke, C. J. (2002) Settling and deformation of a thin elastic shell onto a thin fluid layer overlying a solid surface, *J. Colloid Interface Sci.*, **245**, 187–197

Cho, P. (1991) Stability of the precorneal tear film: a review. *Clin. Exp. Optom.*, **74**, 19–25

Creech, J. L., Do, L. T., Fatt, I. *et al.* (1998) In vivo tear-film thickness determination and implications for tear-film stability. *Curr. Eye Res.*, **17**, 1058–1066

Creech, J. L., Chauhan, A. and Radke, C. J. (2001) Dispersive mixing in the posterior tear film under a soft contact lens. *Ind. Eng. Chem. Res.*, **40**, 3015–3026

Danjo, Y., Nakamura, M. and Hamano, T. (1994) Measurement of the precorneal tear film thickness with a non-contact optical interferometry film thickness measurement system. *Jpn. J. Ophthalmol.*, **38**, 260–266

Doane, M. G. (1980) Interaction of eyelids and tears in corneal wetting and the dynamics of the normal human eye blink. *Am. J. Ophthalmol.*, **89**, 507–526

Doane, M. G. (1981) Blinking and the mechanics of the lacrimal drainage system. *Am. Acad. Ophthalmol.*, **88**, 844–851

Doane, M. G. (1984) Blinking and tear drainage. *Adv. Ophthalmol. Plastic Recon. Surg.*, **3**, 39–52

Doane, M. G. (1994) Abnormalities of the structure of the superficial lipid layer on the in-vivo dry-eye tear film. *Adv. Exp. Med. Biol.*, **350**, 489–493

Dumbleton, K. (2002) Adverse events with silicone hydrogel continuous wear. *CLAO J.*, **25**, 137–146

Fatt, I. (1991) Observations of tear film break up on model eyes. *CLAO J.*, **17**, 267–281

Fatt, I. and Weisman, B. A. (1992) *Physiology of the Eye*. Butterworth-Heinemann, Boston, Ch. 6.

Fleiszig, S. M., Zaidi, T. S., Preston, M. J. *et al.* (1996) Relationship between cytotoxicity and corneal epithelial cell invasion by clinical isolates of *Pseudomonas aeruginosa*. *Infect. Immunol.*, **64**, 2288–2294

Fleiszig, S. M., Lee, E. J., Wu, C. *et al.* (1998) Cytotoxic strains of *Pseudomonas aeruginosa* can damage the intact corneal surface in vitro. *CLAO J.*, **24**, 41–47

Fonn, D., MacDonald, K. E., Richter, D. *et al.* (2002) The ocular response to extended wear of a high *Dk* silicone hydrogel contact lens. *Clin. Exp. Optom.*, **85**, 176–182

Funkenbusch, G. M. T. and Benson, R. C. (1999) Centering mechanism for soft contact lenses. *J. Biomech. Eng.*, **212**, 188–195

Guillon, M. and McGrogan, L. (1997) Post lens particle exchange under hydrogel contact lenses: effects of contact lens characteristics. *Optom. Vis. Sci.*, **74**(12s), 73

Guiot, E., Enescu, M., Arrio, B. *et al.* (2000) Molecular dynamics of biological probes by fluorescence correlation microscopy with two-photon excitation. *J. Fluoresc.*, **10**, 413–419

Holden, B. A., Sweeney, D. F., Vannas, A. *et al.* (1985) Effects of long-term extended contact lens wear on the human cornea. *Invest. Ophthalmol. Vis. Sci.*, **26**, 1489–1501

Holden, B. A., Stephenson, A. and Stretton, S. (2001) Superior epithelial arcuate lesions with soft contact lens wear. *Optom. Vis. Sci.*, **78**, 9–12

Humphreys, J. A., Larke, J. R. and Parrish, S. T. (1980) Microepithelial cysts observed in extended contact-lens wearing subjects. *Br. J. Ophthalmol.*, **64**, 888–889

Kenyon, E., Polse, K. A. and Seger, R. G. (1986) Influence of wearing schedule on extended-wear complications. *Ophthalmology*, **93**, 231–236

Kok, J. H., Boets, E. P., van Best, J. A. *et al.* (1992) Fluorophotometric assessment of tear turnover under rigid contact lenses. *Cornea*, **11**, 515–517

Korb, D. R. and Greiner, J. V. (1994) Increase in tear film lipid layer thickness following treatment of meibomian gland dysfunction. *Adv. Exp. Med. Biol.*, **350**, 293–298

Korb, D. A., Grenier, J. V., Herman, J. P. *et al.* (2002) Lid wiper epitheliopathy and dry eye symptom in contact lens wearers. *CLAO J.*, **28**, 211–216

Latkovic, S. and Nilsson, S. E. (1997) The effect of high and low *Dk/L* soft contact lenses on the glycocalyx layer of the corneal epithelium and on the membrane associated receptors for lectins. *CLAO J.*, **23**, 185–191

Lebow, K. P. K. (1980) Ocular changes associated with extended wear contact lenses. *Int. Cont. Lens Clin.*, 7, 49–55

Lemp, M. A. and Gold, J. B. (1986) The effects of extended-wear hydrophilic contact lenses on the human corneal epithelium. *Am. J. Ophthalmol.*, **101**, 274–277

Lemp, M. A. and Weiler, H. H. (1983) How do tears exit? *Invest. Ophthalmol. Vis. Sci.*, **24**, 619–622

Lin, M. C., Graham, A. D., Polse, K. A. *et al.* (1999) Measurement of post contact lens tear thickness. *Invest. Ophthalmol. Vis. Sci.*, **40**, 2833–2839

Lin, M. C., Soliman, G. N., Song, M. *et al.* (2002a) Extended wear effects on epithelial permeability: hypoxic or mechanical mechanism? *Cont. Lens Ant. Eye.*, **30**, 1–6

Lin, M. C., Graham, A.D., Polse, K. A. *et al.* (2002b) The impact of rigid contact lens extended wear on corneal epithelial barrier function. *Invest. Ophthalmol. Vis. Sci.*, **43**, 1019–1024

Lin, M. C., Duong, A. and Polse K. A. (2002c) The effect of ethnicity on soft lens tear mixing. *Invest. Ophthalmol. Vis. Sci. ARVO Abstracts*, **3076-B60**, 124

Lin, M. C., Chen, Y. Q. and Polse, K. A. (2002d) The effects of soft lens and ocular characteristics on the post-lens tear thickness. *Eye Cont. Lens*, **29**, S33–36

McDonald, J. E. (1969) Surface phenomena of the tear film. *Am. J. Ophthalmol.*, **67**, 56–64

McDonald, J. E. and Brubaker, S. (1971) Meniscus-induced thinning of tear films. *Am. J. Ophthalmol.*, **72**, 139–144

McGrogan, L, Guillon, M., Dilly, N. *et al.* (1997) Particle exchange under hydrogel contact lenses: effect of contact lens characteristics. *Optom. Vis. Sci.*, **74**(12s), 73

McNamara, N. A., Polse, K. A, Fukunaga, S. A. *et al.* (1998) Soft lens extended wear affects epithelial barrier function. *Ophthalmology*, **105**, 2330–2335

McNamara, N. A., Polse, K. A., Brand, R. J. *et al.* (1999) Tear mixing under a soft contact lens: effect of lens diameter. *Am. J. Ophthalmol.*, **127**, 659–665

Mertz, G. and Holden, B. A. (1981) Clinical implications of extended wear research. *Can. J. Optom.*, **43**, 203–205

Miller, K. L. (2002) Tear film considerations with and without contact-lens wear. PhD dissertation, University of California, Berkeley

Miller, K. L., Polse, K. A. and Radke, C. J. (2002) Black-line formation and the 'perched' human tear film. *Curr. Eye Res.*, **25**, 155–162

Miller, K. L., Polse, K. A. and Radke, C. J. (2003) Fenestrations enhance tear mixing under soft contact lenses. *Invest. Ophthalmol. Vis. Sci.*, **44**, 60–67

Nichols, J. J. and King-Smith, P. E. (2000) The thickness of the post-contact lens tear film measured by interferometry. *Optom. Vis. Sci.*, **77**(12s), 264

Nicolson, P. C., Baron, R.C., Charbrecek, P. *et al.* (1999) Extended wear ophthalmic lens. US Patent 5965631

O'Hare, N. A., Naduvilath, T. J., Jalbert, I. *et al.* (2000) A clinical comparison of limbal and paralimbal superior epithelial arcuate lesions (SEALs) in high *Dk* EW. *Invest. Ophthalmol. Vis. Sci., ARVO Abstracts*, **41**, s595

O'Leary, D. J., Wilson, G. and Bergmanson, J. (1985) The influence of calcium in the tear-side perfusate on desquamation from the rabbit corneal epithelium. *Curr. Eye Res.*, **4**, 729–731

Paugh, J. R., Stapleton, F., Keay, L. *et al.* (2001) Tear exchange under hydrogel contact lenses: methodological considerations. *Invest. Ophthalmol. Vis. Sci.*, **42**, 2813–2820

Polse, K. A. (1979) Tear flow under a hydrogel contact lens. *Invest. Ophthalmol. Vis. Sci.*, **18**, 409–413

Polse, K. A., Brand, R. J., Cohen, S. R. *et al.* (1990) Hypoxic effects on corneal morphology and function. *Invest. Ophthalmol. Vis. Sci.*, **31**, 1542–1554

Polse, K. A., Lin, M. C. and Han, S. (2002) Wearing time affects post-lens tear thickness under a soft contact lens. *Invest. Ophthalmol. Vis. Sci., ARVO Abstracts*, 970

Ren, D. H., Yamamoto, K., Ladage, P. M. *et al.* (2002) Adaptive effects of 30-night wear of hyper-O_2 transmissible contact lenses on bacterial binding and corneal epithelium: a 1-year clinical trial. *Ophthalmology*, **109**, 27–39

Sack, R. A., Beaton, A., Sathe, S. *et al.* (2000) Towards a closed eye model of the pre-ocular tear layer. *Prog. Ret. Eye Res.*, **19**, 649–668

Sankaridurg, P. R., Sweeney, D. F., Sharma, S. *et al.* (1999) Adverse events with extended wear of disposable hydrogels: results for the first 13 months of lens wear. *Ophthalmology*, **106**, 1671–1680

Schein, O. D., Glynn, R. J., Poggio, E. C. *et al.* (1989) The relative risk of ulcerative keratitis among users of daily-wear and extended-wear soft contact lenses: a case–control study. Microbial Keratitis Study Group. *N. Engl. J. Med.*, **321**, 773–778

Sharma, A. and Ruckenstein, E. (1990) Energetic criteria for the breakup of liquid films on nonwetting solid surfaces. *J. Colloid Interface Sci.*, **137**, 433–445

Sweeney, D. F., Stern, J., Naduvilath, T. *et al.* (2002) Inflammatory adverse event rates over 3 years with silicone hydrogel lenses. *Invest. Ophthalmol. Vis. Sci., ARVO Abstracts*, 976

Taylor, A. J. and Wilson, S. D. R. (1996) Centration mechanism of soft contact lenses. *Optom. Vis. Sci.*, **73**, 215–221

Thoft, R. A. and Friend, J. (1975) Permeability of regenerated corneal epithelium. *Exp. Eye Res.*, **21**, 409–416

Tsubota, K., Hata, S., Toda, I. *et al.* (1996) Increase in corneal epithelial cell size with extended wear soft contact lenses depends on continuous wearing time. *Br. J. Ophthalmol.*, **80**, 144–147

Wang, J. H., Fonn, D., Simpson, T. L. and Jones L. (2003) Pre-corneal and pre- and post-lens tear film thickness measured indirectly with optical coherence tomography. *Invest. Ophthalmol. Vis. Sci.*, **44**, 2524–2528

Wong, H., Fatt, I. and Radke, C. J. (1996) Deposition and thinning of the human tear film. *J. Colloid Interface Sci.*, **184**, 44–51

Chapter **4**

Inflammation and infection and the effects of the closed eye

Mark Willcox, Padmaja R. Sankaridurg, Hua Zhu,
Emma Hume, Nerida Cole, Tim Conibear, Melissa Glasson,
Najat Harmis and Fiona Stapleton

INTRODUCTION

This chapter will focus on the systems in tears and the cornea that are either antimicrobial and/or inflammatory and changes that occur to these systems during sleep and with contact lens wear. In particular, this chapter focuses on changes in the protein/glycoprotein composition of tears, changes in white blood cell numbers in tears and in the cornea, alterations in the normal microbiota of the eye, and the types of micro-organisms that cause infection or inflammation in the contact-lens-wearing eye and their pathogenic mechanisms. Findings or speculation on the effect of silicone hydrogel lens wear on these systems will be presented throughout the chapter.

THE REGULATED AND CONSTITUTIVE LACRIMAL GLAND PROTEINS AND PLASMA PROTEINS

The tear film performs several essential functions that maintain the clarity of the cornea. The daytime tear film, i.e. open eye or basal tears, washes the cornea, provides an optically clear surface and has several antimicrobial proteins/glycoproteins that protect the cornea from infection. Table 4.1 lists the major antimicrobial proteins in the tears and their source. Lysozyme is present at approximately 30 per cent of total protein in open eye tears. Lysozyme is an enzyme, muramidase, which catalyses the hydrolysis of the bond between N-acetyl muramic acid and N-acetyl glucosamine, the building blocks of the peptidoglycan of bacterial cell walls. Once lysozyme has hydrolysed the bond, bacteria are killed by the inflow of water into their cytoplasm and subsequent osmotic lysis. Lysozyme is thus a bactericidal (i.e. kills bacteria) protein and generally functions more effectively against Gram-positive bacteria (e.g. micrococci, *Corynebacterium* and *Propionibacterium*) than against Gram-negative bacteria (e.g. pseudomonads), as the peptidoglycan of Gram-negative bacteria is hidden from lysozyme by their outer

Table 4.1   Major proteins present in the tears

Protein	Function	Approximate concentration (mg/ml)			Source and type of production
		Reflex tears	Open-eye tears	Closed-eye tears	
Lysozyme[a]	Enzymatic cleavage of bacterial peptidoglycan	1.6	2.0	1.8	Lacrimal gland – regulated synthesis[g]
Lactoferrin[a]	Sequestration of iron and disruption of lipid membranes	1.8	2.6	1.8	Lacrimal gland – regulated synthesis[g]
Lipocalin[b]	A lipid carrier and stabilizer of the tear fluid	1.7[a]	1.4	NK	Lacrimal gland – regulated synthesis[g]
Secretory IgA[a]	Anti-adhesion and opsonin	0.2	0.9	8.4	Lacrimal gland – constitutive synthesis[g]
Secretory phospho-lipase A2[c]	Antimicrobial activity, particularly against Gram-positive bacteria	0.6	NK	NK	Synthesized in the lacrimal gland,[h] and also produced by leucocytes
Specific leucocyte protease inhibitor[d]	Antiprotease and antimicrobial activity	0.008		0.05	Produced by infiltrating PMNs
Mucin[e]	Provides a wettable surface and scaffolding for the tear film; anti-adhesion and binding site for PMNs	0.037[e]	0.07[f]	NK	Conjunctival and corneal epithelial layers

NK, not known; PMNs, polymorphonuclear leucocytes.
[a] Sack et al. (1992).
[b] Lipocalin has been previously called tear-specific pre-albumin.
[c] Saari et al. (2001); Qu and Lehrer (1998).
[d] Sack et al. (2000).
[e] Mucin in the tears is composed of several different species designated MUC1, MUC4, MUC5AC and MUC2 (Inatomi et al., 1995; Gipson and Inatomi, 1998; Jumblatt et al., 1999; Pflugfelder et al., 2000). The concentration of mucin or all of the individual species in tears is currently not known. Nakamura et al. (2001) measured amount of the sugar sialic acid as a measure of amount of total mucin.
[f] Zhao et al. (2001). Amount defined as µg/ml equivalent to porcine stomach mucin. 'Tears' collected using a Schirmer strip (probably composed of open-eye, reflex and ocular surface mucin).
[g] Fullard and Tucker (1991).
[h] Aho et al. (1996).

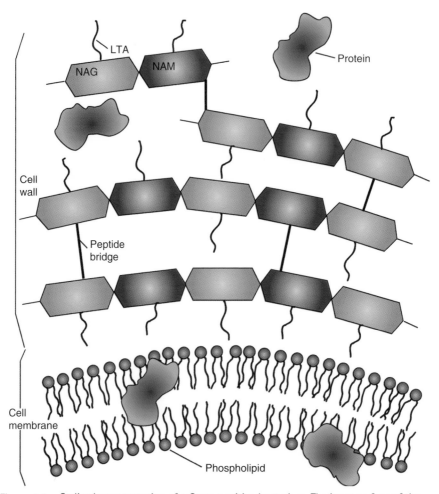

Figure 4.1 Stylized representation of a Gram-positive bacterium. The inner surface of the cell is termed the cell membrane and is composed of a bilayer of phospholipids. The cell wall is composed of N-acetyl glucosamine (NAG) and N-acetyl muramic acid (NAM), which are the building blocks of bacterial peptidoglycan. Peptidoglycan is a large carbohydrate polymer that forms a rigid outer layer of Gram-positive bacteria and prevents them from bursting because of the osmotic pressure inside the cell relative to the outside environment. Peptide bridges give the peptidoglycan its rigidity. Proteins can reside within the cell membrane and cell wall and can be exported into the environment. Attached to the cell wall are teichoic acids and lipoteichoic acids (LTA), which are potent inflammatory molecules of Gram-positive bacteria

lipid membrane. Figures 4.1 and 4.2 show the outer surface of Gram-positive and Gram-negative bacteria, respectively, in a stylized form.

Lactoferrin, also present in open eye tears at approximately 30 per cent of the total protein, has multiple functions in the tears. It is an extremely efficient iron-binding protein and thus sequesters any free iron in the tears, preventing micro-organisms from using this essential ion and therefore limiting their growth. This

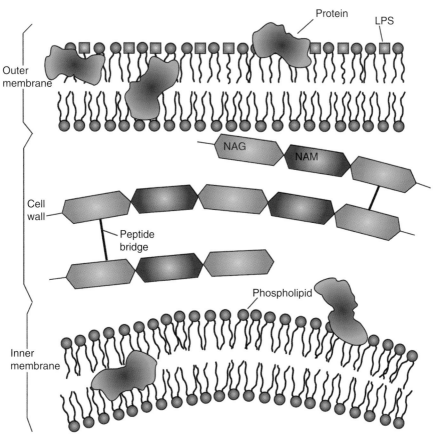

Figure 4.2   Stylized representation of a Gram-negative bacterium. Gram-negative bacteria differ from Gram-positive bacteria in having a reduced amount of peptidoglycan and an outer phospholipid membrane. This outer membrane contains lipopolysaccharide (LPS). LPS is the major inflammatory molecule of Gram-negative bacteria and is probably responsible for some of the inflammation seen when Gram-negative bacteria cause keratitis

effect is bacteriostatic (i.e. does not kill bacteria but prevents them replicating). Lactoferrin has also been shown to be bactericidal. A portion of the lactoferrin molecule, called lactoferricin, is highly positively charged and disrupts the outer membrane of micro-organisms. The exact mechanism of this disruption is not fully known, but lactoferrin can compete with Ca^{2+} and Mg^{2+}, which stabilize the lipopolysaccharide in the outer membrane of bacteria, leading to disruption in the integrity of the membrane, or it may be able to insert directly into the membrane and then form channels (Arnold *et al.*, 1982; Bellamy *et al.*, 1992; Yamauchi *et al.*, 1993) that disrupt essential enzyme activities which occur in the space between the outer and inner membranes and may also cause osmotic distress to the micro-organism. Lactoferrin may also allow the passage of lysozyme into the space between the outer and inner membranes of Gram-negative bacteria so that lysozyme can digest their peptidoglycan. It has been demonstrated that

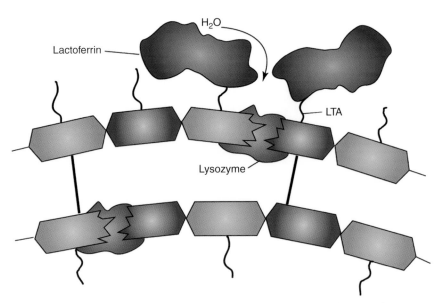

Figure 4.3 The action of lysozyme and lactoferrin on Gram-positive bacteria. Lysozyme is an enzyme that catalyses the hydrolysis of the bond between *N*-acetyl glucosamine and *N*-acetyl muramic acid. This hydrolysis weakens the peptidoglycan layer and cells are burst by water rushing into the cell. Lactoferrin is believed to act in synergy with lysozyme by binding to LTA and facilitating the entry of lysozyme to the peptidoglycan layer

lactoferrin can act in concert with lysozyme to kill staphylococci (which can be resistant to the action of lysozyme alone; Leitch and Willcox, 1999). The molecular basis of this interaction is not fully understood, but it is possible that lactoferrin (which needs to act before the lysozyme) opens up the cell wall of the Gram-positive bacteria, allowing greater access of lysozyme to its peptidoglycan substrate. Figures 4.3 and 4.4 show the action of lactoferrin and lysozyme of Gram-positive and Gram-negative bacteria, respectively.

Immunoglobulins are present in tears and are highly specific proteins that are synthesized by specialized white blood cells to be specific for particular antigens. Secretory immunoglobulin A (sIgA) is the major immunoglobulin in tears and is present in open-eye tears at a concentration of approximately 1 mg/ml in non-lens wearers (Table 4.1). The function of sIgA is thought to be predominantly anti-adhesive. Once sIgA is bound to the surface of micro-organisms (bacteria, fungi or viruses) it prevents their adhesion to surfaces. sIgA may also serve a more active role as, when it is bound to the surface of micro-organisms, it acts as an opsonin (coats substances for engulfment by cells) and so facilitates their removal by specialized phagocytic white blood cells such as polymorphonuclear leucocytes (PMNs; see below). PMNs have been shown to possess sIgA surface receptors (Fanger *et al.*, 1983). Open-eye tears also contain lower levels of other immunoglobulins (IgG, IgM and IgE). These immunoglobulins can act as opsonins in a similar way to sIgA but also perform more inflammatory activities

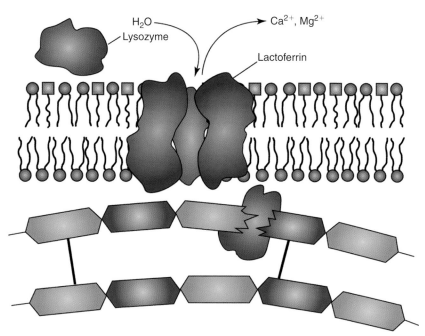

Figure 4.4 The action of lysozyme and lactoferrin on Gram-negative bacteria. Lactoferrin binds to the lipopolysaccharide in the outer membrane of Gram-negative bacteria. This either displaces Ca^{2+} or Mg^{2+} and destabilizes the membrane or forms pores in the membrane. Lysozyme is able, subsequently, to gain access to the peptidoglycan layer of the Gram-negative bacteria. The displacement of Ca^{2+} or Mg^{2+} or pore-forming ability of lactoferrin disrupts essential metabolic systems and can be bactericidal. The hydrolysis of the peptidoglycan by lysozyme results in bursting of the bacteria as a result of osmotic shock

as they act in concert with inflammatory mediators, especially complement, to facilitate phagocytosis and lysis of micro-organisms.

Several groups have demonstrated that secretory phospholipase A_2 ($sPLA_2$) in tears is antibacterial. $sPLA_2$ is produced by the lacrimal gland (in acinar cells distinct from those producing lysozyme; Nevalainen *et al.*, 1994; Aho *et al.*, 1996). $sPLA_2$ hydrolyses phospholipids and has been shown to have antistaphylococcal effects. Indeed, $sPLA_2$ is believed to be the principal bactericide in tears for staphylococci (Qu and Lehrer, 1998). One study has demonstrated increased levels of $sPLA_2$ in tears of subjects with chronic blepharitis (Song *et al.*, 1999) and another study has shown that, in order to achieve corneal infection by *Staphylococcus aureus*, $sPLA_2$ activity needs to be reduced (Moreau *et al.*, 2001).

Other groups of antimicrobials in tears are positively charged proteins, represented by defensins, and specific leucocyte protease inhibitor (SLPI). Alpha- and beta-defensins have been found in tears and the cornea (Haynes *et al.*, 1999), and especially when the cornea is assaulted, for example during microbial keratitis (MK; Gottsch *et al.*, 1998) or corneal wound healing (McDermott *et al.*, 2001). Defensins probably act on bacteria by forming pores in bacterial cell membranes and therefore damaging bacterial metabolism and also helping to burst bacteria due to osmotic

MUC1   Bacterial
                adhesion to MUC1

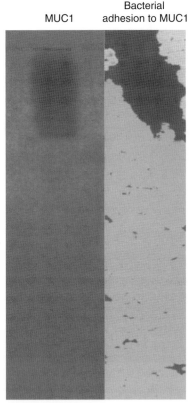

Figure 4.5   Bacterial adhesion to tear mucin. Tears were separated on agarose/polyacryl-
amide gels (which allow separation of high-molecular-weight species), transferred to
nitrocellulose and probed with either peroxidase-conjugated antibodies to mucin MUC1
or ^{125}I-labelled *P. aeruginosa* Paer1. As can be seen, tears contain MUC1. *P. aeruginosa*
Paer1 bound to the mucin spheres tentatively identified as MUC1

shock. SLPI has been shown to be concentrated mostly in closed-eye tears and is
produced from the PMNs that enter the tear film during sleep (Sathe *et al.*, 1998;
Sakata *et al.*, 1999). SLPI has two functions. As the name suggests it has a protease
inhibitor located on one domain, and another domain containing the antimicrobial
activity (Eisenberg *et al.*, 1990; Hiemstra *et al.*, 1996). The mode of action of the
antimicrobial activity of SLPI is unknown.

Other potential antimicrobial proteins/glycoproteins in tears include beta-
lysin, lipocalin and mucin. The molecular basis for the antibacterial function of
beta-lysin is unknown. Lipocalin is probably a lipid-carrying protein and its antibacterial action has not been elucidated.

Along with its lipid-carrying function, there may also be a role for it in tear film
stability. Lipocalin accounts for approximately 30 per cent of the total protein of
reflex tears. Mucin, instead of actively lysing micro-organisms as lysozyme and
lactoferrin do, probably functions to 'bundle up' micro-organisms and thus facilitate
their removal from the eye. Bacteria bind to mucin in the tears (Figure 4.5) and this

interaction may prevent the adhesion of bacteria to the corneal surface. The exact amount of mucin in tears has been difficult to determine partly because of the heterogenic nature of all the mucins in the eye and also for lack or specific high-affinity antibodies. However, $70\,\mu g/ml$ of open-eye tears is the best estimate available.

During sleep active tear flow is stopped and the antimicrobial factors in tears change. Lysozyme and lactoferrin are present in similar concentrations during sleep in closed-eye tears (Table 4.1) as in open-eye conditions. However, because these proteins are regulated (i.e. their production is linked to the production of the fluid component of tears), and during sleep the fluid component of tears is reduced and the total protein content of tears increases, their percentage concentration actually decreases to approximately 10 per cent of total proteins during sleep. We have estimated that mucin concentration, on the other hand, increases fivefold during sleep. The concentration of sIgA increases dramatically during sleep, reaching up to 60 per cent of the total tear protein (Sack *et al.*, 1992). The effect of sleep on $sPLA_2$ and the defensins is not known. The concentration of SLPI increases approximately sevenfold during sleep (Sathe *et al.*, 1998; Sack *et al.*, 2000). During sleep there is also increased leakage of plasma into the tears. Plasma contains several antimicrobial proteins/glycoproteins including the complement cascade. Complement, a series of up to 30 proteins, is bactericidal and opsonic. Complement is in an inactive state normally; however, during complement activation the proteins designated C5 to C9 form pores in the membranes of micro-organisms and thus facilitate their lysis (Rother and Till, 1988). In addition, the complement proteins designated C3 and C5 are opsonins for PMNs (Rother and Till, 1988), i.e. once bound to the surface of micro-organisms they facilitate their ingestion by PMNs. Other consequences of complement activation include the release of potent inflammatory mediators (see below). The concentration of transferrin also increases during sleep. Transferrin is another iron-binding protein and so its antimicrobial action is similar to the bacteriostatic action of lactoferrin.

THE INFLAMMATORY MEDIATORS PRESENT IN TEARS DURING SLEEP

Not only does the relative concentration of the major tear proteins/glycoproteins change during sleep but several new proteins that act as inflammatory mediators appear in the tears. There is an increase in the concentration of immunoglobulin G (IgG; Sack *et al.*, 1996). The complement system appears to be active during sleep (Willcox *et al.*, 1997a) and the activation of this system releases potent inflammatory mediators in the form of small peptides designated C3a and C5a, also known as anaphylatoxins (Rother and Till, 1988). Particular functions of the anaphylatoxins that may be important in the tears during sleep include their chemotactic (attractive) activity for PMNs and other white blood cell types, their vasodilatory effects, which may partly induce the conjunctival chemosis response during sleep, and their ability to activate white blood cells (especially PMNs that are recruited into tears during sleep (see below) and mast cells that are resident in the conjunctiva).

Inflammatory mediators are probably also released from epithelial cells, infiltrating white blood cells and resident mast cells into the tears during sleep (and there may also be a low constitutive expression of them during the day). These mediators are either cytokines (proteins) or arachidonic acid metabolites (lipids). It has been demonstrated that closed-eye tears contain several potent cytokines (Thakur *et al.*, 1998). The function of these cytokines is varied and not clear but one probable function is to recruit PMNs into the tears during sleep and to activate the PMNs for phagocytosis. Interleukin 8 (IL-8) is a potent attractor of PMNs and is known as a chemokine (a protein (cytokine) that attracts white blood cells). The concentration of IL-8 in tears during sleep is very high (150 ng/ml), which in other areas of the body would lead to tissue damage. Interleukin 6 (IL-6) and granulocyte–monocyte colony-stimulating factor (GM-CSF) also increase in closed eye tears (Thakur *et al.*, 1998). IL-6 and GM-CSF activate PMNs and increase their ability to phagocytose particles that are coated with sIgA (Lan *et al.*, 1997). The arachidonic acid metabolites also increase during sleep. The only ones that have been examined extensively in closed-eye tears are leukotriene B$_4$ (LTB$_4$), 12-hydroxy-5,8,14-eicosatrienoic acid (12-HETrE) and platelet activation factor (PAF)-like activity (Husted *et al.*, 1997; Thakur *et al.*, 1998) although others are likely to be present. LTB$_4$ and PAF are chemotactic for PMNs (and other white blood cells) and activate them for phagocytosis. 12-HETrE is inflammatory and angiogenic (i.e. stimulates the growth of blood vessels). Figure 4.6 demonstrates the temporal sequence of proteins entering the tear film during sleep.

Protease activity in tears may also lead to inflammation. The conjunctival and corneal epithelium are likely sources for most of these proteases, although the

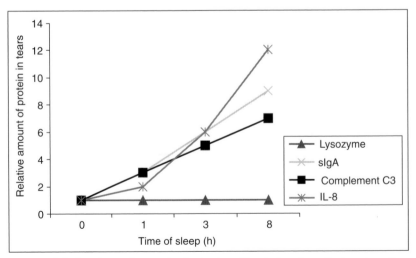

Figure 4.6   Relative change in proteins in the tear film during sleep. During sleep the concentration of lysozyme remains unchanged. There are dramatic increases in the concentration of inflammatory mediators such as complement and C3 and IL-8 and in the immunoglobulin sIgA

source of one of the major proteases, elastase, is believed to be the infiltrating PMN (Sakata *et al.*, 1997). Proteases are inflammatory when they release active peptides during protein degradation. These inflammatory peptides could be derived from tear, plasma or epithelial cell proteins.

THE EFFECT OF HYDROGEL LENS WEAR ON TEAR FILM PROTEINS AND INFLAMMATORY MEDIATORS

Several studies have been conducted into the effect of wearing hydrogel lenses on either a daily-wear (DW) or extended-wear (EW) schedule on tear proteins and inflammatory mediators. It is generally accepted that hydrogel lens wear does not affect the concentrations of lysozyme, lactoferrin or lipocalin in tears (Carney *et al.*, 1997; Glasson, 2001) even when the lenses being worn are Group IV hydrogel lenses that are known to absorb large amounts of lysozyme. Presumably the amount of lysozyme taken up by the Group IV lenses is rapidly replenished during tear turnover/flow. It is less certain whether contact lens wear affects the level of immunoglobulins in tears. The concentration of sIgA in tears has been reported to decrease during contact lens wear (Vinding *et al.*, 1987; Kijlstra *et al.*, 1992; Cheng *et al.*, 1996) but there has also been a report of an increase in the concentration of sIgA/IgA (Mannucci *et al.*, 1984) or the levels of sIgA/IgA remaining constant (Sengor *et al.*, 1990; Temel *et al.*, 1990).

Work in our laboratories has clearly demonstrated that long-term DW and EW of hydrogel Group IV lenses causes decreases in the concentration of sIgA and in the concentration of specific sIgA (with specificity for *Pseudomonas aeruginosa*) in tears (Pearce *et al.*, 1999; Willcox and Lan, 1999) but that short-term wear (6 hours DW) does not change sIgA levels (Glasson, 2001). We were able to monitor the concentration of sIgA in the tears of contact lens wearers who were asked to refrain from wearing lenses for one week and non-wearers who were asked to wear hydrogel Group IV lenses for one week of DW. The concentration of sIgA in the tears of ex-contact lens wearers did not increase to the levels in the tears of non-lens wearers during this time and neither did the levels of sIgA in the tears of the lens wearers decrease (Lan *et al.*, 1998a). These studies demonstrate that the decrease in sIgA in tears was not simply due to the presence of the contact lens or the uptake of sIgA by the lens but that other factors must contribute to the decrease. These factors could include a longer-term effect of the contact lens covering part of the conjunctiva and the cornea and therefore these areas may not be as exposed to antigenic stimulation as the non-lens-wearing eye. The consequence of less sIgA in tears may mean that the eye is more prone to infection. Masinick *et al.* (1997) have shown that IgA can protect the cornea from infection by *P. aeruginosa*.

Other work in our laboratories has examined the effect of contact lens wear on inflammatory mediators in the tears (Thakur and Willcox, 1998). Contact lens wear does not affect the concentration of complement C3 in tears (Thakur *et al.*, 1996). However, wearing lenses during sleep does alter the concentrations of IL-8 in tears. Tears of adapted daily wearers who slept in their lenses for one night

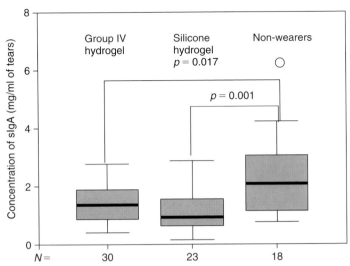

Figure 4.7   The effect of contact lens wear on the concentration of sIgA in tears. Box-plot of levels of IgA alpha chain immunoreactivity in open-eye tears of soft contact lens wearers and non-wearers. Heavy bars represent median values. Box represents the inter-quartile range, with error bars representing extreme values with outliers (shown by ○) excluded. p-Value results from Mann–Whitney statistical tests

during the study had significantly higher levels of IL-8 compared to non-lens wearers. This study demonstrated that contact lens wear has the potential to disrupt the normal homeostatic mechanisms that occur in tears during sleep. Production of the lipid inflammatory mediator 12-HETrE has been shown to be induced by wearing contact lenses (Davis *et al.*, 1992) and the induction was thought to be due to associated hypoxia or to mechanical trauma.

Are silicone hydrogel materials likely to have an effect similar to that of hydrogel lenses? Currently there are only limited studies examining the effect that new silicone hydrogel materials have on tear proteins/glycoproteins and inflammatory mediators. No reports have been forthcoming on the effect silicone hydrogel lenses might have on proteins such as lysozyme, lactoferrin, lipocalin and mucin. It is unlikely the concentrations of lysozyme or lactoferrin would change during wear of silicone hydrogel materials given that there is no change of these proteins during wear of commercially available hydrogels. As the currently available silicone hydrogel lenses are not as negatively charged as etafilcon A hydrogel lenses, they are unlikely to bind lysozyme as avidly as these lenses. Interestingly, our results, using subjects who have worn lenses for at least 12 months, have demonstrated that wearing silicone hydrogel lenses on a 30-night (30N) EW schedule still resulted in decreases in sIgA concentrations in tears compared with no lens wear. However, there was no statistical difference between subjects wearing commercially available Group IV lenses on a six-night (6N) EW schedule compared to the 30N wear of silicone hydrogel lenses (Figure 4.7). It appears that the reduction in the concentration of sIgA in tears results from lens wear in either modality. This reduction in sIgA may mean that eyes wearing lenses are predisposed to colonization by micro-organisms.

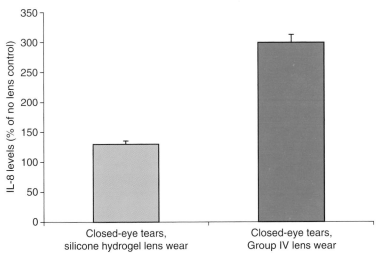

Figure 4.8   IL-8 levels in closed-eye tears of subjects wearing silicone or Group IV hydrogel lenses for 8 hours' sleep. Subjects were the same for each group. Tears in the absence of lens wear were collected on day 1. Subsequently, the tears were collected after 8 hours' sleep in silicone hydrogel lenses. Finally, after a wash-out period of one week, tears were collected after 8 hours' sleep in Group IV lenses. Results are expressed as a percentage of the level of IL-8 in non-lens-wearing closed-eye tears

Studies in our laboratories have examined the effect of wearing silicone hydrogel lenses on the levels of IL-8 in closed eye tears. Subjects who normally do not wear contact lenses were asked to sleep in silicone hydrogel lenses for one night. On a subsequent night the same subjects were asked to sleep in a Group IV contact lens. The level of IL-8 determined by a specific immunosorbent assay was then determined and compared with levels in tears of the same individuals after 8 hours sleep without wearing lenses. Figure 4.8 shows the results of this study. Sleep in silicone hydrogel lenses resulted in significantly more IL-8 appearing in closed-eye tears compared with sleep without a lens ($p < 0.02$). The highest level of IL-8 in tears was seen when the subjects slept in the Group IV lenses and the levels were significantly increased compared with no lens ($p < 0.01$) or the silicone hydrogel lens ($p = 0.01$). These increases were consistent for all subjects ($n = 8$). These results tend to indicate that the silicone hydrogel lenses have a smaller effect on the closed-eye tear homeostasis than the Group IV lenses.

THE EFFECT OF ADSORBED TEAR FILM COMPONENTS ON BACTERIAL ADHESION TO CONTACT LENSES

Several investigators have examined whether deposits on contact lenses, and specifically protein deposits, affect bacterial adhesion. Total protein does not correlate with adhesion of *P. aeruginosa* to lenses (Mowrey-McKee *et al.*, 1992). However, deposits on lenses did increase adhesion in one study (Butrus and Klotz, 1990) and this may be due to increased surface roughness; however, Bruinsma *et al.* (2001) could find no correlation between roughness and bacterial adhesion. Worn lenses did usually increase the adhesion of bacteria (Williams *et al.*, 1997). Albumin coated on to the surface of contact lenses increased the adhesion of *P. aeruginosa* (Taylor *et al.*, 1998; Bruinsma *et al.*, 2001). Similarly, some strains of *Serratia marcescens* adhered better to lenses coated in an artificial tear fluid (Hume and Willcox, 1997). Lysozyme adsorbed to a contact lens increases the adhesion of *S. aureus* to lenses (Thakur *et al.*, 1999) but does not appear to affect the adhesion of *P. aeruginosa* (unpublished data).

How do silicone hydrogel lenses behave? A study by our group (Willcox *et al.*, 2001) has shown that three strains of bacteria (two of *P. aeruginosa* and one of *Aeromonas hydrophila*) adhered in increased numbers to silicone hydrogel lenses compared to hydrogel lenses. This increase may have been due to the more hydrophobic nature of the underlying contact lens material in the high-*Dk* lenses. Interestingly, after wear of silicone hydrogel lenses, the adhesion of *P. aeruginosa*, *A. hydrophila*, *Haemophilus influenzae* and *Stenotrophomonas maltophilia* increased. There is a paucity of information in the literature on the composition of deposits on the silicone hydrogel lenses, although it has been reported that there is more deposition on the surface of balafilcon A lenses compared to etafilcon A lenses (however, no biochemical analysis of the deposits was reported; Franklin, 2000). *In vitro* data have demonstrated that balafilcon A lenses adsorb less total proteins (approximately one-third as much) than Group IV hydrogel lenses (Willis *et al.*, 2001). Furthermore, lysozyme binds to silicone hydrogel lenses at much reduced levels compared to Group IV lenses *in vitro*, but lipids, particularly oleic acid and oleic acid methyl ester, bind at greater levels to silicone hydrogel lenses than Group IV lenses (Jones and Senchyna, 2002).

THE ROLE OF WHITE BLOOD CELLS IN PROTECTION OF THE CORNEA AND EFFECT OF SLEEP AND LENS WEAR

TYPES OF WHITE BLOOD CELLS THAT PROTECT THE CORNEA

The cornea is protected by the concerted effects of various specialized white blood cells. These cells may be either resident in the cornea, limbus, conjunctiva or lacrimal gland, or migratory. The resident white blood cells that protect the cornea include Langerhans cells in the conjunctiva and limbus, stationary macrophages in the conjunctiva and mast cells in the conjunctiva. The main migratory white blood cell type that protects the cornea in the absence of overt infection/inflammation is the PMN.

Langerhans cells are usually located in the conjunctiva and the limbus. They function as antigen-presenting cells; that is, they are able to phagocytose foreign particles, including micro-organisms, and then present parts of these foreign particles to T lymphocytes, which then stimulate either the production of other white blood cells or antibodies. Langerhans cells can also release cytokines and other mediators of inflammation. Langerhans cells use specialized cell surface receptors to present antigens and these receptors are called major histocompatibility complex Class II proteins (MHC II, also known as human leucocyte-associated antigens, HLA). Using a mechanism that is still not fully understood, Langerhans cells engulf foreign particles, break down the particles and then present parts of the material in association with MHC II proteins on their surface. Having engulfed the particles at their site of residence (in our case chiefly the conjunctiva), the Langerhans cells travel to peripheral lymph nodes and present their MHC II-loaded proteins to specialized T lymphocytes called helper T lymphocytes, which possess the cell surface protein CD4. The helper T lymphocytes are then involved in mediating antibody responses and/or cellular immune responses. The type of response elicited by a particular antigen/MHC II combination depends to a large extent on the type of helper T lymphocyte that recognizes the MHC II and the surrounding cytokine milieu. Type 1 helper T lymphocytes elicit an IgG-mediated response and increase killing by phagocytic cells (Ogra *et al.*, 1994). Type 2 helper T lymphocytes elicit an IgA/IgE response (Ogra *et al.*, 1994). The immunoglobulins are manufactured and released by B lymphocytes.

Macrophages are also antigen-presenting cells and can function in a very similar way to the Langerhans cells. In addition, macrophages are able to ingest and destroy foreign particles. Macrophages possess antimicrobial defences in the form of oxygen radicals such as the superoxide anion and hydrogen peroxide and oxygen-independent mechanisms such as lysozyme and cationic proteins. Macrophages can also be involved in the initiation of the inflammatory response as they produce and release several pro-inflammatory cytokines such as IL-1 and tumour necrosis factor-alpha (TNFα) which mediate diverse activities such as activation of white blood cells and production of other cytokines.

Mast cells are the main effectors of IgE-mediated responses in the conjunctiva, i.e. hypersensitivity reactions. They can be activated by a number of stimuli including the cross-linking of surface-associated IgE molecules by antigen and by complement anaphylatoxins. Mast cells contain pre-formed and newly formed mediators of inflammation including the vasoactive molecules histamine and leukotriene C_4, as well as the chemotactic molecules neutrophil chemotactic factor and LTB$_4$ (Ogra *et al.*, 1994).

PMNs are the major cell type that help to protect the cornea during sleep, being selectively recruited into the tear film during sleep (Tan *et al.*, 1993), reaching a peak number after around 8 hours. Recruitment of PMNs probably occurs as a consequence of epithelial cells in the conjunctiva and/or cornea releasing IL-8 into the tears and tissues (Thakur *et al.*, 1998). PMNs are attracted towards a concentration gradient of this and possibly other chemokines and then travel through the blood vessels and epithelial surfaces to emerge into the tears during sleep (Figure 4.9). PMNs are phagocytic cells that contain oxygen-mediated (such as hydrogen peroxide and hydroxyl radicals) and non-oxygen-mediated (such as lysozyme and proteases) killing systems to combat engulfed micro-organisms. PMNs also release inflammatory mediators such as cytokines and arachidonic acid metabolites. PMNs may or may not need to have the foreign particle opsonized with either antibodies (presumably sIgA in tears) or complement in order to phagocytose particles.

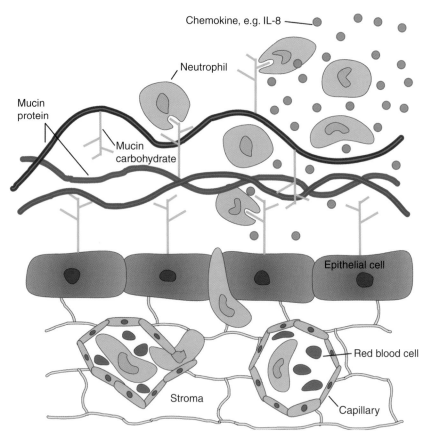

Figure 4.9 Stages in the recruitment of PMNs into the tears. PMNs move through a concentration gradient of chemotactic substances such as IL-8, extravasate through conjunctival capillaries (in the bulbar or palpebral conjunctiva), travel through the stroma and enter the tear film by migrating through the epithelium. Once in tears, PMNs probably migrate around the ocular surfaces using the carbohydrate side chains of mucin molecules as receptor/tether sites

EFFECT OF HYDROGEL LENS WEAR ON WHITE BLOOD CELLS IN THE CONJUNCTIVA AND/OR CORNEA

There have been only a few reported studies on the effect of hydrogel lens wear on the presence or recruitment of white blood cells in the absence of infection or inflammation. Using a guinea-pig model of contact lens wear we have shown that wearing HEMA-based hydrogel lenses on an EW schedule (up to eight nights) resulted in the recruitment of Langerhans cells into the paracentral and central cornea (Sankaridurg *et al.*, 2000; Figure 4.10). This migration of Langerhans cells also occurs when rabbits wear hydrogel lenses on an EW schedule (Hazlett *et al.*, 1999). This is of significance as these cells are not usually present in the cornea but are confined to the limbus. Presumably the recruitment of these cells

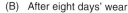
(A) Before wear

(B) After eight days' wear

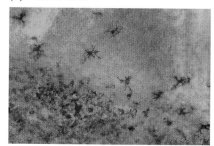
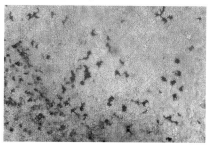

Figure 4.10   Migration of Langerhans cells into the peripheral central corneal epithelium during lens wear. Guinea-pigs wore HEMA-based hydrogel lenses for up to eight nights. Langerhans cells were disclosed by staining to demonstrate ATPase activity. The cells (A) were restricted to the edge of the cornea before wear, but migrated into the mid-peripheral and central cornea during lens wear. During migration the cells lose their normal morphology (B)

to the central cornea would render this area much more prone to inflammatory consequences. It has been demonstrated that the absence of Langerhans cells from the paracentral and central cornea (as well as other factors) maintains anterior chamber-associated immune deviation (ACAID; Niederkorn, 1995). ACAID allows, among other things, the eye as a whole to be fairly recalcitrant to inflammation and to accept corneal grafts. We can speculate that if the recruitment of Langerhans cells into the cornea of guinea-pigs also occurs during lens wear in humans, then corneal grafts from contact lens wearers would be much more likely to be rejected. Also, Hazlett *et al.* (2002) have demonstrated that the progression of *P. aeruginosa* keratitis in mice with Langerhans cells in the central cornea is increased (with certain mouse types), leading to the possibility that the presence of Langerhans cells in the cornea alters the innate immune response during keratitis, worsening the outcome.

We have also been studying the effect of hydrogel lens wear on the recruitment of PMNs into the tears during sleep (Stapleton *et al.*, 1997). Subjects who had worn their contact lenses on a DW schedule for several years had less PMN recruitment when they wore lenses for the first time during the night. This was surprising as the data we had obtained from tears demonstrated that these lens wearers had increased levels of IL-8 in their tears (see above) and might therefore be expected to have increased PMN recruitment. This apparent anomaly is explicable as chemoattractants function optimally over a fairly narrow range, with concentrations falling outside this range (either less or more than the optimal) resulting in less chemoattraction. Also, sIgA in tears has been shown to be partly responsible for PMN chemotaxis (Lan *et al.*, 1998b) and it may be that the differences in PMN chemotaxis that occur during lens wear reflect changes not only in IL-8 but also in sIgA levels in tears. The consequence of this reduced number of PMNs in the tear film would probably be to reduce the effectiveness of this defence system. Thus, any entrapped debris or micro-organisms would be less likely to be removed and, in the case of micro-organisms, could grow to pathogenic levels that might be able to induce inflammation or infection. There is evidence that bacterial numbers attached to contact lenses increase during sleep (Stapleton *et al.*, 1997).

Are silicone hydrogel lenses likely to have a similar effect on Langerhans cell recruitment into the central cornea? As yet no definitive studies have been reported in this area. We can only speculate on the possible causes for the changes in recruitment and then hypothesize if these would be likely to change during EW of silicone hydrogel lenses. It has been reported that the cytokines IL-1β, IL-6, TNFα, interferon-alpha (IFNα), IL-2 and IL-7 induce the migration of Langerhans cells into the central cornea (Dekaris *et al.*, 1998; Ho *et al.*, 1998). Experiments need to be performed to demonstrate whether lens wear upregulates the production of any of these cytokines and whether the presence of the cytokines is responsible for the recruitment of Langerhans cells during lens wear. Hypoxia has been shown to upregulate the expression of IL-6 in lung epithelia (Tamm *et al.*, 1998) and both TNFα and IL-1β in placental tissue (Benyo *et al.*, 1997). Thus, wearing lenses of low oxygen permeability may well result in upregulation of cytokines that are chemotactic for Langerhans cells. Conversely, the new high-oxygen-permeable lenses might not result in upregulation of cytokines and therefore would not result in movement of Langerhans cells to the central cornea. The significance of Langerhans cell migration into the cornea during contact lens wear is that Langerhans cells in the cornea predispose to infections (Hazlett *et al.*, 2002) and that corneas of lens wearers may then not be useful for grafting.

The effect of silicone hydrogel lenses on the recruitment of PMNs into the tears during sleep has received some attention (Stapleton *et al.*, 1996). A group of five neophytes either wore an experimental silicone hydrogel lens or a Group IV hydrogel in one eye on successive nights, or wore no lens. There was no statistical difference between numbers of PMNs collected from the ocular surface/tears between these test conditions, even though in other experiments the concentration of IL-8 in tears increased dramatically (Figure 4.8). This suggests that the lenses offer a barrier to PMNs reaching the corneal surface. It remains to be seen whether wearing silicone hydrogels over a longer period results in the decrease in PMN numbers seen with hydrogel lens wear (see above). If PMN recruitment is still altered this may predispose the cornea to infection or inflammation as a deficit of PMNs would probably allow micro-organisms to grow to levels that would be pathogenic.

THE NORMAL OCULAR MICROBIOTA

We have discussed the defence systems in the tears and effects that lens wear may have on these systems. These systems prevent excessive colonization of the cornea and conjunctiva by either the normal microbiota or potential pathogens.

The conjunctiva and lids contain a normal microbiota. The conjunctiva may be colonized by several bacterial genera, the most common of which are the Gram-positive coagulase-negative staphylococci, *Corynebacterium* sp. and *Propionibacterium* sp. (Perkins *et al.*, 1975; Fleiszig and Efron, 1992). Approximately

50 per cent of the population harbour one or more of the above bacterial types on their conjunctiva at any given time (Perkins *et al.*, 1975; Stapleton *et al.*, 1995a). Other micro-organisms may be isolated from the conjunctiva, but at much lower rates (e.g. *S. aureus*, *Micrococcus* sp., *Bacillus* sp. and certain Gram-negative pseudomonads; Perkins *et al.*, 1975; Fleiszig and Efron, 1992). The lids usually harbour a microbiota similar to the normal skin microbiota and harbour more bacteria of more species than the conjunctiva (Stapleton *et al.*, 1995a). Again the predominating types of bacteria are coagulase-negative staphylococci, *Corynebacterium* sp. and *Propionibacterium* sp. During sleep the number of bacteria colonizing the conjunctiva and lid increases (Ramachandran *et al.*, 1995).

THE EFFECT OF LENS WEAR ON THE NORMAL OCULAR MICROBIOTA

An increase in the number of bacteria isolated from the conjunctiva and lids during daily lens wear has been reported (Larkin and Leeming, 1991; Stapleton *et al.*, 1995a), although the types of micro-organisms were not found to differ from non-lens-wearing eyes. In a mixed group of lens wearers an alteration in the types of micro-organisms was seen with lens wear (more Gram-negative bacteria being isolated) along with an increase in the frequency of cultures growing no micro-organisms (Hovding, 1981). This finding has been confirmed for EW disposable hydrogel lens users in a more recent study where the ocular microbiota was sampled on seven occasions during 12 months of lens wear (Stapleton *et al.*, 1995a). This is significant as Gram-negative organisms are common ocular pathogens associated with contact lens-related corneal infections (Schein *et al.*, 1989). Other studies, however, have reported no differences between wearers and non-lens wearers although an increase in positive ocular cultures was found in former lens users and in association with certain modes of lens wear and types of disinfection systems (Fleiszig and Efron, 1992).

Lens contamination during asymptomatic lens wear appears to be infrequent and involves small numbers of organisms (Hart *et al.*, 1993). The most common bacteria isolated from contact lenses are coagulase-negative staphylococci (Hovding, 1981; Fleiszig and Efron, 1992; Hart *et al.*, 1993; Gopinathan *et al.*, 1997). Occasional isolation of *S. aureus*, streptococci and a variety of Gram-negative bacteria has also been noted (Fleiszig and Efron, 1992; Gopinathan *et al.*, 1997). Contact lens contamination commonly occurs through lens handling (Mowrey-McKee *et al.*, 1992) but it appears that during uncomplicated lens wear these organisms are readily cleared from the lens surface by the ocular defence mechanisms. Other sources of contamination of lenses by the normal microbiota include the eyelids of wearers (Willcox *et al.*, 1997b). However, during lens-related corneal infection and inflammation, high numbers of Gram-negative bacteria are frequently recovered from the contact lens (Stapleton *et al.*, 1995b; Holden *et al.*, 1996). Gram-negative bacteria on the lens may be derived from the contact lens storage case, contaminated lens care systems or from other exogenous sources. We have reported that Gram-negative bacteria are likely to be derived from domestic water supplies (Willcox *et al.*, 1997b). Under certain circumstances organisms may adhere to and form a glycocalyx on the posterior lens surface in close proximity to the corneal epithelium. This may prolong the retention time of organisms at the ocular surface, enhance bacterial resistance and inhibit normal clearing mechanisms. Bacteria encased within a biofilm on the posterior surface of the contact lens have been demonstrated in wearers with *Pseudomonas* infection of the cornea (Stapleton and Dart, 1995). Other data from our laboratories have shown that contamination of lenses during wear is sporadic. Subjects sampled on successive days of EW lens wear, from one night to 13 nights, were as likely to have contaminated lenses on day 1 as on day 13 (Sweeney *et al.*, 1994). In other words, wearing lenses for increasing lengths of time did not result in increasing microbial contamination. Thus, silicone hydrogel lenses which can be worn for up to 30 nights are unlikely to have more bacteria associated with them than those used for six nights' wear.

THE EFFECT OF SILICONE HYDROGEL LENSES ON THE NORMAL OCULAR MICROBIOTA

Wearing silicone hydrogel lenses on a 30-night (30N) EW schedule did not greatly alter the types of bacteria that colonized the lids or conjunctiva (Table 4.2). The only significant differences between the colonization rates on the two lens types/wear schedules was a slightly greater frequency of colonization by *Corynebacterium* spp.

Table 4.2   The frequency of microbial contamination of either the lid margin or conjunctiva for subjects wearing hydrogel or silicone hydrogel lenses on two different wear schedules

Bacteria	Frequency of microbial contamination of ocular surfaces (%)			
	Hydrogel lens wear 6N EW ($n = 53$)		Silicone hydrogel lens wear 30N EW ($n = 171$)	
	Lid microbiota	Conjunctiva microbiota	Lid microbiota	Conjunctiva microbiota
Corynebacterium spp.	9*	6	27*	10
Micrococcus spp.	11	4	8	4
Propionibacterium spp.	83	42	79	46
Staphylococcus epidermidis	94	36	87	46
Staphylococcus hyicus	11	4	14	8
Staphylococcus saprophyticus	26	15	30	18

*Differences between the frequency of isolation were statistically significant ($p < 0.02$). No other statistically significant differences were found. Other micro-organisms, e.g. Gram-negatives, *S. aureus* or fungi, were found very infrequently and there was no difference in isolation rates between the lens types. *S. epidermidis*, *S. hyicus* and *S. saprophyticus* are coagulase-negative staphylococci.

Table 4.3   Frequency of microbial colonization of hydrogel and silicone hydrogel lenses worn on two different EW schedules

Bacteria	Frequency (%)		
	Hydrogel lens wear 6N EW ($n = 64$)	Silicone hydrogel lens wear 6N EW ($n = 32$)	Silicone hydrogel hydrogel lens wear 30N EW ($n = 183$)
Coagulase-negative staphylococci	47	41	54
Propionibacterium spp.	31	13[a]	43[a]
Gram-negative bacteria	2	9	2
Staphylococcus aureus	0	0	2

[a] The only significant differences seen were between the frequency of colonization of *Propionibacterium* sp. from 6N versus 30N silicone hydrogel lens wear, with 30N being colonized more frequently that 6N. However, the frequencies of colonization by *Propionibacterium* spp. of 6N hydrogel lens wear and 30N silicone hydrogel lens wear were not different. No other significant differences were seen between the bacterial types above and any other bacterial or fungal types isolated from the different lens types.

on the lids of silicone hydrogel wearers. As *Corynebacterium* spp. are considered part of the normal ocular microbiota and the number of colonies from the lids was not different, this finding is likely to be clinically unimportant. In addition to the colonization rates of micro-organisms on the lid margin or conjunctiva of subjects, we have also monitored the colonization rates of hydrogel (Group IV) lenses worn on a 6N schedule and silicone hydrogel lenses worn on either a 6N or 30N schedule (Table 4.3; Keay *et al.*, 1998). The only difference noted was a decrease in the frequency of isolation of *Propionibacterium* spp. from the six-night silicone hydrogel group. Again, as these bacteria are normal ocular microbiota, the significance of this is not known but may not be high. This indicates that, from a microbiological point of view, 30N EW would not change the predisposition of the cornea to inflammation or infection compared with six nights' EW.

MICRO-ORGANISMS AND ADVERSE EVENTS

Chapter 7 will describe in detail the types of adverse responses that can occur during contact lens wear. Several types of micro-organisms cause adverse events associated with wearing hydrogel contact lenses. Corneal infection, or MK, is a rare but severe complication of contact lens use. EW of lenses poses the highest risk of corneal infection and use of current commercially available hydrogel lenses appears to have a greater risk compared with rigid lens use (Dart *et al.*, 1991). The risk of corneal infection to the individual has been estimated to be one in 500 for EW lens users and one in 2500 DW users per year developing the disease in a US population (Poggio *et al.*, 1989). The spectrum of causative organisms in lens-related infections differs from that associated with non-lens-related infections, with up to 70 per cent of culture-proved cases attributable to *P. aeruginosa* (Schein

Table 4.4   Summary of the bacteria isolated from cases of MK with silicone hydrogels and HEMA-based hydrogel lenses

Causative bacteria	Silicone hydrogel	HEMA-based hydrogel
Total culture-positive cases	12	100[a]
Gram-negatives	75%	73%
P. aeruginosa or spp.	42%	66%
S. marcescens	8%	4%
Alcaligenes xylosidans	8%	–
Acinetobacter spp.	8%	–
H. influenzae	–	1%
Morganella morgani	–	1%
Escherichia coli	–	1%
Unidentified	8%	–
Gram-positives	25%	25%
Streptococcus viridans	17%	–
Coagulase-negative staphylococci	–	13%
S. aureus	–	6%
Corynebacterium spp.	8%	3% (mixed)
Propionibacterium spp.	–	3%
Bacillus cereus	–	1%
Unidentified	–	1%

[a] Weissman et al. (1984); Patrinely et al. (1985); Mondino et al. (1986); Cohen et al. (1987); Donnenfeld et al. (1986); Schein et al. (1989).

et al., 1989), in contrast with non-contact lens wearers where S. aureus is the predominant bacterium. Other Gram-negative rods such as Serratia spp., Proteus spp. and other Pseudomonas spp. have also been reported to cause MK during lens wear. Of the Gram-positive species, Staphylococcus spp. are the most prevalent. Other micro-organisms that have been reported to cause corneal infections during contact lens use include Acanthamoeba spp., fungi (yeasts and moulds) and viruses (although whether contact lens use increases the rate of viral keratitis remains uncertain). Chapter 7 lists in more detail the micro-organisms that have been isolated from cases of MK. Table 4.4 provides a summary of the main bacteria isolated from MK in both silicone hydrogel and HEMA-based hydrogel lenses. Although the cases of MK with silicone hydrogels is low, similar trends in types of bacteria causing MK are seen in comparison with the HEMA-based hydrogel lenses, with Gram-negatives predominating and P. aeruginosa being the most common of the Gram-negatives.

Other adverse responses that have been associated with micro-organisms include contact lens induced acute red eye (CLARE), contact lens peripheral ulcers (CLPU), infiltrative keratitis (IK) and asymptomatic infiltrative keratitis (AIK). CLARE, CLPU, IK and AIK are probable inflammatory responses of the cornea and conjunctiva caused by the presence of bacteria colonizing the contact lens and are not considered to be infections of the cornea or conjunctiva (refer to

Table 4.5   Microbes associated with inflammatory non-infectious keratitis

Microbial type	Associated adverse response
Gram-negative	
Abiotrophia defectiva	IK
Acinetobacter spp.	CLARE, IK, AIK
Aeromonas hydrophilia	CLARE
Alcaligenes xylosoxidans subsp. *denitrificans*	IK
Branhamella catarrhalis	IK
Enterobacter cloacae	IK, AIK
Escherichia coli	CLARE, IK
Haemophilus influenzae	CLARE, IK, AIK
Haemophilus parainfluenzae	CLARE, IK
Klebsiella oxytoca	CLARE, IK, AIK
Klebsiella pneumoniae	CLARE
Neisseria spp.	IK
Pseudomonas aeruginosa	CLARE, CLPU
Pseudomonas paucimobilis	AIK
Serratia liquefaciens	CLPU, IK
Serratia marcescens	CLARE, IK
Stenotrophomonas maltophilia	CLARE, AIK
Vibrio holisae	AIK
Gram-positive	
Non-haemolytic *Streptococcus* spp.	IK
Staphylococcus aureus	CLPU, IK
Streptococcus pneumoniae	CLARE, CLPU, IK, AIK
Streptococcus viridans	CLARE, IK, AIK
Fungus	
Yeast	IK
Mould	IK

Data from Holden *et al.* (1996); Sankaridurg *et al.* (1996); Sankaridurg *et al.* (1999); unpublished. Cultures returning members of the normal microbiota (coagulase-negative staphylococci, *Propionibacterium* spp. and *Corynebacterium* spp.) are not included as these would have been cultured in the absence of an adverse response.

Chapter 7; Holden *et al.*, 1996; Grant *et al.*, 1998). The bacteria that have been shown to cause these adverse responses are listed in Table 4.5.

We have shown that large numbers (over 28 million/lens) of Gram-negative bacteria need to be present on a contact lens before a CLARE is produced in an animal model (Table 4.6). This correlates with the large numbers of bacteria that are cultured from the contact lenses from CLARE eyes during the acute phase of the response in humans (Holden *et al.*, 1996; Sankaridurg *et al.*, 1996). On the other hand, CLPU can be produced by a lower number (approximately 11 000/lens) of bacteria attached to the lenses (Figure 4.11). Again, this correlates with the low numbers of bacteria isolated during an acute response in humans (Jalbert *et al.*, 1999).

The pathogenic mechanisms involved in MK and the less severe inflammatory reactions are likely to have overlapping characteristics. All events will have a bacterial

Table 4.6 Numbers of *P. aeruginosa* on lenses required to produce a CLARE-like response in a guinea-pig's eye

Number of animals	3	4	4	4
Bacterial count on lenses (cells/mm² of lens)	94 000	23 000	12 000	10 000
Number of eyes showing CLARE-like response (% eyes with infiltrates)	67	50	33	0

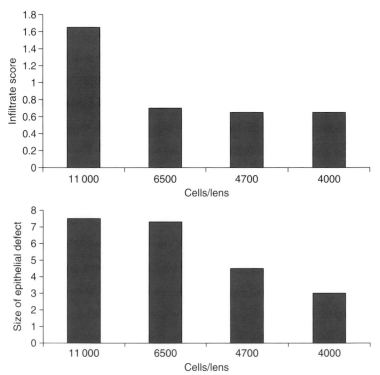

Figure 4.11 Number of *S. aureus* adhered to a contact lens required to produce a CLPU-like response in a rabbit model; 11 000 cells/lens gave a CLPU-like response in 100% of animals. Numbers of bacteria/lens below 11 000 cells gave either a lower percentage of animals with the responses and/or a less severe response

component that induces inflammation. All events probably require metabolically active bacteria but we believe that only MK is a truly infectious process and so this event is likely to be the only one displaying rapid growth of bacteria in tissues.

Most work on MK and bacterial pathogenic properties has focused on *P. aeruginosa*. There are potentially many traits of this bacterium that contribute to the infectious and inflammatory processes (Table 4.7). It is possible that all of these contribute to some extent to the production of the tissue destruction and

Table 4.7 Potential pathogenic products of *P. aeruginosa* involved in the production of MK and non-infectious keratitis

Bacterial component	Mechanism	Role in keratitis
Structural		
Lipopolysaccharide	Activates complement, immunogenic, stimulates production of cytokines (IL-1, TNF and IL-6 in particular); binds to galectin 3 in human corneas and asialo GM_1 in mouse corneas (Gupta *et al.*, 1994, 1997); LPS of serotypes I, G and E more adherent to corneal epithelial cells (Thuruthyil *et al.*, 2001); activates metalloproteinase-9 (Miyajima *et al.*, 2001)	Potent inflammatory agent; potential adhesin
Pili/fimbriae	Adhesion to corneal epithelial proteins (Wu *et al.*, 1995)	Allows bacteria to adhere to corneal surface
Type IV pili	Specialized form of motility called twitching motility, which facilitates colonization of surfaces (Wall and Kaiser, 1999)	May facilitate entry into cornea
Type IV secretion system	Acts like a gun to fire toxins into mammalian cells. Bacteria-to-mammalian cell contact required (Christie, 2001)	Destruction of resident and recruited mammalian cells
Extracellular		
Elastase	Degrades proteins including collagen and IgA (Heck *et al.*, 1990); degrades IL-2 (Theander *et al.*, 1988), IFNα and TNFα (Parmely *et al.*, 1990); activates corneal matrix metalloproteinase (Matsumoto *et al.*, 1993; Twining *et al.*, 1993)	Destroys corneal integrity and tear proteins
Alkaline protease	Degrades proteins including collagen; degrades IFNγ and TNFα (Parmely *et al.*, 1990); is involved in adhesion to cornea (Gupta *et al.*, 1996); activates metalloproteinase 9 (Miyajima *et al.*, 2001)	Destroys corneal integrity and tear proteins; allows bacteria to adhere to corneal surface; but may not be essential for corneal pathology (Pillar *et al.*, 2002)

(continued)

Table 4.7   (*continued*)

Bacterial component	Mechanism	Role in keratitis
Protease IV	Degrades gelatin (and perhaps collagen; Engel *et al.*, 1997)	Destroys corneal stroma (O'Callaghan *et al.*, 1996)
Phospholipase C	Hydrolyses phosphorylcholine (Cota-Gomez *et al.*, 1997)	Destroys mammalian cells (erythrocytes)
Exoenzyme S	ADP-ribosylates mammalian proteins including Ras (McGuffie *et al.*, 1998), which affects cell multiplication, immunoglobulins (Knight and Barbieri, 1997)	Destroys protein functions
Exoenzyme T	Similar to exoenzyme S but lower activity	Similar to exoenzyme S
Exoenzyme U	Cytotoxic enzyme associated with certain epidemic clones of *P. aeruginosa* (Lomholt *et al.*, 2001)	May damage resident and recruited mammalian cells
Exotoxin A	Inhibits protein synthesis in cornea (Twining *et al.*, 1993); helps to prolong survival of bacteria in eye (Pillar and Hobden, 2002)	Prevents adequate corneal healing
Porins (allow passive diffusion of solutes across outer membrane)	Induce release of IL-6 and TNFα (Cusumano *et al.*, 1997)	Initiates inflammatory cascade
Acylated homoserine lactones	Function as signalling molecules to tell the bacteria that a quorum has developed and results in expression of many virulence factors (Miller and Bassler, 2001; Zhu *et al.*, 2001)	Regulates the expression of many virulence factors such as proteases and toxins
Intracellular		
PepB/PopB	Unknown but may allow entry of putative cytotoxin into mammalian cells (Hauser *et al.*, 1998; Yahr *et al.*, 1997)	Associated with induction of cytotoxicity in mammalian cells
PepD/PopD	Unknown but may allow entry of putative cytotoxin into mammalian cells (Hauser *et al.*, 1998; Yahr *et al.*, 1997)	Associated with induction of cytotoxicity in mammalian cells

inflammation seen in MK and the loss of one trait may not render the bacterium unable to infect the cornea. It is also possible that lipopolysaccharide (LPS, endo-toxin; Figure 4.2) leaching from the bacteria colonizing the contact lens is the factor chiefly responsible for the inflammation seen during CLARE. Indeed it has been demonstrated in a rabbit model that LPS alone can produce a CLARE-like response (Schultz *et al.*, 1997).

More recent work has examined the factors involved in *S. aureus*-induced MK. A collagen adhesin of *S. aureus* promotes, but is not essential for, MK production (Rhem *et al.*, 2000). Another adhesin of *S. aureus*, the fibronectin-binding protein, appears to be essential for the internalization (invasion) of this bacterium into corneal epithelial cells (Jett and Gilmore, 2002). Several lysogenic toxins are produced by *S. aureus*. Alpha-toxin and gamma-toxin have been implicated in MK. Alpha-toxins appear to be involved in mediating corneal erosions (in a rabbit model; Hume *et al.*, 2001; Dajcs *et al.*, 2002a) but the role of gamma-toxin has yet to be defined. Also, beta-toxin appears to mediate ocular oedema during MK (Dajcs *et al.*, 2002b). Elastase production by *S. aureus* correlates with isolation from CLPU (Wu *et al.*, 1999).

In our laboratories a mouse model of *S. aureus* keratitis has been developed. Like the well-characterized *P. aeruginosa* model of this disease, we have found that the outcome of corneal challenge with *S. aureus* is dependent on both the characteristics of the infecting strain of bacteria and the genetic background of the host. Our preliminary findings suggest that *S. aureus* induces a muted cytokine response in the cornea that differs from that induced during *P. aeruginosa* challenge in both profile and kinetics.

We have been studying the fact that strains of the same species, notably *P. aeruginosa* or *Serratia marcescens*, are able to cause MK or CLARE and we have been trying to ascertain whether it is differences in pathogenic potential of the bacteria that predicts if they will cause CLARE or MK, or whether it is predisposing factors in the contact lens wearer (or animal model).

Using a mouse scratch model of corneal infection we have shown that there are differences in the ability of certain strains isolated from human MK or CLARE to produce disease (Cole *et al.*, 1998; Cowell *et al.*, 1998; Table 4.8). Infection or non-infectious inflammation (e.g. a response such as CLARE) was not predicted from the ability of strains to adhere to corneal epithelial cells or contact lenses or their ability to produce protease. If strains either produce corneal epithelial cell cytotoxicity or invade human corneal epithelial cells *in vitro* they may be more likely to cause infection. More recently, we have assessed, using a guinea-pig contact lens-wearing model, whether, after adhesion to the contact lens, strains of *P. aeruginosa* could infect the cornea in the presence or absence of an epithelial defect (Table 4.8; Figures 4.12 and 4.13). Our results confirm that there needs to be an epithelial break prior to an infection, even in the presence of bacteria that are known either to invade or produce cytotoxicity in *in vitro* and *ex vivo* assays. Furthermore, in studies using prolonged contact lens wear in rabbits, we have shown that *S. aureus* does not cause MK but can cause IK after three weeks of hydrogel lens wear (Wu *et al.*, 2000).

These results demonstrate some important points regarding the production of MK or non-infectious keratitis, e.g. CLARE. First, not all bacteria of the same genera and species are the same – some may be potentially more pathogenic than others (and this has been corroborated by us and others with both *P. aeruginosa* and *Serratia marcescens*; Hazlett *et al.*, 1991; Hume *et al.*, 1999; Willcox and

Table 4.8   Differences between bacteria isolated from MK or CLARE in *in vivo* and *in vitro* tests

Test	*Pseudomonas aeruginosa* (condition from which the strain was isolated)				*Serratia marcescens* (condition from which the strain was isolated)	
	Paer1 (CLARE)	6294 (MK)	Paer24 (MK)	Paer25 (CLARE)	Smar5 (CLARE)	SVH (MK)
Mouse model with epithelial scratch[a]	Non-infectious	Infectious	Infectious	Infectious	Non-infectious	Non-infectious
Guinea-pig contact lens-wearing model[b]	Non-infectious	Infectious only in presence of epithelial break	NK	NK	NK	NK
Adhesion to Group IV contact lenses[c]	8000 cells/mm^2	15 000 cells/mm^2	NK	NK	100 cells/mm^2	300 cells/mm^2
Initial adhesion to corneal epithelium (mouse model)[d]	1×10^6 cells/cornea	3×10^5 cell/cornea	NK	NK	3×10^5 cells/cornea	1×10^6 cells/cornea
Cytotoxicity of human corneal epithelial cells[e]	−	+++	±	±	NK	NK
Invasion of human corneal epithelial cells[f]	−	−	++	++	−	NK
Protease production[g]	+	+	++	++	++	+

−, not produced; ±, little produced; +, produced; ++, moderate amount produced; +++, large amount produced; NK, not known.
[a]Data from Cole *et al.* (1998) or Cowell *et al.* (1998) or previously unpublished data.
[b]Previously unpublished data.
[c]Data from Williams *et al.* (1997), Hume and Willcox (1997).
[d]Previously unpublished data.
[e]Data from Cole *et al.* (1998) or previously unpublished.
[f]Data from Cole *et al.* (1998) or previously unpublished.
[g]Data from Cowell *et al.* (1998) or previously unpublished.

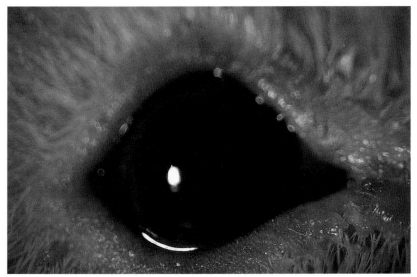

Figure 4.12   Corneal response in a guinea-pig after fitting a contact lens soaked in *P. aeruginosa* 6206 (an MK-causing strain in the mouse scratch model; Table 4.8) to a normal healthy cornea. After 24 hours there was no evidence of any infection or ulceration

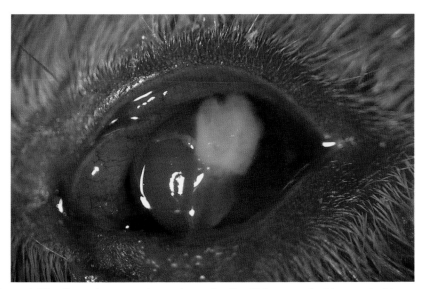

Figure 4.13   Corneal response in a guinea-pig after fitting a contact lens soaked in *P. aeruginosa* 6206 (an MK-causing strain in the mouse scratch model; Table 4.8) to a cornea that had been scratched with a needle. After 24 hours there was severe conjunctival chemosis, dense corneal infiltration involving the entire stromal depth, with ulceration and necrosis. Note discharge attached to the infiltrate, which is a feature of pseudomonal keratitis

Hume, 1999). Secondly, it is likely that there needs to be a predisposing corneal epithelial trauma before infection occurs, even though some bacteria are able to invade or cause epithelial cells to die. With these findings in mind we can speculate on the effect of silicone hydrogel lenses on the incidence of MK and non-infectious keratitis. We believe that the current silicone hydrogel lenses have not been designed with any antimicrobial characteristics in mind. Thus, we believe that the new silicone hydrogel lenses will still give rise to MK and non-infectious keratitis such as CLARE, CLPU and IK (refer to Chapter 7). However, the silicone hydrogel lenses do give vastly superior performance in terms of preventing hypoxic stress of the cornea. Therefore, while there is likely to be infection and inflammation, their severity or frequency may be reduced with silicone hydrogel lenses. A healthier epithelium should mean there is less compromise of the surface integrity and ocular surface defence mechanisms and therefore less chance of infection.

CONCLUSIONS

In summary, several changes occur during lens wear that disrupt the normal corneal homeostasis. These include reductions in the concentration of sIgA in tears, perturbations in the amounts of cytokines in tears and changes in the number of PMNs in tears as well as location of Langerhans cells in the cornea. These changes may allow bacteria to proliferate, especially during sleep, to levels that are potentially pathogenic. Lens wear does alter the types or numbers of bacteria that can be isolated from the ocular surfaces but the lenses themselves may provide a niche for colonization of the eye by unusual bacteria, especially Gram-negative bacteria. The Gram-negative bacteria cause the majority of the adverse responses seen during hydrogel lens wear. Animal model work has enabled us to define characteristics of the bacteria and/or lens that predispose to some of these adverse responses. Clearly, there are bacteria that are unable to infect the eye and those that have the potential to cause MK. However, preliminary findings indicate that there needs to be compromise to the corneal surface in order for bacteria to infect the cornea. Whether the highly oxygen-permeable silicone hydrogel lenses will produce the same frequency or types of adverse responses remains to be seen. It is only after controlled prospective clinical trials and/or data collected from subjects in the field that we will be able to identify clearly risk factors associated with silicone hydrogel lens wear and determine whether these lenses provide a safer alternative to hydrogel lenses for use on an EW schedule.

REFERENCES

Aho, H. J., Saari, K. M., Kallajoki, M. *et al.* (1996) Synthesis of group II phospholipase A_2 and lysozyme in lacrimal glands. *Invest. Ophthalmol. Vis. Sci.*, **37**, 1826–1832

Arnold, R. R., Russell, J. E., Champion, W. J. *et al.* (1982) Bactericidal activity of human lactoferrin: differentiation from the stasis of iron deprivation. *Infect. Immun.*, **35**, 792–797

Bellamy, W., Takase, M., Wakabayashi, H. *et al.* (1992) Antibacterial spectrum of lactoferricin B, a potent antibacterial peptide derived from the N-terminal region of bovine lactoferrin. *J. Appl. Bacteriol.*, **73**, 472–479

Benyo, D. F., Miles, T. M. and Conrad, K. P. (1997) Hypoxia stimulates cytokine production by villous explants from human placenta. *J. Clin. Endocrinol. Metab.* **82**, 1582–1588

Bruinsma, G. M., van der Mei, H. C. and Busscher, H. J. (2001) Bacterial adhesion to surface hydrophilic and hydrophobic contact lenses. *Biomaterials*, **22**, 3217–3224

Butrus, S. I. and Klotz, S.A. (1990) Contact lens surface deposits increase the adhesion of *Pseudomonas aeruginosa*. *Curr. Eye Res.*, **9**, 717–724

Carney, F. P., Morris, C. A. and Willcox, M. D. P. (1997) The effect of hydrogel lens wear on the major tear proteins during extended wear. *Aust. NZ J. Ophthalmol.*, **25**, s36–s38

Cheng, K. H., Spanjaard, L., Rutten, H. *et al.* (1996) Immunoglobulin A antibodies against *Pseudomonas aeruginosa* in the tear fluid of contact lens wearers. *Invest. Ophthalmol. Vis. Sci.*, **37**, 2081–2088

Christie, P. J. (2001) Type IV secretion: intracellular transfer of macromolecules by systems ancestrally related to conjugation machines. *Mol. Microbiol.*, **40**, 294–301

Cohen, E. J., Laibson, P. R., Arentsen, J. J. and Clemons, C. S. (1987) Corneal ulcers associated with cosmetic extended wear soft contact lenses. *Ophthalmology*, **94**, 109–114

Cole, N., Willcox, M. D. P., Fleiszig, S. M. J. *et al.* (1998) Different strains of *Pseudomonas aeruginosa* isolated from ocular infections or inflammation display distinct corneal pathologies in an animal model. *Curr. Eye Res.*, **17**, 730–735

Cota-Gomez, A., Vasil, A. I., Kadurugamuwa, J. *et al.* (1997) PlcR1 and PlcR2 are putative calcium-binding proteins required for secretion of the hemolytic phospholipase C of *Pseudomonas aeruginosa*. *Infect. Immun.*, **55**, 2904–2913

Cowell, B. A., Willcox, M. D. P., Hobden, J. A. *et al.* (1998) An ocular strain of *Pseudomonas aeruginosa* is inflammatory but not virulent in the scarified mouse model. *Exp. Eye Res.*, **67**, 347–356

Cusumano, V., Tufano, M. A., Mancuso, G. *et al.* (1997) Porins of *Pseudomonas aeruginosa* induce release of tumor necrosis factor alpha and interleukin-6 by human leukocytes. *Infect. Immun.*, **65**, 1683–1687

Dajcs, J. J., Austin, M. S., Sloop, S. D. *et al.* (2002a) Corneal pathogenesis of *Staphylococcus aureus* strain Newman. *Invest. Ophthalmol. Vis. Sci.*, **43**, 1109–1115

Dajcs, J. J., Thibodeaux, B. A., Girgis, D. O. *et al.* (2002b) Corneal virulence of *Staphylococcus aureus* in an experimental model of keratitis. *DNA Cell Biol.*, **21**, 375–382

Dart, J. K. G., Stapleton, F. and Minassian, D. (1991) Contact lenses and other risk factors in microbial keratitis. *Lancet*, **338**, 650–653

Davis, K. L., Conners, M. S., Dunn, M. W. and Schwartzman, M. L. (1992) Induction of corneal epithelial cytochrome P-450 arachidonate metabolism by contact lens wear. *Invest. Ophthalmol. Vis. Sci.*, **33**, 291–297

Dekaris, I., Yamada, J., Zhu, S. N. and Dana, M. R. (1998) The TNF-α receptor mediates centripetal Langerhans cell migration after corneal stimulation. *Invest. Ophthalmol. Vis. Sci.*, **39**, s1120

Donnenfeld, E. D., Cohen, E. J., Arentsen, J. J. *et al.* (1986) Changing trends in contact lens associated corneal ulcers: an overview of 116 cases. *CLAO J.*, **12**, 145–149

Eisenberg, S. P., Hale, K. K., Heimdal, P. and Thompson, R. C. (1990) Location of the protease-inhibitory region of secretory leukocyte protease inhibitor. *J. Biol. Chem.*, **265**, 7976–7981

Engel, L. S., Hobden, J. A., Moreau, J. M. *et al.* (1997) *Pseudomonas* deficient in protease IV has significantly reduced corneal virulence. *Invest. Ophthalmol. Vis. Sci.*, **38**, 1535–1542

Fanger, M. W., Goldstine, S. N. and Shen, L. (1983) Cytofluorographic analysis of receptors for IgA on human polymorphonuclear cells and monocytes and the correlation of receptor expression with phagocytosis. *Mol. Immunol.*, **20**, 1019–1027

Fleiszig, S. M. J. and Efron, N. (1992) Microbial flora in the eyes of current and former contact lens wearers. *J. Clin. Microbiol.*, **30**, 1156–1161

Franklin, V. (2000) A study of the spoilation profiles of high *Dk* fluorosilicone hydrogel lenses. In *British Contact Lens Association 24th Annual Clinical Conference and Exhibition*, Birmingham, UK, 2000

Fullard, R. J. and Tucker, D. L. (1991) Changes in human tear protein levels with progressively increasing stimulus. *Invest. Ophthalmol. Vis. Sci.*, **32**, 2290–2301

Gipson, I. K. and Inatomi, T. (1998) Cellular origin of mucins of the ocular surface tear film. *Adv. Exp. Med. Biol.*, **438**, 221–227

Glasson, M. J. (2001) The determination of tear film characteristics that lead to contact lens wear intolerance. PhD thesis, University of New South Wales, Sydney, Australia

Gopinathan, U., Stapleton, F., Sharma, S. *et al.* (1997) Microbial contamination of hydrogel contact lenses during extended wear. *J. Appl. Bacteriol.*, **82**, 653–658

Gottsch, J. D., Li, Q., Ashraf, M. F. *et al.* (1998) Defensin gene expression in the cornea. *Curr. Eye Res.*, **17**, 1082–1086

Grant, T., Chong, M. S., Vajdic, C. *et al.* (1998) Contact lens induced peripheral ulcers (CLPUs) during hydrogel contact lens wear. *J. Cont. Lens Assoc. Ophthalmol.*, **24**, 145–151

Gupta, S. K., Berk, R. S., Masinick, S. and Hazlett, L. D. (1994) Pili and lipopolysaccharide of *Pseudomonas aeruginosa* bind to the glycolipid asialo GM1. *Infect. Immun.*, **62**, 4572–4579

Gupta, S. K., Masinick, S.A ., Hobden, J. A. *et al.* (1996) Bacterial proteases and adherence of *Pseudomonas aeruginosa* to mouse cornea. *Exp. Eye Res.*, **62**, 641–650

Gupta, S. K., Masinick, S., Garrett, M. and Hazlett, L. D. (1997) *Pseudomonas aeruginosa* lipopolysaccharide binds galectin-3 and other human corneal epithelial proteins. *Infect. Immun.*, **65**, 2747–2753

Hart, D. E., Reindel, W., Proskin, H. M. and Mowrey-McKee, M. F. (1993) Microbial contamination of hydrophilic contact lenses: quantitation and identification of microorganisms associated with contact lenses while on the eye. *Optom. Vis. Sci.*, **70**, 185–191

Hauser, A. R., Fleiszig, S., Kang, P. J. *et al.* (1998) Defects in type III secretion correlate with internalisation of *Pseudomonas aeruginosa* by epithelial cells. *Infect. Immun.*, **66**, 1413–1420

Haynes, R. J., Tighe, P. J. and Dua, H. S. (1999) Antimicrobial defensin peptides of the human ocular surface. *Br. J. Ophthalmol.*, **83**, 737–741

Hazlett, L. D., Moon, M. M., Singh, A. *et al.* (1991) Analysis of adhesion, piliation, protease production and ocular infectivity of several *P. aeruginosa* strains. *Curr. Eye Res.*, **10**, 351–362

Hazlett, L. D., McClellan, S. M., Dacjs, J. D. *et al.* (1999) Extended wear contact lens usage induces Langerhans cell migration in cornea. *Exp. Eye Res.*, **69**, 575–577

Hazlett, L. D., McClellan, S. A., Rudner, X. L. *et al.* (2002) The role of Langerhans cells in *Pseudomonas aeruginosa* infection. *Invest. Ophthalmol. Vis. Sci.*, **43**, 189–197

Heck, L. W., Alarcan, P. G., Kulhavy, R. M. *et al.* (1990) Degradation of IgA proteins by *Pseudomonas aeruginosa* elastase. *J. Immunol.*, **144**, 2253–2257

Hiemstra, P. S., Maassen, R. J., Stolk, J. *et al.* (1996) Antibacterial activity of antileukoprotease. *Infect. Immun.*, **64**, 4520–4524

Ho, J. J., Epstein, S. P. and Asbell, P. A. (1998) Chemotaxis by cytokines of Ia$^+$ Langerhans cells into the central cornea of mice. *Invest. Ophthalmol. Vis. Sci.*, **39**, s774

Holden, B. A., La Hood, D., Grant, T. *et al.* (1996) Gram negative bacteria can induce contact lens related acute red eye (CLARE) responses. *J. Cont. Lens Assoc. Ophthalmol.*, **22**, 47–52

Hovding, G. (1981) The conjunctival and contact lens bacterial flora during lens wear. *Acta Ophthalmol.*, **59**, 387–401

Hume, E. B. H. and Willcox, M. D. P. (1997) Adhesion and growth of *Serratia marcescens* on artificial closed eye tears (ATF) soaked hydrogel contact lenses. *Aust. NZ J. Ophthalmol.*, **25**, s39–s41

Hume, E. B. H., Conerly, L. L., Moreau, J. M. *et al.* (1999) *Serratia marcescens* keratitis: strain-specific corneal pathogenesis in rabbits. *Curr. Eye Res.*, **19**, 525–532

Hume, E. B. H., Dajcs, J. J., Moreau, J. M. *et al.* (2001) *Staphylococcus* corneal virulence in a new topical model of infection. *Invest. Ophthalmol. Vis. Sci.*, **42**, 2904–2908

Husted, R. C., Conners, M. S., Connors, R. A. *et al.* (1997) Quantitative analysis of 12-hydroxy-5,8,14-eicosatrienoic acid (12-HETrE) in rabbit aqueous humor and corneal extracts and in human tears. *Invest. Ophthalmol. Vis. Sci.*, **38**, s285

Inatomi, T., Spurr-Michaud, S., Tisdale, A. S. and Gipson, I. K. (1995) Human corneal and conjunctival epithelial express MUC1 mucin. *Invest. Ophthalmol. Vis. Sci.*, **36**, 1818–1827

Jalbert, I., Willcox, M. D. P. and Sweeney, D. F. (1999) Isolation of *Staphylococcus aureus* from a contact lens at the time of a contact lens induced peripheral ulcer: case report. *Cornea*, **19**, 116–120

Jett, B. D. and Gilmore, M. S. (2002) Internalization of *Staphylococcus aureus* by human corneal epithelial cells: role of bacterial fibronectin-binding protein and host cell factors. *Infect. Immun.*, **40**, 4697–4700

Jones, L. and Senchyna, M. (2002) Protein and lipid deposition of silicone-hydrogel contact lens materials. http://www.siliconehydrogel.org/editorials

Jumblatt, M. M., McKenzie, R. W. and Jumblatt, J. E. (1999) MUC5AC mucin is a component of the human precorneal tear film. *Invest. Ophthalmol. Vis. Sci.*, **40**, 43–49

Keay, L. J., Harmis, N., Corrigan, K. *et al.* (1998) Comparison of bacterial populations on worn contact lenses following 6 nights extended wear of Acuvue and 30 nights extended wear of investigational hydrogel lenses. *Aust. Ophthalmol. Vis. Sci.*, Abstracts, 61

Kijlstra, A., Polak, B. C. and Luyendijk, L. (1992) Transient decrease of secretory IgA in tears during rigid gas permeable contact lens wear. *Curr. Eye Res.*, **11**, 123–126

Knight, D. A. and Barbieri, J. T. (1997) Ecto-ADP-ribosyltransferase activity of *Pseudomonas aeruginosa* exoenzyme S. *Infect. Immun.*, **65**, 3304–3309

Lan, J., Willcox, M. D. P. and Jackson, G. D. F. (1997) The role of tear sIgA in ocular immune defence. *Invest. Ophthalmol. Vis. Sci.*, **38**, 518

Lan, J., Willcox, M. D. P. and Jackson, G. D. F. (1998a) Effect of tear secretory IgA on chemotaxis of polymorphonuclear leukocytes. *Aust. NZ J. Ophthalmol.*, **26**(s), 36–39

Lan, J., Willcox, M. D. P. and Jackson, G. D. F. (1998b) The effect of contact lens wear on the level of tear secretory IgA and specific IgA. *Invest. Ophthalmol. Vis. Sci.*, **39**, 786

Larkin, D. F. P. and Leeming, J. P. (1991) Quantitative alterations in the commensal eye bacteria in contact lens wear. *Eye*, **5**, 70–74

Leitch, E. C. and Willcox, M. D. P. (1999) Elucidation of the antistaphylococcal action of lactoferrin and lysozyme. *J. Med. Microbiol.*, **48**, 867–871

Lomholt, J. A., Poulsen, K. and Kilian, M. (2001) Epidemic population structure of *Pseudomonas aeruginosa*: evidence for a clone that is pathogenic for the eye and that has a distinct combination of virulence factors. *Infect. Immun.*, **69**, 6284–6295

Mannucci, L. L., Pozzau, M., Fregona, I. and Secchi, A. G. (1984) The effect of extended wear contact lenses on tear immunoglobulins. *J. Cont. Lens Assoc. Ophthalmol.*, **10**, 163–165

Masinick, S. A., Montgomery, C. P., Montgomery, P. C. and Hazlett, L. D. (1997) Secretory IgA inhibits *Pseudomonas aeruginosa* binding to cornea and protects against keratitis. *Invest. Ophthalmol. Vis. Sci.*, **38**, 910–918

Matsumoto, K., Shams, N. B. K., Hanninen, L. A. and Kenyon, K. R. (1993) Cleavage and activation of corneal matrix metalloproteases by *Pseudomonas aeruginosa* proteases. *Invest. Ophthalmol. Vis. Sci.*, **34**, 1945–1953

McDermott, A. M., Redfern, R. L., Zhang, B. (2001) Human beta-defensin 2 is upregulated during re-epithelialization of the cornea. *Curr. Eye Res.*, **22**, 64–67

McGuffie, E. M., Frank, D. W., Vincent, T. S. and Olson, J. C. (1998) Modification of Ras in eukaryotic cells by *Pseudomonas aeruginosa* exoenzyme S. *Infect. Immun.*, **66**, 2607–2613

Miller, M. B. and Bassler, B. L. (2001) Quorum sensing in bacteria. *Annu. Rev. Microbiol.*, **55**, 165–169

Miyajima, S., Akaike, T., Matsumoto, K. *et al.* (2001) Matrix metalloproteinases induction by pseudomonal virulence factors and inflammatory cytokines in vitro. *Microb. Pathogen.*, **31**, 271–281

Mondino, B. J., Weissman, B. A., Farb, M. D. and Pettit, T. H. (1986) Corneal ulcers associated with daily-wear and extended-wear contact lenses. *Am. J. Ophthalmol.*, **102**, 58–65

Moreau, J. M., Grigis, D. O., Hume, E. B. *et al.* (2001) Phospholipase A(2) in rabbit tears: a host defense against *Staphylococcus aureus. Invest. Ophthalmol. Vis. Sci.*, **42**, 2347–2354

Mowrey-McKee, M. F., Sampson, H. J. and Proskin, H. M. (1992) Microbial contamination of hydrophilic contact lenses. Part II: quantitation of microbes after patient handling and after aseptic removal from the eye. *J. Cont. Lens Assoc. Ophthalmol.*, **18**, 240–244

Nakamura, Y., Yokoi, N, Tokushige, H. *et al.* (2001) Sialic acid in normal human tear fluid. *Jpn J. Ophthalmol.*, **45**, 327–331

Nevalainen, T. J., Aho, H. J. and Peuravuori, H. (1994) Secretion of group 2 phospholipase A_2 by lacrimal glands. *Invest. Ophthalmol. Vis. Sci.*, **35**, 417–421

Niederkorn, J. Y. (1995) Effects of cytokine-induced migration of Langerhans cells on corneal allograft survival. *Eye*, **9**, 215

O'Callaghan, R. J., Engel, L. S., Hobden, J. A. *et al.* (1996) *Pseudomonas* keratitis: the role of an uncharacterised exoprotein, protease IV, in corneal virulence. *Invest. Ophthalmol. Vis. Sci.*, 534–543

Ogra, P. L., Mestecky, J., Lamm, M. E. *et al.* (1994) *Handbook of Mucosal Immunology.* Academic Press, London

Parmely, M., Gale, A., Clabaugh, M. *et al.* (1990) Proteolytic inactivation of cytokines by *Pseudomonas aeruginosa. Infect. Immun.*, **58**, 3009–3014

Patrinely, J. R., Wilhelmus, K. R., Rubin, J. M. and Key, J. E. (1985) Bacterial keratitis associated with extended wear soft contact lenses. *CLAO J.*, **11**, 234–236

Pearce, D. J., Demirci. G. and Willcox, M. D. (1999) Secretory IgA epitopes in basal tears of extended-wear soft contact lens wearers and non-lens wearers. *Aust. NZ J. Ophthalmol.*, **27**, 221–223

Perkins, R. E., Kundsin, R. B., Pratt, M. V. *et al.* (1975) Bacteriology of normal and infected conjunctiva. *J. Clin. Microbiol.*, **1**, 147–149

Pflugfelder, S. C., Liu, Z., Monroy, D. *et al.* (2000) Detection of sialomucin complex (MUC4) in human ocular surface epithelium and tear fluid. *Invest. Ophthalmol. Vis. Sci.*, **41**, 1316–1326

Pillar, C. M. and Hobden, J. A. (2002) *Pseudomonas aeruginosa* exotoxin A and keratitis in mice. *Invest. Ophthalmol. Vis. Sci.*, **43**, 1437–1444

Pillar, C. M., Hazlett, L. D. and Hobden, J. A. (2002) Alkaline protease-deficient mutants of *Pseudomonas aeruginosa* are virulent in the eye. *Curr. Eye Res.*, **21**, 730–739

Poggio, E. C., Glynn, R. J., Schein, O. D. *et al.* (1989) The incidence of ulcerative keratitis among users of daily wear and extended-wear soft contact lenses. *New Engl. J. Med.*, **321**, 779–783

Qu., X. D. and Lehrer, R. I. (1998) Secretory phospholipase A_2 is the principal bactericide for staphylococci and other Gram-positive bacteria in human tears. *Infect. Immun.*, **66**, 2791–2797

Ramachandran, L., Sharma, S., Sankaridurg, P. R. *et al.* (1995) Examination of the conjunctival microbiota after 8 hours of eye closure. *J. Cont. Lens Assoc. Ophthalmol.*, **21**, 195–199

Rhem, M. N., Lech, E. M., Patti, J. M. *et al.* (2000) The collagen-binding adhesin is a virulence factor in *Staphylococcus aureus* keratitis. *Infect. Immun.*, **68**, 3776–3779

Rother, K. and Till, G. O. (1988) *The Complement System*. Springer, Berlin

Saari, K. M., Aho, V. V., Paavilainen, V. *et al.* (2001) Group II PLA$_2$ content of tears in normal subjects. *Invest. Ophthalmol. Vis. Sci.*, **42**, 318–320

Sack, R. A., Tan, K. O. and Tan, A. (1992) Diurnal tear cycle: evidence for a nocturnal inflammatory constitutive tear fluid. *Invest. Ophthalmol. Vis. Sci.*, **33**, 626–640

Sack, R. A., Sathe, S., Hackworth, L. A. *et al.* (1996) The effect of eye closure on tear flow, protein and complement deposition on Group IV hydrogel contact lenses. *Curr. Eye Res.*, **15**, 1092–1100

Sack, R. A., Beaton, A., Sathe, S. *et al.* (2000) Towards a closed eye model of the pre-corneal tear layer. *Prog. Ret. Eye Res.*, **19**, 649–668

Sakata, M., Sack, R. A., Sathe, S. *et al.* (1997) Polymorphonuclear leukocyte cells and elastase in tears. *Curr. Eye Res.*, **16**, 810–819

Sakata, M., Shinmura, S. and Tsubota K. (1999) Localisation of secretory leukocyte protease inhibitor in the human ocular surface. *Invest. Ophthalmol. Vis. Sci.*, **40**, s338

Sankaridurg, P. R., Willcox, M. D. P., Sharma, S. *et al.* (1996) *Haemophilus influenzae* adherent to contact lenses is associated with the production of acute ocular inflammation. *J. Clin. Microbiol.*, **34**, 2426–2431

Sankaridurg, P. R., Sharma, S., Willcox, M. *et al.* (1999) Colonization of hydrogel lenses with *Streptococcus pneumoniae*: risk of development of corneal infiltrates. *Cornea*, **18**, 289–295

Sankaridurg, P. R., Rao, G. N., Rao, H. N. *et al.* (2000) ATPase-positive dentritic cells in the limbal and corneal epithelium of guinea pigs after extended wear of hydrogel lenses. *Cornea*, **19**, 374–377

Sathe, S., Sakata, M, Beaton, A. R. and Sack, R. A. (1998) Identification, origin and the diurnal role of the principal serine protease inhibitors in human tear fluid. *Curr. Eye Res.*, **17**, 348–362

Schein, O. D., Ormerod, L. D., Barraquer, E. *et al.* (1989) Microbiology of contact lens-related keratitis. *Cornea*, **8**, 281–285

Schultz, C. L., Morck, D. W., McKay, S. G. *et al.* (1997) Lipopolysaccharide induced acute red eye and corneal ulcers. *Exp. Eye Res.*, **64**, 3–9

Sengor, T., Gurgul, S., Ogretmenoglu, S. *et al.* (1990) Tear immunology in contact lens wearers. *Contactologia*, **12**, 43–45

Song, C. H., Choi, J. S., Kim, D. K. *et al.* (1999) Enhanced secretory group II PLA$_2$ in the tears of blepharitis patients. *Invest. Ophthalmol. Vis. Sci.*, **40**, 2744–2748

Stapleton, F. and Dart, J. K. G. (1995) *Pseudomonas* keratitis associated with biofilm formation on a disposable soft contact lens. *Br. J. Ophthalmol.*, **79**, 864–865

Stapleton, F., Willcox, M. D. P., Fleming, C. M. *et al.* (1995a) Changes in the ocular biota with time in extended and daily wear disposable contact lens use. *Infect. Immun.*, **63**, 4501–4505

Stapleton, F., Dart, J. K. G., Seal, D. V. and Matheson, M. (1995b) Epidemiology of *Pseudomonas aeruginosa* in contact lens wearers. *Epidemiol. Infect.*, **114**, 395–402

Stapleton, F., Sansey, N., Willcox, M. D. P. and Holden, B. A. (1996) Recruitment of polymorphonuclear leukocytes into the tear film during overnight contact lens wear. *Invest. Ophthalmol. Vis. Sci.*, **37**, s1024

Stapleton, F., Willcox, M. D. P., Sansey, N. and Holden, B. A. (1997) Ocular microbiota and polymorphonuclear leucocyte recruitment during overnight contact lens wear. *Aust. NZ J. Ophthalmol.*, **25**, s33–s35

Sweeney, D. F., Stapleton, F., Leitch, C. *et al.* (1994) The microbial colonization of soft contact lenses over time. *Invest. Ophthalmol. Vis. Sci.*, **35**, 1779

Tamm, M., Bihl, M., Eickelberg, O. *et al.* (1998) Hypoxia-induced interleukin-6 and interleukin-8 production is mediated by platelet-activating factor and platelet-derived growth factor in primary human lung cells. *Am. J. Resp. Cell Mol. Biol.*, **19**, 653–661

Tan, K. O., Sack, R. A., Holden, B. A. and Swarbrick, H. A. (1993) Temporal sequence of changes in tear film composition during sleep. *Curr. Eye Res.*, **12**, 1001–1007

Taylor, R. L., Willcox, M. D., Williams, T. J. *et al.* (1998) Modulation of bacterial adhesion to hydrogel contact lenses by albumin. *Optom. Vis. Sci.*, **75**, 23–29.

Temel, A., Kazokoglu, H. and Taga, Y. (1990) The effect of contact lens wear on tear immunoglobulins. *Contactologia*, **12**, 39–42

Thakur, A. and Willcox, M. D. P. (1998) Cytokines and lipid inflammatory mediator profile of human tears of contact lens associated inflammatory diseases. *Exp. Eye Res.*, **67**, 9–19

Thakur, A., Willcox, M. D. P., Morris, C. A. and Holden, B. A. (1996) Inflammatory components of human tear fluid. *Aust. NZ J. Ophthalmol.*, **24**, s13–s16

Thakur, A., Willcox, M. D. P. and Stapleton, F. (1998) The proinflammatory cytokines and arachidonic acid metabolites in human overnight tears: homeostatic mechanisms. *J. Clin. Immunol.*, **18**, 61–70

Thakur, A., Chauhan, A. and Willcox, M. D. P. (1999) Effect of lysozyme on adhesion and toxin release by *Staphylococcus aureus*. *Aust. NZ J. Ophthalmol.*, **27**, 224–227

Theander, T. G., Kharzami, A., Pedersen, B. K. *et al.* (1988) Inhibition of human leukocyte proliferation and cleavage of interleukin-2 by *Pseudomonas aeruginosa* proteases. *Infect. Immun.*, **56**, 1673–1677

Thuruthyil, S., Zhu, H. and Willcox, M. D. P. (2001) Serotype and adhesion of *Pseudomonas aeruginosa* isolated from contact lens wearers. *Clin. Exp. Ophthalmol.*, **29**, 147–149

Twining, S. S., Kirschner, S. E., Mahnke, L. A. and Frank, D. W. (1993) Effect of *Pseudomonas aeruginosa* elastase, alkaline protease, and exotoxin A on corneal proteinases and proteins. *Invest. Ophthalmol. Vis. Sci.*, **34**, 2699–2712

Vinding, T., Eriksen, J.S. and Nielsen, N. V. (1987) The concentration of lysozyme and secretory IgA in tears from healthy persons with and without contact lens use. *Acta Ophthalmol.*, **65**, 23–26

Wall, D. and Kaiser, D. (1999) Type IV pili and cell motility. *Mol. Microbiol.*, **32**, 1–10

Weissman, B. A., Mondino, B. J., Pettit, T. H. and Hofbauer, J. D. (1984) Corneal ulcers associated with extended-wear soft contact lenses. *Am. J. Ophthalmol.*, **97**, 476–481

Willcox, M. D. P. and Hume, E. B. H. (1999) Differences in the pathogenesis of bacteria isolated from contact-lens induced infiltrative conditions. *Aust. NZ J. Ophthalmol.*, **27**, 231–233

Willcox, M. D. P. and Lan, J. (1999) Secretory immunoglobulin A in tears: functions and changes during contact lens wear. *Clin. Exp. Optom.*, **82**, 1–3

Willcox, M. D. P., Morris, C. A., Sack, R. A. *et al.* (1997a) Complement and complement regulatory proteins in human tears. *Invest. Ophthalmol. Vis. Sci.*, **38**, 1–8

Willcox, M. D. P., Power, K. N., Stapleton, F. *et al.* (1997b) Potential sources of bacteria that are isolated from contact lenses during wear. *Optom. Vis. Sci.*, **74**, 1030–1038

Willcox, M. D. P., Harmis, N. Y., Cowell, B. A. *et al.* (2001) Bacterial interactions with contact lenses: effects of lens material, lens wear and microbial physiology. *Biomaterials*, **22**, 3235–3247

Williams, T. J., Willcox, M. D. P. and Schneider, R. P. (1997) The role of tear fluid in the growth of Gram-negative bacteria on contact lenses. *Aust. NZ J. Ophthalmol.*, **25**, s30–s32

Willis, S. L., Court, J. L., Reman, R. P. *et al.* (2001) A novel phosphorylcholine-coated contact lens for extended wear use. *Biomaterials*, **22**, 3261–3272

Wu, X., Gupta, S. K. and Hazlett, L. D. (1995) Characterisation of *P. aeruginosa* pili binding human corneal epithelial proteins. *Curr. Eye Res.*, **14**, 969–977

Wu, P. Z., Zhu, H., Thakur, A. *et al.* (1999) Comparison of potential pathogenic traits of staphylococci that may contribute to corneal ulceration and inflammation. *Aust. NZ J. Ophthalmol.*, **27**, 234–236

Wu, P. Z., Thakur, A., Stapleton, F. *et al.* (2000) *Staphylococcus aureus* causes acute inflammatory episodes in the cornea during contact lens wear. *Clin. Exp. Ophthalmol.*, **28**, 194–196

Yahr, T., Mende-Mueller, L. M., Friese, M. B. and Frank, D. W. (1997) Identification of type III secreted products of the *Pseudomonas aeruginosa* exoenzyme S regulon. *J. Bacteriol.*, **179**, 7165–7168

Yamauchi, K., Tomita, M., Giehl, T. J. and Ellison, R. T. III (1993) Antibacterial activity of lactoferrin and a pepsin-derived lactoferrin fragment. *Infect. Immun.*, **61**, 719–728

Zhao, H., Jumblatt, J. E., Wood, T. O. *et al.* (2001) Quantification of MUC5AC protein in human tears. *Cornea*, **20**, 873–877

Zhu, H., Thuruthyil, S. and Willcox, M. D. P. (2001) Production of *N*-acetyl homoserine lactones by Gram-negative bacteria isolated from contact lens wearers. *Clin. Exp. Ophthalmol.*, **29**, 150–152

Chapter 5

Corneal hypoxia

Noel A. Brennan and Desmond Fonn

INTRODUCTION

The cornea is a unique biological tissue with regard to its optical function and aerobic metabolism. Through the requirement of transparency, the tissue has evolved to obtain an oxygen supply via diffusion across its limiting layers rather than via an opaque vascular system. It uses the oxygen in aerobic catabolism to prevent hydration, which leads to loss of tissue transparency.

The placement of hydrogel contact lenses and to some extent rigid gas-permeable (RGP) lenses on to the eye can place the cornea under hypoxic stress. This weakness has had a much greater impact on extended wear (EW), but many patients wearing hydrogel lenses (now considered 'low Dk/t') on a daily wear (DW) basis have developed ocular changes that are caused by chronic hypoxia. The advent of silicone hydrogel lenses, whose oxygen transmissibility ranges from 110 to 175×10^{-9} barrers/cm, has effectively eliminated or significantly minimized the hypoxic effects on the cornea and other ocular structures. In this chapter we will review the state of research into corneal oxygenation by considering the basics of cellular physiology, techniques for assessing the corneal physiological response and the influence of lens wear on this response.

Holden and Mertz (1984) hypothesized that if lenses have an oxygen Dk/t in excess of 87×10^{-9} then overnight corneal swelling with the lens should not exceed the swelling of a non-lens-wearing eye. This criterion was established on the basis that the non-wearing eye swelled approximately 4 per cent overnight (Mertz, 1980). If overnight corneal swelling was lower, however, the oxygen transmissibility of the lens would have to be proportionally higher. Mertz's overnight corneal swelling value appears to be slightly high, as we will show later in this chapter. Independently, Harvitt and Bonanno have suggested that the critical value is 125×10^{-9} Dk/t, which would be in agreement with the Holden and Mertz predicted value if the overnight corneal swelling is 3.2 per cent. The availability of highly permeable silicone hydrogel lenses has enabled us to test the Holden and Mertz hypothesis.

PHYSIOLOGY OF HYPOXIA

CELLULAR RESPONSE TO HYPOXIA

When the oxygen supply is interrupted there are a number of possible outcomes from cell damage and death to adaptive responses. These occur at the local cellular level or can affect parts of tissue or the entire organ. Many of these events are universal in aerobically respiring cells. However, some tissues have unique responses, such as the cornea.

The partial oxygen pressure (pO_2) within most cells falls within narrow physiological constraints, the supply remarkably matching consumption under a wide variety of conditions. The consequences of departure from this concentration can be dramatic. High oxygen levels can lead to the formation of reactive oxygen species which can be toxic and cause oxidative damage. In most body tissues, the intracellular micro-environment is far removed from atmospheric oxygen pressure; however, corneal tissue is subject to extremes of oxygen tension. Epithelial cellular pO_2 may be as high as 155 mmHg or fall to zero during closed-eye wear of contact lenses. To cope with the high oxygen levels, the cornea has strong antioxidant activity.

On the other hand, low concentrations can produce responses which can range from adaptation to cellular, tissue, organ and entire animal damage or death. Some tissues, such as the brain and heart, may only tolerate low oxygen for a matter of minutes before severe adverse cellular events arise. These include failure of energy-dependent membrane ion channels, breakdown of cellular calcium equilibrium and disruption of cellular enzymes, ultimately leading to loss of cellular homeostasis. Traditionally, hypoxia-induced cell death was considered to be necrotic but recently there has been overwhelming evidence that apoptosis also plays a major role in hypoxically induced cell death.

The critical oxygen supply to different cell types varies widely but is difficult to quantify simply as the damage is dependent not only on the pO_2 but also duration of exposure and pre-adaptation. To a certain extent, pO_2 for normal function can be determined by the pressure that allows the mitochondria to maintain aerobic metabolism. Figure 5.1 shows the best-fit curve of oxygen flux into the mitochondria as a function of pO_2 for rat heart mitochondria, and these are similar to those for many other tissues (Gnaiger *et al.*, 2000). The p_{50} value, at which oxygen flux into the mitochondria is half the maximum, is equal to approximately 0.25 mmHg. This partial pressure is $1/600$ of atmospheric pressure, showing that respiration of cells is maintained despite great restriction to oxygen supply. Other cellular activities are more sensitive to oxygen restriction and Table 5.1 lists the K_mO_2 (pO_2 at which half maximum activity is maintained) for a number of different enzymes (Leach and Treacher, 2002).

In many cases restricted oxygen supply does not mean tissue death or permanent damage, and adaptational changes are important. Cellular tolerance to hypoxia may involve 'hibernation' strategies that reduce metabolic rate, increased extraction of oxygen from surrounding tissues and adaptations of enzymes to allow metabolism at low pO_2. High energy functions like ion transport and protein production are downregulated to balance supply and demand. Anaerobic

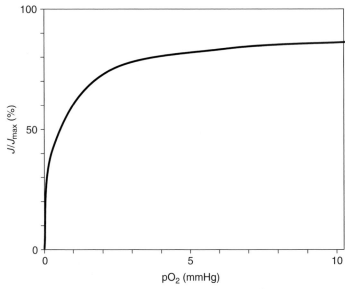

Figure 5.1   Relative oxygen flux into mitochondria versus pO_2 (after data for rat heart mitochondria, Gnaiger, 2001)

Table 5.1   Oxygen affinities of cellular enzymes expressed as the partial pressure of oxygen in mmHg at which the enzyme rate is half maximum (K_mO_2)

Enzyme	Substrate	K_mO_2 (mmHg)
Glucose oxidase	Glucose	57
Xanthine oxidase	Hypoxanthine	50
Tryptophan oxygenase	Tryptophan	37
Monoamine oxidase	Catecholamines	30
Nitric oxide synthase	L-Arginine	25
NADPH oxidase	Oxygen	23
Cytochrome aa$_3$	Oxygen	0.05

energy production is important to the survival of some tissues despite its ineffi-ciency. Skeletal muscle increases glucose uptake by 600 per cent during hypoxia and bladder smooth muscle can generate up to 60 per cent of total energy requirement by anaerobic glycolysis.

ANAEROBIC PREDISPOSITION

Despite the emphasis in research on aerobic corneal metabolism, the extent to which the cornea is predisposed to survive anaerobically is remarkable. To illus-trate the reliance on non-aerobic pathways, consider the following:

■ The cornea undergoes and withstands greater fluctuations in oxygen concen-tration than most body tissues.

- It is avascular, thus deriving nutrients and oxygen exogenously in lieu of an extensive vascular bed to provide these substrates at a consistent rate and constant level.

- It has been estimated that only 15 per cent of corneal glucose substrate is metabolized aerobically (Riley, 1969).

- The corneal epithelium has an inhibitory protein to prevent vascularization in the absence of oxygen (Makino *et al.*, 2001).

- The epithelium does not show ultrastructural changes to prolonged systemic hypoxic threat where the stroma and endothelium do (Mastropasqua *et al.*, 1998).

- Human corneal epithelial cells are resistant to apoptosis for five days of hypoxia (15 mmHg) in culture and poly-ADP-ribose polymerase cleavage (signalling initiation of the apoptotic pathway) is not evident for seven days (Esco *et al.*, 2001).

- *In vivo*, the cornea can withstand long periods (over 8 hours) of zero oxygen tension at its anterior surface.

- During these periods of prolonged hypoxia, it loses neither transparency nor shape and maintains its barrier functions.

- A strong 'Pasteur effect' has also been noted in the endothelium (Riley and Winkler, 1990).

- In keeping with a low organelle count to maintain transparency, corneal epithelial cells have a low count of mitochondria, the site of aerobic respiration.

- Its partner tissue, the lens, has no mitochondria.

Although Sloan (1965) demonstrated that corneas are somewhat resilient to hypoxia, it has been hypothesized that hypoxia with EW renders the cornea susceptible to infection. In reality, Sloan's report has been contradicted by a more recent report (Sweeney, 1992) of corneal warpage and exhaustion syndrome, particularly with wear of oxygen-impermeable polymethyl methacrylate (PMMA) or thick hydrogel lenses.

CORNEAL RESPONSE TO HYPOXIA

CORNEAL ADAPTIVE RESPONSES

The corneal response to hypoxia demonstrates that it has the capacity to undergo adaptation, and current molecular biology theory suggests that these responses occur in a controlled manner. It is presumed that certain changes associated with contact lens wear are hypoxic in origin but it is not feasible to study long-term hypoxic influences in isolation. More information in this regard is coming to light since the usage of silicone hydrogel materials, which enables the influence of hypoxia and the mechanical presence of the contact lens to be isolated.

ALTERED CORNEAL EPITHELIAL METABOLISM

In response to hypoxia, the corneal epithelium is known to undergo a range of short- and long-term changes as anaerobic metabolism becomes the predominant energy-producing pathway. Changes in the levels of various enzymes have been noted, although both hypoxia and mechanical effects may play a role in producing this finding (Uniacke *et al.*, 1972; Hill *et al.*, 1974; Fullard and Carney, 1985; Ichijima *et al.*, 1992; Bonazzi *et al.*, 2000). Genetic expression upregulating anaerobic metabolism in the cornea is presumed rather than documented, but corneal ATP levels observed during hypoxia can most likely be attributed to compensatory ATP generation by enhanced glycolysis (Masters *et al.*, 1989).

Harvitt and Bonanno (1998) found an increase in rabbit corneal oxygen consumption with decreasing corneal pH. During contact lens-induced hypoxia, corneal pH falls, and the consumption rate is paradoxically predicted to rise. The authors have used this effect to explain in part differences in anterior oxygen tension between measured and modelled values (see below for more details; Harvitt and Bonanno, 1999). More information regarding control of corneal metabolic homeostasis is necessary to ascertain the role of the regulatory mechanism in promoting increased consumption in the short-term response to hypoxia.

Longer-term studies have shown decreased corneal oxygen consumption as measured by a polarographic oxygen sensor (Farris and Donn, 1972; Holden *et al.*, 1985; Carney and Brennan, 1988). One can hypothesize the basis of this as being decreased total epithelial tissue or direct regulation of respiratory activity. Bonanno *et al.* (2003), however, were recently unable to replicate this finding using phosphorescence spectroscopy with a sample of soft lens wearers. The difference in these studies may be the degree of hypoxic stress between the wearing groups.

REDUCED CORNEAL SWELLING RESPONSE

Lactate accumulation results from the shutdown in aerobic pathways leading to the classic corneal swelling response (for more detail on this response, see below). However, the cornea appears to adapt in that the swelling response changes with time of wear. Numerous studies have found that prolonged exposure to low-Dk/t contact lenses reduces the oedema response by about 2 per cent with DW and by about 3–4 per cent with EW (Bradley and Schoessler, 1979; Hirji and Larke, 1979; Lowther and Tomlinson, 1979; Lebow and Plishka, 1980; Schoessler and Barr, 1980; Cox *et al.*, 1991). This effect includes a reduction in the overnight oedema response without lens wear (Cox *et al.*, 1991). The reduction in the corneal swelling response is directly related to hypoxia, as shown by the absence of such an effect with wear of high-Dk/t lenses (Cornish *et al.*, 2001). The mechanism behind this adaptation is yet to be elucidated, but it may be related to altered oxygen consumption.

ALTERED CORNEAL EPITHELIAL MITOSES, THICKNESS AND EXFOLIATION

Under normal conditions, an unknown control mechanism maintains a stable equilibrium in which cell production, size, movement and exfoliation are coordinated to achieve a stable corneal epithelial architecture. Cells at the basal epithelium may undergo mitosis several times before terminally differentiating, advancing towards the surface, undergoing apoptosis and finally sloughing into the tears. The general population of cells is renewed from stem cells, which seems to be located at the limbus (Sangwan, 2001). As a result, there is both a centripetal and forward movement of cells. Contact lens wear impacts proliferation in the basal layers of the corneal epithelium (Hamano *et al.*, 1983). All types of contact lens wear, including soft or RGP, low Dk/t or high Dk/t, lead to decreased cellular division. Reduced mitosis with contact lens wear must be followed by at least one of the following three occurrences: increased cell life, cell enlargement or epithelial thinning (Bergmanson and Chu, 1982; Bergmanson *et al.*, 1985; Holden *et al.*, 1985; Lemp and Gold, 1986; Tsubota and Yamada, 1992; Wilson, 1994; Tsubota *et al.*, 1996). Oxygen supply definitely plays a role in epithelial architectural homeostasis, as low-Dk/t lenses suppress proliferation more than high-Dk/t lenses (Ladage *et al.*, 2003). It seems, however, that the mechanical presence of the lens or reduced flow in the post-lens tear film also plays a role. All contact lenses decrease surface cell sloughing rate, possibly as a result of reduced blink shear pressure, and this may signal the basal layer to reduce mitotic activity. Control of epithelial architectural equilibrium by mechanical forces is critical to vision, as the effect of orthokeratology is produced at least in part by redistribution of the epithelial volume (Alharbi and Swarbrick, 2003).

SHORT-TERM EPITHELIAL THICKNESS AND LIGHT-SCATTER RESPONSES

There are dichotomous reports of how the corneal epithelium responds to hypoxia. Early studies using microdensitometry to examine rabbit eyes *in vitro* found that glycogen depletion resulting from anoxia was accompanied by epithelial swelling (Uniacke *et al.*, 1972). Lowther and Hill (1973) also found thickening of the rabbit epithelium with anoxia, but further *in vitro* studies, using a specular microscope to measure corneal changes (Wilson *et al.*, 1973; Lambert and Klyce, 1981) in response to hypoxia, did not find any increase in epithelial thickness, though they did document stromal swelling. Specular microscopy was also used to examine the eyes of live rabbits (Wilson and Fatt, 1980) finding, again, that corneal swelling was due to swelling of the stroma and not the epithelium. Bergmanson *et al.* (1985) also studied the effect of different contact lens thicknesses on live primate corneas and did not find epithelial thickening.

O'Leary *et al.* (1981) developed a micropachometer to measure epithelial thickness of a living, human cornea and found that epithelial thickness remained constant regardless of how long the cornea was deprived of oxygen. A more

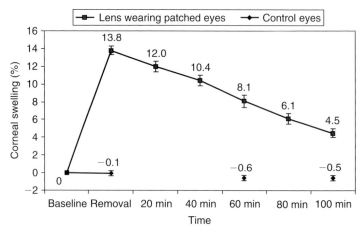

Figure 5.2 Percentage change (mean ± SE) of corneal thickness in patched eyes compared to control eyes in 20 subjects. Baseline refers to the measurements taken before soft contact lens (SCL) wear and eye closure. Removal point refers to the measurements taken immediately after SCL removal following 3 hours of lens wear (reprinted with permission from Wang *et al.*, 2002c)

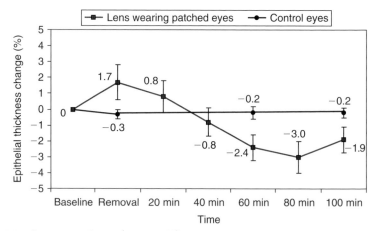

Figure 5.3 Percentage change (mean ± SE) of epithelial thickness of patched eyes compared to control eyes in 20 subjects. Baseline refers to the measurements taken before SCL wear and eye closure. Removal point refers to the measurements taken immediately after SCL removal following 3 hours of lens wear (reprinted with permission from Wang *et al.*, 2002a)

recent study performed by Wang *et al.* (2002a) used optical coherence tomography (OCT) to measure central corneal and epithelial thickness of human eyes. The results of this study support the findings that corneal thickness increases in response to oxygen deprivation caused by a contact lens and eye closure (Figure 5.2), but the increase is due to swelling of the stroma and not the epithelium (Figure 5.3). Although the graph shows thickening of the epithelium, it was not statistically significant. Wang *et al.* (2003a) also measured corneal and epithelial thickness

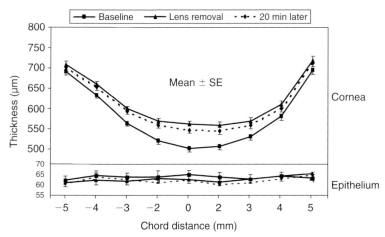

Figure 5.4 Topographical thickness of the corneal epithelium and total cornea of 18 eyes after 3 hours of PMMA lens wear with eye closure. The change in corneal thickness was greater centrally than peripherally and epithelial thickness across the cornea did not change significantly (reprinted with permission from Wang *et al.*, 2003a)

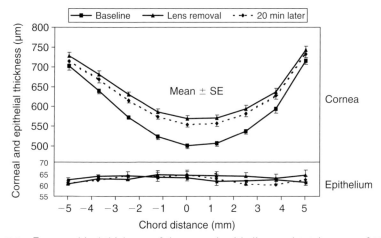

Figure 5.5 Topographical thickness of the corneal epithelium and total cornea of 18 eyes after 3 hours of SCL wear with eye closure. The change in corneal thickness was greater centrally than peripherally and epithelial thickness across the cornea did not change significantly (reprinted with permission from Wang *et al.*, 2003a)

across a 10 mm horizontal chord and demonstrated that epithelial thickness did not increase in response to wearing PMMA and thick hydrogel lenses with 3 hours of eye closure (Figures 5.4 and 5.5).

Although hypoxia can cause light scatter of the epithelium resulting in halos, glare and loss of visual acuity (Wilson and Fatt, 1980; Lambert and Klyce, 1981), it paradoxically does not cause epithelial swelling. Lambert and Klyce (1981) have suggested that the tissue in a living epithelium avoids oedema by regulating itself, relying on metabolic energy as a means of compensating for the effects of hypoxia. Feng *et al.* (2001) did report an increase in epithelial thickness after sleep. They attributed this increase to hypotonicity of the tear film during eye closure.

Though swelling does not occur, the epithelium appears to thin significantly during recovery from hypoxia (O'Leary *et al.*, 1981; Wang *et al.*, 2002a) as shown in Figure 5.3. O'Leary *et al.* (1981) suggest that this shrinkage is due to the electrolyte leaving the cell at a faster rate than it can leak back in during the recovery period. Wang *et al.* (2002a) offer a similar explanation, suggesting that the cornea may regulate itself in this case as well, continuing to expel fluid (and thin) beyond its baseline thickness.

Epithelial thickness has not been measured following overnight wear of silicone hydrogel contact lenses but it is doubtful that any measurable increase will occur due to the lens, as corneal swelling with these lenses is very similar to that with no lens wear (Fonn *et al.*, 1999).

EFFECTS OF ORTHOKERATOLOGY

Orthokeratology or corneal refractive therapy (CRT) has had a resurgence in the last five years because of the development of reverse geometry lens designs and the process has been accelerated with these new designs in overnight wear (Horner and Richardson, 1992; Dave and Ruston, 1997; Day *et al.*, 1997; Swarbrick *et al.*, 1998; Mountford, 1997, 1998; Nichols *et al.*, 2000). The designs are distinctive in that the centre of the lens is flatter than the central corneal curvature, thus applying physical pressure to the centre of the cornea which is accentuated with eye closure. The mid-periphery of the lens contains a secondary curve radius that is steeper than the central curve, which creates a tear reservoir through localized clearance from the cornea. The effect of this design is to reduce myopia by altering the shape of the cornea. Studies such as those described by Swarbrick *et al.* (1998), Wang *et al.* (2002b) and Alharbi and Swarbrick (2003) have added insight to this procedure by examining the changes in corneal tissue that accompany the reduction in myopia.

Swarbrick *et al.* (1998) and Alharbi and Swarbrick (2003) found that a reduction in refractive myopic error was accompanied by a flattening of the central cornea, although their study designs were different. In Swarbrick's study the subjects wore the lenses during the day and Alharbi's subjects only wore the lenses during the night. Using optical pachometry they both found thinning of the central cornea occurring primarily in the epithelium. Both studies revealed a significant thickening of the mid-peripheral stroma of the cornea, but no thickening of the mid-peripheral epithelium. Alharbi's study showed an alarming 35 per cent thinning of the central corneal epithelium, which is of concern as the epithelium serves to protect the cornea. The thinning could be either a compression of epithelial cells or the loss of one or more cell layers, as described by Greenberg and Hill (1973).

Wang *et al.* (2002b) studied the effects of overnight wear (one night only) of CRT RGP lenses using OCT to measure epithelial and total corneal thickness across a 10 mm horizontal chord diameter. The oxygen *Dk/t* of these lenses was approximately 65×10^{-9}. The results of this study also showed significant central and even greater mid-peripheral corneal swelling immediately following sleep, as would be expected with these lenses. They also found central thinning (5 per cent) and mid-peripheral thickening (2 per cent) of the epithelium. They continued the measurements for 12 hours after waking but found that both epithelial and corneal thickness returned to baseline levels within 3 hours of lens removal, as would be expected.

Swarbrick *et al.*'s (1998) hypothesis is that orthokeratology does not change the structure of the overall cornea, but rather causes a redistribution of the cornea's anterior stromal and epithelial tissue, resulting in a temporary alteration in refractive error. Further work is needed to determine whether the tissue changes are permanent and how these changes will affect the stability of refractive error. The work described in this section demonstrates that the epithelium alters when subjected to mechanical pressure from a lens but not from hypoxia, as described in the previous section.

THE CORNEAL SWELLING RESPONSE

The prime measure of the cornea's physiological status is its thickness. The corneal stroma swells in response to hypoxia as well as disease. Understanding factors influencing this response potentially enables the practitioner to avert long-term adverse physiological effects. The study of this phenomenon has therefore been a cornerstone of contact lens research. Before considering the patterns of corneal swelling in contact lens wearers it is worth considering the techniques available for measuring corneal thickness.

TECHNIQUES FOR MEASUREMENT

Optical pachometry

Optical pachometry is generally regarded as the gold standard for pachometry. When performed by experienced individuals, measurements are reproducible to approximately 4 µm.

Optical pachometry is able to achieve a low degree of error because of the high degree of accuracy with which alignment can be achieved, the ease of calibration against RGP contact lenses with well-defined parameters and the high degree of confidence in the parameters used in the calculations.

Numerous pachometric configurations have been proposed which enable various mathematical solutions relating true corneal thickness to apparent corneal thickness. Brennan *et al.* (1989) published a universal solution, by adopting a configuration in which the angle of incidence and the angle of observation are independent, allowing greater flexibility. When these angles are maximized and the angle of incidence of the observation and illumination beams are set large and approximately equal, a bright image can be observed, both surfaces can be viewed in focus simultaneously and the apparent image size is maximized, increasing the accuracy. Furthermore, epithelial thickness can be measured. The technique and calibration can be laborious, however, and the accuracy of the measurement relies upon a number of assumptions, including the uniformity of corneal refractive index.

Ultrasound pachometry

Ultrasound pachometry has been very popular in refractive surgical practice but has been less commonly used for corneal swelling measurements during contact lens wear. The technique shares an accuracy similar to that of optical pachometry, but it is considerably simpler to use. The procedure requires contact with the eye, which may cause discomfort or apprehension on the part of the subject or make anaesthesia necessary, which may influence the phenomenon under study. Furthermore, the measurement is dependent on knowledge of the acoustic index of the cornea and localization of corneal position can only be approximated. Ultrasound pachometry enables measurements of corneal thickness to be achieved with an accuracy similar to optical pachometry. Recently, high-frequency ultrasound has enabled increasing accuracy of measurement.

Optical coherence tomography

OCT is a relatively new, non-invasive and non-contact optical imaging technique which uses infrared light and an image mapping process to display high-resolution micrometre-scale, cross-sectional imaging of ocular tissue (Huang *et al.*, 1991; Hrynchak and Simpson, 2000). OCT is based on Michelson interferometry. The instrument (Figure 5.6) has a longitudinal or axial resolution of 10–20 μm and

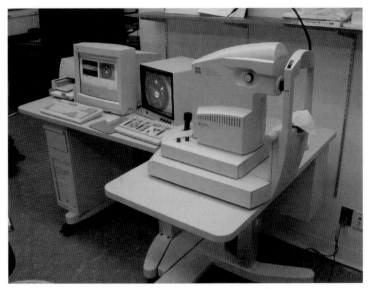

Figure 5.6 Humphrey–Zeiss optical coherence tomographer (reprinted with permission of L. Jones in *Contact Lens Practice*, edited by N. Efron, 2002, published by Butterworth-Heinemann)

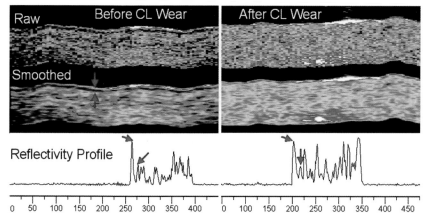

Figure 5.7　OCT images of before and after closed-eye wear of a low-*Dk* hydrogel lens. The lower images are smoothed versions of the upper pixelated images. The plots represent the reflectivity profiles of the images and the red arrow delineated peaks (highest reflectivity) in this example represent epithelial thickness (reprinted with permission of L. Jones in *Contact Lens Practice*, edited by N. Efron, 2002, published by Butterworth-Heinemann)

works on the principle of reflected or back-scattered light (Fujimoto *et al.*, 1995). Haag-Streit has recently announced the launch of a one-dimensional low-coherence optical pachometer with an accuracy of 1 μm. The OCT technique is analogous to ultrasound B-mode imaging, except that light is used rather than sound. Reflections occur at boundaries of the tissue or within the tissue if the refractive indices are different. OCT two-dimensional scans are processed by a computer and the scans are displayed using a false colour representation scale, in which warm colours (red to white) represent high optical reflectivity and cool colours (blue to black) represent minimal reflectivity (Ripandelli *et al.*, 1998). The resultant image (Figure 5.7) is a cross-sectional view of the tissue and is similar in appearance to a histological section (Hrynchak and Simpson, 2000).

OCT was originally designed to measure thickness of the different layers of the retina (Toth *et al.*, 1997; Bowd *et al.*, 2000). Recently, OCT has been used to measure corneal and epithelial thickness in normal living corneas (Izatt *et al.*, 1994; Wang *et al.*, 2002a, 2002b) and it has been demonstrated that the instrument is highly repeatable for both epithelial and total corneal thickness (2.7 and 2.8 μm respectively) measured on two different occasions (Fonn *et al.*, 2000). Maldonado *et al.* (2000) used OCT to measure the thickness of the corneal cap and stromal bed after laser *in situ* keratomileusis (LASIK).

OCT measurements of corneal thickness and swelling are greater than optical pachometry (Wang *et al.*, 2002c), as shown in Figure 5.8. Although the measurements of corneal and epithelial thickness include the pre-corneal tear film (Hitzenberger *et al.*, 1992), this should not affect the thickness measurements significantly as recent pre-corneal tear film thickness measurements are of the order of 3 μm (King-Smith *et al.*, 2000; Wang *et al.*, 2003b). OCT is unable to resolve the tear film because of the axial resolution limit of the instrument. OCT has some

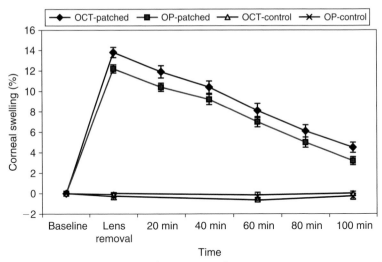

Figure 5.8 Central corneal swelling (mean ± SE %) measured with OCT and optical pachymetry (OP) in 20 unadapted subjects after 3 hours of lens wear and eye closure shows that there was significant corneal swelling induced by 3 hours of lens wear and eye closure with both instruments. The difference between instruments was significant (reprinted with permission from Wang *et al.*, 2002c)

advantages over optical pachometry in that the measurements are objective, quick and can be performed in normal room lighting. Simple fixation devices can be used in order to measure thickness over large chords of the cornea. Another very useful component of OCT is the information that can be derived from the scanned image (Figure 5.7). This particular example shows how back-scattered light has altered, which is indicative of increased light scatter due to corneal oedema.

Confocal and specular microscopy

Confocal microscopy enables *in vivo* examination of thin sections of tissue in a plane perpendicular to the line of observation. Stacks of images can be accumulated and imaged to produce a three-dimensional view of the cornea. These images make it possible to make detailed estimates of the thickness of the various corneal layers. Specular microscopy allows thin sections of tissue to be examined in much the same way as a slit-lamp beam, but with the specular reflection being constantly observed. There is more scattered light than with confocal microscopy. Reproducibility is of the order of the other techniques.

Orbscan

The Orbscan instrument (Bausch & Lomb, Rochester) allows determination of corneal shape and thickness by gathering images of a series of slit beams projected

Table 5.2   Estimates of central corneal thickness by various authors with various techniques

		Optical	Ultrasound	Orbscan	Specular/ Confocal Mic.	OCT/partial coherence interferometry
Mandell and Polse	1969	506				
Koretz et al.	1989		470			
Nissen et al.	1991	531	524			
Reinstein et al.	1994		514			
Patel and Stevenson	1994	553	506			
Li et al.	1997				532	
Yaylali et al.	1997		543	571		
Harper et al.	1996		546			
Bechmann et al.	2001		581			530
Modis et al.	2001		570		542	
Doughty et al.	2002		533			
Wirbelauer et al.	2002		549			541
Wang et al.	2002c	490				523
Rainer et al.	2002		541			519
Wong et al.	2002		555	556		523
Myrowitz et al.	2002			546		
Phillips et al.	2003		554			
Cosar and Sener	2003			538		

on to the cornea. In this way it uses smoothing algorithms to build a three-dimensional model of the cornea, which enables topographical estimation of thickness. This instrument offers the great advantage of being objective, easy to use, providing topographical thickness estimation and allowing estimation of angles kappa and alpha and positioning of the thinnest corneal point. Details of the algorithms used in Orbscan calculations are not publicly available, however, so it is essentially a black box. Calibration of thickness measurement has not been available until recently and details of the accuracy of such calibration are not yet available. Reliability of the Orbscan is of the order of 4 µm at the central site and 9 µm at 3 mm from the corneal centre.

Comparison of techniques

The principal techniques for assessing corneal thickness all provide approximately the same degree of accuracy. Consistent differences have been found between the techniques, however. Table 5.2 shows the results of various studies which have measured the central corneal thickness of subjects. The average of all of these results places the mean central corneal thickness in the population at slightly over 530 µm. In a meta-analysis of corneal thickness measures, Doughty and Zaman (2000) found a mean corneal thickness of 534 µm, with optical pachometry producing slightly lower values than ultrasound values, as is evident from Table 5.2.

PATTERNS OF CORNEAL SWELLING

Typically, corneal oedema is expressed as a percentage swelling from baseline corneal thickness, which is usually judged to be the thickness of the cornea prior to sleep. Subjects show a range of corneal thickness values (typically standard deviation of population estimates of corneal thickness are between 30 and 40 μm) and also individual swelling responses. Variation in swelling between subjects is probably determined by a complex combination of anatomical and functional factors, including endothelial cellular density. Furthermore, the cornea does not show uniform swelling; the greatest degree of swelling occurs centrally.

Overnight response

Corneal thickness exhibits considerable diurnal variation, increasing during sleep and returning to its original level during the day. Various estimates of the amount of overnight corneal swelling in the absence of contact lens wear have been made (see Table 5.3). It was originally believed that overnight swelling in unadapted wearers was of the order of 4 per cent. The figures provided in Table 5.3, however, reveal that many studies have found lower values. Probably the most significant factor influencing the mean values for overnight swelling estimates is the level of adaptation to contact lens wear. Cox *et al.* (1991) found that the cornea of a subject adapted to DW of traditional hydrogels swells by some 2 per cent less than observed in an unadapted wearer, with adapted extended wearers swelling less, by a further 1 per cent.

Table 5.3   Overnight central corneal swelling in the absence of contact lens wear by various authors

Author	Year	Estimate (%)
Mertz	1980	4.3
Koers	1982	1.8
Kiely *et al.*	1982	2.1
Holden *et al.*	1983	3.0
La Hood *et al.*	1988	3.2
Cox *et al.*	1991	0.7[a]
Cox *et al.*	1991	2.0[a]
Cox *et al.*	1991	3.8[a]
Harper *et al.*	1996	5.5
Fonn *et al.*	1997	1.8
Fonn *et al.*	1999	2.3 and 1.4[b]
du Toit *et al.*	2003	2.9

[a]Cox's data showed 0.7%, 2.0% and 3.8% overnight swelling in EW- and DW-adapted wearers and non-lens wearers respectively.
[b]Fonn *et al.*'s (1999) data showed differences in response according to the lens type worn in the contralateral eye.

Response to contact lenses

As previously noted, the principal factor causing corneal swelling during overnight lens wear is hypoxia. Temperature, tear osmolarity and tear pH may also vary under the closed eye but these effects contribute only a portion of the overall oedema effect. The presence of a contact lens between the palpebral conjunctiva and the cornea during closed-eye contact lens wear can be a substantial barrier to oxygen flow into the cornea.

Holden *et al.* (1983) plotted the corneal swelling response over a period of wear of low-*Dk/t* contact lenses. Mean overnight corneal swelling ranged from 9.7 to 15.1 per cent in a manner dependent on the average *Dk/t* of the contact lenses worn. The corneas returned in part to their original thickness during the course of the day, but did not necessarily return to baseline, demonstrating a maximum capacity to deswell that was consistent between lenses despite *Dk/t* and averaging 8.2 per cent. From this knowledge, Holden and Mertz (1984) estimated that the minimum *Dk/t* required to avoid daytime oedema was 34×10^{-9} (cm/s)(mlO$_2$/ml·mmHg).

CONUNDRUMS

Sympathetic response

Corneal thickness can be affected by eye closure and the oxygen transmissibility of the contact lens being worn. One of the most common tests to determine the effect of the lens is to measure corneal swelling and an accepted paradigm is to have the individual wear one lens and to leave the other eye free as a control (Holden *et al.*, 1983; Holden and Mertz, 1984; La Hood *et al.*, 1988; Cox *et al.*, 1991; Sakamoto *et al.*, 1991). This paradigm, which is designed to eliminate inter-subject variability, was used by Fonn *et al.* (1999) to compare the swelling response of a high-*Dk* silicone hydrogel lens and low-*Dk* hydrogel lens when worn overnight. The two lenses were worn on alternate nights and the non-lens-wearing eye was used as the control. Corneal swelling increased predictably in the lens-wearing eye but, surprisingly, swelling also increased in the lens-free eye, as shown in Table 5.4. It would be common practice to pool the results of the non-wearing eyes (the controls of the low-*Dk* lens-wearing eyes and the controls of the high-*Dk* lens-wearing eyes), but that could not be done in this case because they were statistically different.

Table 5.4   Overnight corneal swelling (%)

	High–yoked response		Low–yoked response	
	Acuvue	Control	Lotrafilcon	Control
Mean	8.7	2.3	2.7	1.4
SD	2.8	1.3	1.9	0.9

It appears that the amount of swelling in the control eye is yoked with the swelling induced by the lens worn in the test eye; low-Dk lenses produced more swelling in the lens-wearing eye and the control eye showed a relatively higher swelling response, while high-Dk lenses produced significantly less swelling in the lens-wearing eye and the control eye swelled less. This appears to be a sympathetic effect. Exactly the same results were documented by Guzey *et al.* (2002) in rabbits.

This hypothesis is supported by the results of a study (Drubaix *et al.*, 1997) in which excimer laser photoablation induced an increase in the hyaluronan content of treated and untreated contralateral rabbit corneas. The authors also used an untreated second control and found a significant increase of hyaluronan in the contralateral control compared to the untreated control. Another interesting finding of the Drubaix *et al.* study was stromal swelling of the control corneas, which they attributed to the increased content of hyaluronan. There are many other examples of contralateral effects after surgery or injury (Hara and Hara, 1987; Ménasche *et al.*, 1988; You *et al.*, 1993; Dunham *et al.*, 1994; Franck *et al.*, 1994; Rask and Jensen, 1995; Ribari and Sziklai, 1995). Ladage *et al.* (2003) studied the effects of eyelid closure with high- and low-Dk contact lenses on rabbit corneal epithelial proliferation and found that the cell proliferation rate of the control cornea was significantly affected by a lens in the contralateral eye.

According to Drubaix *et al.* (1997), the process of ablation involves transecting corneal nerves and keratocytes, which may play a role in signalling hyaluronan production, and it is possible that swelling in the contralateral eye is induced by the production of hyaluronan. To the best of our knowledge this is a new concept in the aetiology of corneal swelling as a response to contact lens wear.

Drubaix has proposed that researchers should not use the contralateral cornea as a control when conducting these types of studies because of the sympathetic response. It would be extremely useful to copy Drubaix's experimental design (using additional untreated control subjects and contralateral controls) in the context of corneal swelling due to contact lens wear.

Diurnal variation of corneal thickness and the 'overshoot' phenomenon of corneal deswelling

The literature contains a number of reports on diurnal variation of corneal thickness (Kiely *et al.*, 1982; Holden *et al.*, 1983; Sakamoto *et al.*, 1991; Harper *et al.*, 1996). More recently, Feng *et al.* (2001) documented diurnal variation of epithelial and total corneal thickness using OCT, and du Toit *et al.* (2003) measured diurnal variation of corneal thickness (Figure 5.9) and sensitivity over a 24-hour cycle using optical pachometry and a prototype pneumatic aesthesiometer. Despite differences in instrumentation, time course and measurements taken at varying times of the day, all the studies showed that the cornea was thickest immediately after eye opening in the morning and decreased through the day and in some cases into the evening. Unfortunately, inconsistencies in the time course of measurements resulted in discrepancies as to when the cornea was thinnest. It is important to establish the point at which the cornea is thinnest because this is the baseline value that is used to calculate overnight swelling.

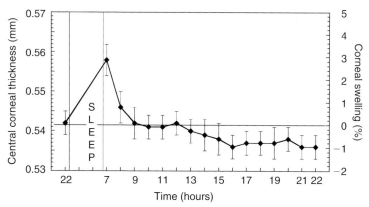

Figure 5.9   Mean measurements of central corneal thickness from 22:00 prior to 8 hours of sleep, the following day on eye opening, and at hour intervals between 7:00 and 22:00 (reprinted with permission from du Toit *et al.*, 2003)

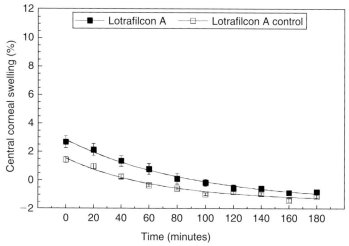

Figure 5.10   The overnight corneal swelling response and deswelling functions induced by overnight wear of lotrafilcon A lenses in one eye and the contralateral non-wearing controls. Note that the corneas continue to thin beyond baseline (zero on the *y*-axis) (reprinted with permission from Fonn *et al.*, 1999)

du Toit *et al.* (2003) measured an overnight corneal swelling response of 2.9 per cent, which is within the range of values recorded in Table 5.3, and the continued hourly measurements after eye opening showed a steady decrease until minimum thickness was recorded approximately 9 hours after eye opening, as shown in Figure 5.9. However, the recovery time to baseline (zero on the ordinate scale) occurred approximately 2 hours after eye opening and thinning continued, which infers that the previous day's baseline thickness was overestimated.

Thinning of the cornea beyond baseline, termed 'overshoot', has been reported (Holden *et al.*, 1983; O'Neal and Polse, 1985; Sakamoto *et al.*, 1991) but is still a largely unexplained aspect of the dynamics of corneal hydration. Figure 5.10 is a typical example. Additionally, Figures 5.2 and 5.10 illustrate the thinning of the control eye while the treated eye deswells. In light of the earlier description of sympathetic effect, 'overshoot' of the control eye may be that or simply diurnal variation.

O'Neal and Polse (1985) ascribed 'overshoot' to the disparity between the rate of fluid loss due to tear film evaporation and the imbibition of fluid through the endothelium. Odenthal *et al.* (1999) suggested that 'overshoot' results when the pump rate of the endothelium is actively or passively regulated as opposed to dissipation of residual swelling after sleep, or diurnal variation. Hypoxic stress may activate a functional reserve in ion pump capacity and 'overshoot' may be caused by a time lag in the deswelling process. In addition to 'overshoot', environmental factors may indirectly influence corneal thickness by exacerbating the evaporation of the pre-corneal tear film. Liu and Pflugfelder (1999) found a reduction in corneal thickness with dry eye. Finally du Toit *et al.* (2003) also found the same 'overshoot' effect of corneal sensitivity and a high correlation between corneal sensitivity and thickness.

How does the oedema response relate to contact lens complications?

Another important corollary to the finding of high intersubject variability in corneal swelling is the question of how this variability impacts long-term wear. One study has shown that subjects prone to higher amounts of oedema are more likely to discontinue lens wear and experience adverse ocular effects (Solomon, 1996). Another study found no effect in that subjects experiencing infiltrative keratitis show the same degree of swelling as subjects without complications (Stapleton *et al.*, 1998). It can also be argued that the cornea adapted to EW, which shows the least amount of swelling, has a reduced metabolic rate and thus has less healing capacity and lower reserves for defences against potential threats. Thus, the patient with a cornea that shows a high degree of swelling may be intolerant to contact lens wear, but at the same time more resilient to threats against corneal health. Further research is needed to resolve this question.

CRITICAL OXYGEN LEVELS

CORNEAL SWELLING

In 1984 Holden and Mertz conducted a landmark study in which they used various criteria to study the oxygen levels required to avoid corneal swelling. The authors investigated overnight wear of a range of lenses made from traditional hydrogel materials and a silicone elastomer lens by 10 neophyte subjects. They determined that the lens Dk/t required to prevent overnight corneal swelling of greater than 4 per cent was 87×10^{-9} (cm/s)(mlO$_2$/ml·mmHg). Although this figure has stood the test of time, the introduction of lenses that meet this criterion, such as silicone hydrogels, has refocused attention on the accuracy of this value. As such, it is appropriate to revisit the methodology used in the Holden–Mertz experiment; the following points are noteworthy. The range of lenses was restricted with only one test lens having a Dk/t of greater than 40×10^{-9} (cm/s)(mlO$_2$/ml·mmHg), making interpretation outside this range somewhat speculative. The subject sample size was relatively low given the variability between individuals in overnight corneal swelling. The subjects were unadapted wearers, which may not be appropriate population for considering the effects on experienced contact lens wearers. Finally, standards for Dk/t measurement had not been written, which means that the Dk/t estimates of lenses used in that study may be inaccurate. These criticisms should not detract from the importance of the Holden–Mertz study or from the importance that this study had in setting goals for the industry to achieve.

To overcome some of the methodological problems, Brennan and Coles (2003, unpublished data) have reanalysed data from a series of overnight studies to reassess the Holden–Mertz criteria, using lenses with a broader range of Dk/t values (Figure 5.11). Twenty-five subjects, previously adapted to DW of low-Dk/t soft lenses, are included in the group, although not every subject wore every lens type. Four lenses of -3.00 D power were worn. These lenses and the number of subjects wearing each lens were as follows:

■ Acuvue (Johnson & Johnson, Jacksonville, FL), $n = 25$
■ PureVision (Bausch & Lomb, Rochester, NY), $n = 24$

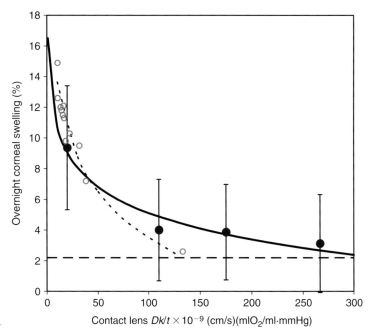

Figure 5.11 Overnight corneal swelling versus contact lens Dk/t. The open red circles are data from Holden and Mertz (1984), and the dotted curve is the best-fit curve. The blue circles are the mean ($\pm$SD) from the data of Brennan and Coles (2003, unpublished) and the solid line is the fitted logarithmic curve to this data. The dashed line represents overnight swelling in the absence of lens wear

- Focus Night & Day (CIBA Vision, Atlanta, GA), $n = 16$
- Silflex (Bausch & Lomb, Rochester, NY), $n = 20$.

Individual variation was taken into account to compensate for the different sample sizes used for each lens; where the sample group for a lens consisted of higher or lower 'swellers', numerical compensation was made for the result for that lens. Corneal thickness measurements were made with the Orbscan (except for the 'no lens wear' situation, in which optical pachometry data were used, $n = 15$). Group mean overnight swelling in the absence of contact lens wear was 2.2 per cent. This lower value is perhaps not surprising given other estimates of overnight swelling with adapted daily wearers (Table 5.2). Figure 5.11 shows the limitations in the Dk/t range of the Holden–Mertz data. It also shows that the two sets of data are not dissimilar. This repeat investigation suggests that the critical Dk/t to avoid overnight corneal oedema of more than that normally encountered without contact lens wear is of the order of 300×10^{-9} (cm/s)(mlO$_2$/ml·mmHg).

OXYGEN CONSUMPTION

During the first 25 years of hydrogel lens wear it was appropriate to use Dk/t as a measure of lens oxygenation, as there was a linear relation between many measures of the corneal response and the Dk/t value. Despite the great pioneering work and advocacy of Fatt, it sadly took the industry nearly this entire time to embrace the concept of Dk/t. In 1996, Professor Fatt realized that the Dk/t concept had run its course when he commented that the Dk/t term 'used by itself as a measure of lens performance has been a disappointment'. He pointed out that the Dk/t term by itself does not allow calculation of the oxygen flux into the cornea, that it gives no indication of how closely oxygen flux into the cornea under a lens matches that when no lens is in place, and that it does not give an indication of the proportionate change in oxygen flux between lenses of different Dk/t values. The Dk/t figure is a benchtop measurement with a modest link to on-eye performance. As usual, Professor Fatt was ahead of the field in recognizing an important paradigm shift. It will be interesting to see whether the industry takes another 20 years to appreciate the significance of these statements and abandon the Dk/t measure as the index for corneal oxygenation.

The more important parameters to consider are corneal oxygen flux and consumption. The flux of oxygen provides an exact indication of the amount of oxygen entering the cornea per unit time and the oxygen consumption provides a direct indication of metabolic activity. In the late 1960s and early 1970s, Fatt and coworkers modelled the steady-state (time-independent) distribution of oxygen in the cornea (Fatt, 1968a, 1968b; Fatt and St Helen, 1971; Fatt et al., 1974). The parameters necessary to make these calculations include the permeability, thickness and consumption rates of the various corneal layers and knowledge of the boundary conditions. A differential equation for the steady-state oxygen diffusion and consumption is written for each layer of the cornea. Since the flux values and partial pressure values at the interfaces of adjoining layers must be equal,

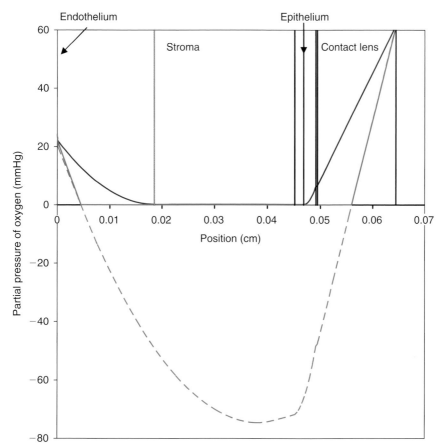

Figure 5.12   Predicted steady-state corneal oxygen tension distribution for closed-eye wear of an Acuvue lens ($Dk/t = 18$) according to the model of Harvitt and Bonanno (1999) in red and Brennan (2003, unpublished data) in blue (thicknesses of tear layer, epithelium and stroma are 3, 40 and 450 μm, respectively). The dashed red line is the predicted oxygen tension when oxygen consumption is not set to zero and the solid red line sets the negative values to zero

a set of simultaneous equations can be constructed. The solution provides details of the oxygen tension across the cornea, which can also be used to assess all other parameters concerned in corneal oxygenation. This format was originally used by Fatt and coworkers to investigate the oxygen tension distribution underneath contact lenses. Fatt and Ruben (1993) used a more simplified model in which the cornea was considered as a single layer.

More recently Harvitt and Bonanno (1999) have incorporated a correction for altered corneal oxygen consumption with varying degrees of acidosis of the cornea into the oxygen profile model and concluded that Dk/t values of 84 and 125×10^{-9} (cm/s)(mlO$_2$/ml·mmHg) were required to avoid epithelial and stromal anoxia respectively. These results should be interpreted with caution, however. Harvitt and Bonanno's model set negative modelled values to zero to account for the clearly impossible scenario of a negative oxygen tension. Figure 5.12 plots

Table 5.5   Estimates of post-lens tear film thickness

Author	Year	Estimate (μm)
Lin et al.	1999	11–12
Nichols and King–Smith	2003	2.3
Wang et al.	2003b	4.6

Table 5.6   Epithelial thickness estimates from various studies

Author	Year	Estimate (μm)
Holden et al.	1985	61
Ladage et al.	2003	49
Wang et al.	2002a	58
Cavanagh et al.	2002	50
Perez et al.	2003	48
Wang et al.	2003a	62

their uncorrected and corrected curves for closed-eye wear of an Acuvue lens of Dk/t equal to 18×10^{-9} (cm/s)(mlO$_2$/ml·mmHg). Their corrected curve shows that the oxygen tension falls to zero within the contact lens and that the oxygen tension and oxygen flux at the corneal surface are zero, which is not possible as neither the contact lens nor the tears consume oxygen. They have also used post-lens tear layer thickness value of 45 μm, which is probably more representative of what might be expected with an RGP lens than a soft lens, and inspection of the graphs in their paper shows values of approximately 40 μm and 455 μm for the epithelial and stromal thicknesses respectively, giving a total corneal thickness of just over 490 μm. Tables 5.2, 5.5 and 5.6 present more recent literature estimates of the values of the thicknesses of various layers used in the model. The average estimate of total corneal thickness from Table 5.2 is just over 530 μm (compared to about 490 μm in the Harvitt–Bonanno paper), Table 5.5 suggests that tear layer thickness is probably around 3 μm but certainly no greater than 12 μm for a soft lens and Table 5.6 provides data to show that epithelial thickness is probably in excess of 50 μm. These differences in thickness can make profound differences to the modelled oxygen tension profiles.

To illustrate the degree to which errors in estimating layer thickness will influence the critical Dk/t values, a simple resistors-in-series equation may be used for the estimate required to avoid stromal oedema (Fatt and Chaston, 1982). A tear layer with Dk of 75×10^{-11} (cm^2/s)(mlO$_2$/ml·mmHg) and thickness of 45 μm provides close to the same resistance to oxygen flow as a lens with Dk/t of 125×10^{-9} (cm/s)(mlO$_2$/ml·mmHg). In combination, they will provide the same resistance as a tear layer thickness of 3 μm plus a lens of Dk/t of 80×10^{-9} (cm/s)(mlO$_2$/ml·mmHg). Might this be a more appropriate estimate of the critical Dk/t to avoid stromal hypoxia?

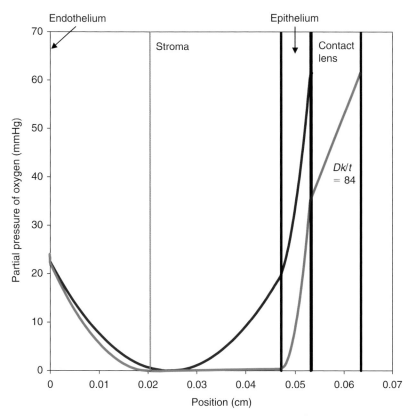

Figure 5.13   Predicted steady-state corneal oxygen tension distribution during eye closure for a cornea with epithelial and total thickness of 60 µm and approximately 530 µm. Without a contact lens, the value falls to zero in the stroma (blue curve). A contact lens with Dk/t of 84 × 10^{-9} (cm/s)(mlO$_2$/ml·mmHg) is required to avoid epithelial anoxia (red line). Correction for acidosis is included

Brennan (2003, unpublished data) has expanded on the Harvitt–Bonanno model, correcting for spurious consumption when the oxygen tension falls to zero at any position within the cornea. This requires an eight-layer model but uses the same basic paradigm. Figure 5.12 plots the curve for the Acuvue lens, as described above, according to Brennan's model. In line with expectations, this improvement gives positive values for both the anterior oxygen tension and the anterior oxygen flux. Correcting for the thickness of the various corneal layers, as listed above, produces altered estimates of the corneal oxygen profiles. For example, the introduction of any contact lens into the model for a corneal thickness of 530 µm with an epithelial layer of 60 m produces anoxia in the stroma (Figure 5.13).

Oxygen profile models potentially provide a comprehensive picture of corneal oxygenation, supplying the values of key indicators of corneal physiology, such as total corneal oxygen consumption, anterior corneal oxygen flux and anterior corneal oxygen tension for lenses of different oxygen transmissibilities. Inconsistencies

Table 5.7   Anterior corneal oxygen pO_2 and flux under closed-eye conditions for a range of lenses from the model of Brennan (2001); for comparison, anterior corneal oxygen fluxes are calculated from the paper by Harvitt and Bonanno (1999), without correction for acidosis

Dk/t (barrer/cm)	Anterior corneal pO_2 (mmHg)	Corneal oxygen flux ($\mu l/cm^2$ per h)	
		Brennan (2001)	Harvitt–Bonanno (1999)
10	6	1.9	[a]
20	12	3.4	[a]
30	17	4.3	[a]
50	26	5.1	5.4
75	34	5.5	5.6
100	39	5.7	5.7
150	44	5.8	5.8
200	51	5.9	5.8

[a] Oxygen flux is not calculable for the reasons demonstrated in Figure 5.12; see text for details

between model-derived values and empirically derived physiological data remain to be addressed, however. A number of sources may be responsible for these discrepancies. Within the profile models, errors and variation between individuals in estimates of closed-eyelid oxygen tension, anterior chamber oxygen tension, consumption by the individual corneal layers, thickness of individual corneal layers and total cornea and oxygen transmissibility of the various layers may be responsible. Further research into this area is important, as continuous wear (CW) becomes a standard part of contact lens practice. High-power negative and positive-power high-Dk/t lenses may fall short of meeting corneal demands.

Finally, to illustrate the importance of using oxygen flux as the measure of corneal oxygenation during contact lens wear, Table 5.7 presents estimates of oxygen flux and oxygen tension provided by Brennan's (2001) model, and also for comparison calculated values of anterior corneal oxygen flux derived from the model developed by Harvitt and Bonanno (1999). As Dk/t increases from 50 to 100 to 200×10^{-9} (cm/s)(mlO$_2$/ml·mmHg), anterior corneal oxygen tension is calculated to rise from 26 to 39 to 51 mmHg. The movement of oxygen into the cornea does not increase so dramatically, however, rising by less than 10 per cent and 6 per cent with these changes. It should be noted that the influence of acidosis is not included in the Harvitt–Bonanno estimations. Despite the potential importance of this influence, the Harvitt–Bonanno model was produced from lenses with Dk/t less than 60×10^{-9} (cm/s)(mlO$_2$/ml·mmHg), and is linked to Dk/t rather than anterior oxygen tension. These aspects of the methodology can provide spurious results.

MICROCYSTS

In the same way that corneal hypoxia has become the classic index of the short-term corneal physiological response, microcyst count is the standard for assessing medium-term corneal hypoxia. The presentation, basis and characterization of microcysts have been described elsewhere (Sweeney *et al.*, 2000). Holden *et al.* (1987a) have suggested that the degree of microcyst development during EW is related to the oedema response on a lens-by-lens basis, but Jaworski *et al.* (2001) have found that within a single lens type the individual's corneal swelling response is not necessarily predictive of the microcystic count. In the absence of lens wear, patients rarely show more than 10 microcysts per cornea. The data from Holden *et al.* (1987a) can be used to calculate that a Dk/t of approximately 50×10^{-9} $(cm/s)(mlO_2/ml \cdot mmHg)$ is required during soft lens wear to prevent the development of an average of 10 microcysts or more per cornea.

LIMBAL INJECTION

Papas (1998) has outlined the nature of the relationship between limbal injection and contact lens-related hypoxia. The association is strong, with contact lens peripheral Dk/t accounting for 81 per cent of the variance in limbal redness in a series of short-term wearing studies. The mean peripheral Dk/t required to avoid a change in limbal redness was determined to be 125×10^{-9} $(cm/s)(mlO_2/ml \cdot mmHg)$, although the highest peripheral Dk/t among the lenses used was 71 and the 95 per cent confidence interval stretches from 56 to 274. Nonetheless, this result has important consequences for negative-power lenses. Typically, lens Dk/t values are quoted for central lens thickness. The periphery of lenses for correcting myopic prescriptions may be considerably thicker than these values, resulting in a high point-to-point loss of Dk/t (in the article by Papas, Dk/t in the periphery was reduced by as much as 80 per cent in one lens). This result is also significant because, as noted above, the stem cells which are the source of new corneal epithelial cells are believed to exist only at the limbus. Hypoxic damage to stem cells may have serious long-term consequences for corneal health.

SUMMARY OF DATA OF CRITICAL OXYGEN LEVELS

It is apparent that there are widely varying estimates of the critical oxygen tension when oxygen transmissibility is used as the measure. When the critical levels are considered on the basis of oxygen flux with reference to Table 5.7, it would appear that provided the total volume of oxygen reaching the cornea per unit time during eye closure does not decrease by more than about 10 per cent, corneal function will remain normal. Decreases in flux by more than this amount will lead to visible alterations in corneal appearance and function, although it remains to be determined to what degree these changes are adaptations versus detrimental changes in function. Given that currently available silicone hydrogel lenses do not seem to decrease oxygen flux by more than 10 per cent in the closed eye, it seems reasonable that corneal health should be maintained during CW of such lenses. The following discussion will focus on the clinical reality of this expectation.

HOW DO SILICONE HYDROGEL LENSES MEASURE UP?

In this section we will discuss the physiological changes that occur during contact lens wear, excluding adverse changes such as microbial keratitis, contact lens-induced acute red eye, contact lens-induced peripheral ulcers and superior epithelial arcuate lesions. Contact lens wear, and in particular EW, produces an extensive list of structural and functional changes in the anterior eye. Most of these findings are considered physiological rather than pathological, since they are non-inflammatory, do not threaten vision and have minimal or unknown significance for eye health. These physiological effects have minimal impact on rate of discontinuation from lens wear. Nonetheless, the potential relationship between corneal hypoxic compromise and microbial keratitis suggests that monitoring the physiological changes may be clinically beneficial.

Physiological changes which have been noted during contact lens wear include the following: reduced corneal sensitivity, limbal injection, eye redness, altered corneal shape, reduced epithelial oxygen consumption, increased epithelial cell size, decreased epithelial cell sloughing rate, altered epithelial permeability, increased epithelial fragility, epithelial thinning, microcyst development, corneal staining, stromal thinning, vascularization, endothelial polymegethism and altered endothelial cell shape. Corneal exhaustion, a syndrome characterized by lens intolerance and ongoing changes in corneal refraction and astigmatism, may be considered a physiological imbalance. Animal studies have also shown changes in epithelial mitoses, epithelial adhesion, epithelial cellular junctional integrity, epithelial healing rate and cellular reserves of glycogen. Hypoxia is the proven cause of many of these changes and the prime candidate in circumstances where the mechanism has not been conclusively identified. Here we will discuss the most important of these changes and consider the impact that high-Dk/t silicone hydrogel contact lenses have from an ocular physiological standpoint.

The Gothenburg study by Holden and coworkers (Holden *et al.*, 1985, 1987b) is considered to be an outstanding investigation of long-term physiological changes with contact lens wear. The authors investigated the effects of five years of unilateral EW in a sample of 27 patients using the contralateral eyes as a control. Physiological markers investigated included epithelial oxygen uptake, epithelial thickness, epithelial microcysts, acute stromal oedema, chronic stromal thinning, endothelial polymegethism and limbal and bulbar conjunctival hyperaemia. Compared to the control eyes, the cornea of the lens-wearing eyes showed a 15 per cent reduction in oxygen consumption, a 6 per cent reduction in epithelial thickness, a 2.3 per cent reduction in stromal thickness and a 22 per cent increase in endothelial polymegethism. Epithelial metabolism recovered one month after wear, but the stromal and endothelial changes persisted for over six months. Patients with thinner corneas and higher endothelial cell density and lower polymegethism in the contralateral, non-lens-wearing eyes showed fewer effects from contact lens wear. Factors identified in minimizing the physiological effects were more frequent lens removal, greater mobility of the lens on the eye, shorter duration between lens replacements and a greater Dk/t of the lens being worn. These features

Table 5.8 Estimates of overnight corneal swelling judged by the appearance of striae at a given time after awakening (data are calculated from equations of La Hood and Grant, 1990, and Polse *et al.*, 1991, using a deswelling coefficient [*D*-value] of 0.115 (l/min) and assuming independence of swelling extent and deswelling rate)

Time after awakening (min)	1 stria	5 striae	10 striae
0	4.2	7.6	11.6
5	4.6	8.0	12.2
30	6.0	10.6	16.4
60	8.4	15.0	23.0
90	11.8	21.0	
120	16.8		

dominated developments in the contact lens industry in the following years. Silicone hydrogels address many of these problems.

CORNEAL OEDEMA AND VISIBLE STRIAE

When worn during eye closure, the original hydrogel lenses induced corneal oedema, observable clinically on awakening as striae and folds. The effects persisted for some time following eye opening and, in some cases, throughout the day. Under some circumstances, visual disturbance in the form of haze and blur was noted. Although the acute effects on corneal oedema resolve rapidly, wearing a traditional hydrogel contact lens in EW produced a recurring pattern of oedema during the night followed by partial resolution during the day (Holden *et al.*, 1983). Chronic exposure to this potentially hostile environment is considered to be unfavourable for long-term corneal health. Clinical assessment of overnight corneal oedema can be made by counting the number of striae and folds in the cornea at a known period after eye opening (Table 5.8).

The introduction of silicone hydrogel lenses has resulted in a dramatic decrease in the appearance of clinical signs of corneal oedema. In a 12-month global study of silicone hydrogel lens wear, there was a significant difference in the percentage of patients showing signs of clinical oedema between low-Dk/t and high-Dk/t lenses (Brennan *et al.*, 2002). The clinical findings are in accord with the data presented above and published studies of overnight swelling (Fonn *et al.*, 1999).

MICROCYSTS

As discussed above, the microcyst response is the most distinctive medium-term clinical indicator of corneal hypoxia. A transitory increase, lasting one to three months, in microcyst count may occur after discontinuation of EW of low-Dk/t lenses, and this effect should be ignored in the early stages of high-Dk/t lens wear

(Holden and Sweeney, 1991). A count of 10 microcysts per eye is an appropriate threshold to differentiate between an acceptable and non-acceptable corneal oxygen environment. High-Dk/t lenses do not produce an appreciable microcyst response and produce a significantly lower number of microcysts over a period of wear than low-Dk/t lenses (Keay *et al.*, 2001; Brennan *et al.*, 2002).

VASCULAR RESPONSE

Contact lens wear induces limbal redness and bulbar conjunctival hyperaemia and may be associated with corneal vascularization. Papas *et al.* (1997) reported results from a short-term clinical study which showed that high-Dk/t soft lenses do not produce significant levels of limbal injection, where low-Dk/t lenses do. The same differentiation was observed by du Toit *et al.* (2001). Longer-term studies have borne this out. Dumbleton *et al.* (2001) have assessed limbal hyperaemia and vascularization during nine months' EW of high- and low-Dk/t lenses and found a lower vascular response on both indices with the high-Dk/t lenses. The high-Dk/t wearers showed no change over the time period. In a 12-month multi-site CW study, both limbal injection and bulbar conjunctival hyperaemia were lower in high-Dk/t wearers than a standard, mid-water, thin hydrogel lens (Brennan *et al.*, 2002). In the only three-year study of CW of high-Dk/t lenses to date, limbal injection was reduced compared to baseline levels with high-Dk/t lenses. The likely scenario for the finding is a significant level of chronic limbal redness associated with DW of low-Dk/t hydrogels prior to entering the study which subsided with wear of the higher-Dk/t lenses (Coles *et al.*, 2001).

REFRACTIVE CHANGES

Soon after the development of soft contact lenses, when lenses were thick and manufactured from low-water-content hydroxyethyl methacrylate (HEMA) materials, resulting in very low oxygen transmissibility, and patients were wearing their lenses predominantly on a DW basis, investigators were reporting a 'myopic shift' (increase) (Grosvenor, 1975; Harris *et al.*, 1975; Hill, 1975; Stone, 1976; Barnett and Rengstorff, 1977). Some of these studies also reported a concurrent steepening of corneal curvature. Increased myopia has also been reported with EW of low-Dk hydrogel lenses (Miller *et al.*, 1980; Binder, 1983).

A number of authors (Dumbleton *et al.*, 1999; Pritchard and Fonn, 1999; Jalbert *et al.*, 2001; Fonn *et al.*, 2002) have documented a significant increase in myopia with low-Dk lenses compared to no increase in myopia with high-Dk silicone hydrogel lenses from prospective EW/CW clinical trials. These studies had subjects wearing low-Dk and high-Dk lenses in contralateral eyes in the same subjects and compared the lenses in different groups of subjects. The low-Dk hydrogel lenses were worn for six nights and the high-Dk silicone hydrogel lenses were worn for up 29 nights continuously. These reports reflect the results of up to six months of wear. These studies found that eyes wearing low-Dk lenses became

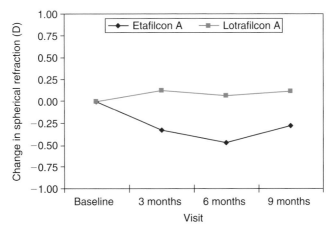

Figure 5.14 Mean change in refractive error over time for high-*Dk* (lotrafilcon A, *n* = 39) and low-*Dk* (etafilcon A, *n* = 23) wearers (reprinted with permission from Dumbleton *et al.*, 1999).

more myopic by as much as 0.50 D compared to the eyes wearing high-*Dk* lenses, which showed little or no increase in refractive error. Figure 5.14 is an example of the comparative change. The significance of this myopic shift becomes even clearer when compared to the results of a study performed by Nizam *et al.* (1996), which found that the refractive error of adult myopic eyes without contact lens wear increased by only 0.30 D over 11 years compared to eyes wearing low-*Dk* lenses on a DW basis, which increased by 1.12 D over the same time period.

Dumbleton *et al.*'s (1999) nine-month study was extended to investigate the effect of switching a subset of the subjects who became more myopic from low- to high-*Dk* lenses. This was done after the subjects had reverted to DW of their low-*Dk* lenses and in that period their refractive error remained stable, as shown in Figure 5.15. After three months of wearing the high-*Dk* silicone hydrogels on a CW basis (29 nights), however, their myopia decreased by 0.37 D (returned to baseline).

The increase in myopia has been attributed to the effects of chronic hypoxia on the cornea from the low-*Dk* lenses, and the decrease that occurred when subjects switched to silicone hydrogels was due to the relief of the hypoxic load from the cornea just as effectively as if lens wear had been terminated. The assumption is that the cornea has altered in some way. Another logical cause is that lens wear produces a change in corneal curvature where steepening would result in increased myopia but the association between refractive error and corneal curvature has been inconsistent. Silicone hydrogels are stiffer lenses than hydrogels and it is possible that these lenses cause corneas to flatten and, therefore, prevent eyes from becoming more myopic. To date, however, no such relationship has been established so it would appear that lens-specific characteristics, such as design or modulus of elasticity, are not risk factors.

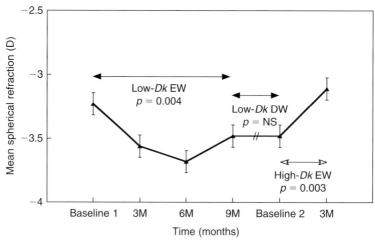

Figure 5.15   Change in refractive error over time. Subset of 13 subjects crossed-over from low-*Dk* (etafilcon A) to high-*Dk* (lotrafilcon A) lenses (reprinted with permission from Dumbleton *et al.*, 1999)

ADVERSE EVENTS

Despite the profound influence of short- and long-term hypoxia on the appearance and function of the cornea, the role of hypoxia in the induction of adverse events with contact lens wear remains hypothetical. High-Dk/t lenses produce similar rates of contact lens-induced acute red eye, contact lens-induced peripheral ulcers and superior arcuate epithelial lesions to conventional hydrogel lens wear (Dumbleton *et al.*, 2000). This suggests that these events are not related to hypoxia. However, the most significant adverse event, microbial keratitis, does appear to be reduced by wear of high-Dk/t silicone hydrogel soft lenses. Further evidence from epidemiological studies is required to confirm this hypothesis.

CONCLUSIONS

This chapter has demonstrated some advances in our understanding of ocular and corneal function and appearance through the development of technology. We have also described how high-*Dk* silicone hydrogel lenses have minimized the physiological response compared to low-*Dk* lenses. These technological developments have given rise to questions such as the re-examination of the critical oxygen requirements for both short- and long-term corneal health, the role of the epithelium in contact lens wear and the value of oxygen transmissibility.

REFERENCES

Alharbi, A. and Swarbrick, H. A. (2003) The effects of overnight orthokeratology lens wear on corneal thickness. *Invest. Ophthalmol. Vis. Sci.*, **44**, 2518–2523

Barnett, W. A. and Rengstorff, R. H. (1977) Adaptation to hydrogel contact lenses: variations in myopia and corneal curvature measurements. *J. Am. Optom. Assoc.*, **48**, 363–366

Bechmann, M., Thiel, M. J., Neubauer, A. S. *et al.* (2001) Central corneal thickness measurement with a retinal optical coherence tomography device versus standard ultrasonic pachymetry. *Cornea*, **20**, 50–54

Bergmanson, J. and Chu, L. (1982) Corneal response to rigid contact lens wear. *Br. J. Ophthalmol.*, **66**, 667–675

Bergmanson, J., Ruben, C. and Chu, L. (1985) Epithelial morphological response to soft hydrogel contact lenses. *Br. J. Ophthalmol.*, **69**, 373–379

Binder, P. S. (1983) Myopic extended wear with Hydrocurve II soft contact lens. *Ophthalmology*, **90**, 623–626

Bonanno, J. A., Nyguen, T., Biehl, T. *et al.* (2003) Can variability in corneal metabolism explain the variability in corneal swelling? *Eye Contact Lens*, **29**, S7–9

Bonazzi, A., Mastyugin, V., Mieyal, P. A. *et al.* (2000) Regulation of cyclooxygenase-2 by hypoxia and peroxisome proliferators in the corneal epithelium. *J. Biol. Chem.*, **275**, 2837–2844

Bowd, C., Weinreb, R. N., Williams, J. M. and Zangwill, L. M. (2000) The retinal nerve fiber layer thickness in ocular hypertensive, normal, and glaucomatous eyes with optical coherence tomography. *Arch. Ophthalmol.*, **118**, 22–26

Bradley, W. and Schoessler, J. (1979) Corneal response to thick and thin hydrophilic lenses. *Am. J. Optom. Physiol. Opt.*, **56**, 414–421

Brennan, N. A. (2001) A model of oxygen flux through contact lenses. *Cornea*, **20**, 104–108

Brennan, N. A, Smith, G., McDonnell, J. and Bruce, A. (1989) Theoretical principles of pachometry. *Ophthalmol. Physiol. Opt.*, **9**, 247–254

Brennan, N. A., Coles, M. L., Levy, B. *et al.* (2002) One-year prospective clinical trial of balafilcon A (PureVision) silicone-hydrogel contact lenses used on a 30-day continuous wear schedule. *Ophthalmology*, **109**, 1172–1177

Carney, L. G. and Brennan, N. A. (1988) Time course of corneal oxygen uptake during contact lens wear. *CLAO J.*, **14**, 151–154

Cavanagh, H. D., Ladage, P. M., Li, S. L. *et al.* (2002) Effects of daily and overnight wear of a novel hyper oxygen-transmissible soft contact lens on bacterial binding and corneal epithelium: a 13-month clinical trial. *Ophthalmology*, **109**, 1957–1969

Coles, M., Brennan, N., Jaworski, A. *et al.* (2001) Ocular signs and symptom in patients completing 3 years with silicone-hydrogel contact lenses in 30-day continuous wear. *Optom. Vis. Sci.*, **78** (suppl.)

Cornish, R., Jaworski, A. and Brennan, N. (2001) Overnight corneal swelling before and after 6 months of extended wear of high and low *Dk* hydrogel contact lenses. *Invest. Ophthalmol. Vis. Sci., ARVO abstracts*, **42** (suppl.), Abstract no. 3168

Cosar, C. B. and Sener, A. B. (2003) Orbscan corneal topography system in evaluating the anterior structures of the human eye. *Cornea*, **22**, 118–121

Cox, I., Zantos, S. and Orsborn, G. (1991) The overnight corneal swelling response of non-wear, daily wear and extended wear soft lens patients. *Int. Cont. Lens Clin.*, **17**, 134–137

Dave, T. and Ruston, D. (1997) Current trends in modern orthokeratology. *Ophthalmic Physiol. Opt.*, **18**, 224–233

Day, J., Reim, T., Bard, R., McGonagill, P. and Gambino, M. (1997) Advanced orthokeratology using custom lens designs. *Cont. Lens Spectrum*, **12**, 34–40

Doughty, M. J. and Zaman, M. L. (2000) Human corneal thickness and its impact on intraocular pressure measures: a review and meta-analysis approach. *Surv. Ophthalmol.*, **44**, 367–408

Doughty, M. J., Laiquzzaman, M., Muller, A. *et al.* (2002) Central corneal thickness in European (white) individuals, especially children and the elderly, and assessment of its possible importance in clinical measures of intra-ocular pressure. *Ophthalmic Physiol. Opt.*, **22**, 491–504

Drubaix, I., Legeais, J. M., Robert, L. and Renard, G. (1997) Corneal hyaluronan content during post-ablation healing: evidence for a transient depth-dependent contralateral effect. *Exp. Eye Res.*, **64**, 301–304

du Toit, R., Simpson, T., Fonn, D. and Chalmers, R. (2001) Recovery from hyperemia after overnight wear of low and high transmissibility hydrogel lenses. *Curr. Eye Res.*, **22**, 68–73

du Toit, R., Vega, J. A., Fonn, D. *et al.* (2003) Diurnal variation of corneal sensitivity and thickness. *Cornea*, **22**, 205–209

Dumbleton, K. A., Chalmers, R. L., Richter, D. B. and Fonn, D. (1999) Changes in myopic refractive error with nine months' extended wear of hydrogel lenses with high and low oxygen permeability. *Optom. Vis. Sci.*, **76**, 845–849

Dumbleton, K., Fonn, D., Jones, L. *et al.* (2000) Severity and management of CL related complications with continuous wear of high *Dk* silicone hydrogel lenses. *Optom. Vis. Sci.*, **77**, 216

Dumbleton, K. A., Chalmers, R. L., Richter, D. B. *et al.* (2001) Vascular response to extended wear of hydrogel lenses with high and low oxygen permeability. *Optom. Vis. Sci.*, **78**, 147–151

Dunham, C. N., Spaide, R. F. and Dunham, G. (1994) The contralateral reduction of intra-ocular pressure by timolol. *Br. J. Ophthalmol.*, **78**, 38–40

Esco, M. A., Wang, Z., McDermott, M. L. *et al.* (2001) Potential role for laminin 5 in hypoxia-mediated apoptosis of human corneal epithelial cells. *J. Cell Sci.*, **114**, 4033–4040

Farris, R. and Donn, A. (1972) Corneal respiration with soft contact lenses. *J. Am. Optom. Assoc.*, **43**, 292–294

Fatt, I. (1968a) Steady-state distribution of oxygen and carbon dioxide in the in vivo cornea II. The open eye in nitrogen and the covered eye. *Exp. Eye Res.*, **7**, 413–423

Fatt, I. (1968b) The oxygen electrode: some special applications. *Ann. NY Acad. Sci.*, **148**, 81–92

Fatt, I. and Chaston, J. (1982) Measurement of oxygen transmissibility and permeability of hydrogel lenses and materials. *Int. Cont. Lens Clin.*, **9**, 76–88

Fatt, I. and Ruben, C. (1993) New oxygen transmissibility concept for hydrogel contact lenses. *J. Br. Cont. Lens Assoc.*, **16**, 141–149

Fatt, I. and St Helen, R. (1971) Oxygen tension under an oxygen permeable contact lens. *Am. J. Optom. Arch. Am. Acad. Optom.*, **48**, 545–555

Fatt, I., Freeman, R. and Lin, D. (1974) Oxygen tension distributions in the cornea: a re-examination. *Exp. Eye Res.*, **18**, 357–365

Feng, Y., Varikooty, J. and Simpson, T. (2001) Diurnal variation of corneal and corneal epithelial thickness measured using optical coherence tomography. *Cornea*, **20**, 480–483

Fonn, D., Vega, J. and du Toit, R. (1997) High *Dk* versus approved 7-day extended wear hydrogel lenses: the overnight corneal swelling response. *Optom. Vis. Sci.*, **74**, 76

Fonn, D., du Toit, R., Simpson, T. L. *et al.* (1999) Sympathetic swelling response of the control eye to soft lenses in the other eye. *Invest. Ophthalmol. Vis. Sci.*, **40**, 3116–3121

Fonn, D., Wang, J. H. and Simpson, T. (2000) Topographical thickness of the epithelium and total cornea using optical coherence tomography. *Invest. Ophthalmol. Vis. Sci.*, **41**, S675

Fonn, D., MacDonald, K. E., Richter, D. and Pritchard, N. (2002) The ocular response to extended wear of a high *Dk* silicone hydrogel contact lens. *Clin. Exp. Optom.*, **85**, 176–182

Franck, C. B., Loitz, B., Bray, R. *et al.* (1994) Abnormality of the contralateral ligament after injuries of the medial collateral ligament: an experimental study. *J. Bone Joint Surg.*, **76A**, 403–412

Fujimoto, J. G., Brezinski, M. E., Tearney, G. J. *et al.* (1995) Optical biopsy and imaging using optical coherence tomography. *Natl Med.*, **1**, 970–972

Fullard, R. J. and Carney, L. G. (1985) Human tear enzyme changes as indicators of the corneal response to anterior hypoxia. *Acta Ophthalmol. (Copenh.)*, **63**, 678–683

Gnaiger, E. (2001) Bioenergetics at low oxygen: dependence of respiration and phosphorylation on oxygen and adenosine diphosphate supply. *Respir. Physiol.*, **128**, 277–297

Gnaiger, E., Mendez, G. and Hand, S. C. (2000) High phosphorylation efficiency and depression of uncoupled respiration in mitochondria under hypoxia. *Proc. Natl Acad. Sci. USA*, **97**, 11080–11085

Greenberg, M. H. and Hill, R. M. (1973) The physiology of contact lens imprints. *Am. J. Optom. Arch. Am. Acad. Optom.*, **50**, 699–702

Grosvenor, T. (1975) Changes in corneal curvature and subjective refraction of soft contact lens wearers. *Am. J. Optom. Physiol. Opt.*, **52**, 405–413

Guzey, M., Satici, A., Kilic, A. and Karadede, S. (2002) Oedematous corneal response of the fellow control eye to Lotrafilcon A and Vifilcon A hydrogel contact lenses in the rabbit. *Ophthalmologica*, **216**, 139–143

Hamano, H., Hori, M., Hamano, T. *et al.* (1983) Effects of contact lens wear on mitosis of corneal epithelium and lactate content in aqueous humor of rabbit. *Jpn J. Ophthalmol.*, **27**, 451–458

Hara, T. and Hara, T. (1987) Postoperative change in the corneal thickness of the pseudophakic eye: amplified diurnal variation and consensual increase. *J. Cat. Refract. Surg.*, **13**, 325–329

Harper, C. L., Boulton, M. E., Bennett, D., *et al.* (1996) Diurnal variations in human corneal thickness [published erratum appears in *Br. J. Ophthalmol.* (1997) **81**(2), 175]. *Br. J. Ophthalmol.*, **80**, 1068–1072

Harris, M. G., Sarver, M. D. and Polse, K. A. (1975) Corneal curvature and refractive error changes associated with wearing hydrogel contact lenses. *Am. J. Optom. Physiol. Opt.*, **53**, 313–319

Harvitt, D. M. and Bonanno, J. A. (1998) pH dependence of corneal oxygen consumption. *Invest. Ophthalmol. Vis. Sci.*, **39**, 2778–2781

Harvitt, D. M. and Bonanno, J. A. (1999) Re-evaluation of the oxygen diffusion model for predicting minimum contact lens Dk/t values needed to avoid corneal anoxia. *Optom. Vis. Sci.*, **76**, 712–719

Hill, J. F. (1975) A comparison of refractive and keratometric changes during adaptation to flexible and non-flexible contact lenses. *J. Am. Optom. Assoc.*, **46**, 290–294

Hill, R., Rengstorff, R., Petrali, J. *et al.* (1974) Critical oxygen requirement of the corneal epithelium as indicated by succinic dehydrogenase reactivity. *Am. J. Optom. Physiol. Opt.*, **51**, 331–336

Hirji, N. and Larke, J. (1979) Corneal thickness in extended wear of soft contact lenses. *Br. J. Ophthalmol.*, **63**, 274–276

Hitzenberger, C. K., Drexler, W. and Fercher, A. F. (1992) Measurement of corneal thickness by laser Doppler interferometry. *Invest. Ophthalmol. Vis. Sci.*, **33**, 98–103

Holden, B. A. and Mertz, G. (1984) Critical oxygen levels to avoid corneal edema for daily and extended wear contact lenses. *Invest. Ophthalmol. Vis. Sci.*, **25**, 1161–1167

Holden, B. A. and Sweeney, D. F. (1991) The significance of the microcyst response: a review. *Optom. Vis. Sci.*, **68**, 703–707

Holden, B. A., Mertz, G. and McNally, J. (1983) Corneal swelling response to contact lenses worn under extended wear conditions. *Invest. Ophthalmol. Vis. Sci.*, **24**, 218–226

Holden, B. A., Sweeney, D., Vannas, A. *et al.* (1985) Effects of long-term extended contact lens wear on the human cornea. *Invest. Ophthalmol. Vis. Sci.*, **26**, 1489–1501

Holden, B. A., La Hood, D. and Sweeney, D. F. (1987a) Prediction of extended wear micro-cyst response on the basis of mean overnight corneal response in an unrelated sample of non-wearers. *Am. J. Optom. Physiol. Opt.*, **64**, 83

Holden, B. A., Swarbrick, H., Sweeney, D. *et al.* (1987b) Strategies for minimising the effects of extended contact lens wear: a statistical analysis. *Am. J. Optom. Physiol. Opt.*, **64**, 781–789

Horner, D. G. and Richardson, L. E. (1992) Reduction of myopia with contact lenses. *Pract. Optom.*, **3**, 64–68

Hrynchak, P. and Simpson, T. (2000) Optical coherence tomography: an introduction to the technique and its use. *Optom. Vis. Sci.*, **77**, 347–356

Huang, D., Swanson, E. A., Lin, C. P. *et al.* (1991) Optical coherence tomography. *Science*, **254**, 1178–1181

Ichijima, H., Ohashi, J. and Cavanagh, H. D. (1992) Effect of contact-lens-induced hypoxia on lactate dehydrogenase activity and isozyme in rabbit cornea. *Cornea*, **11**, 108–113

Izatt, J. A., Hee, M. R., Swanson, E. A. *et al.* (1994) Micrometer-scale resolution imaging of the anterior eye *in vivo* with optical coherence tomography. *Arch. Ophthalmol.*, **112**, 1584–1589

Jalbert, I., Holden, B. A., Keay, L. and Sweeney, D. F. (2001) Refractive and corneal power changes associated with overnight wear: differences between low Dk/t hydrogel and high Dk/t silicone hydrogel lenses. *Optom. Vis. Sci.*, **78**, S234

Jaworski, A., Cornish, R. and Brennan, N. (2001) The relationship between an individual's overnight corneal swelling and the microcyst response for a low Dk contact lens worn in extended wear. *Optom. Vis. Sci.*, **78** suppl.

Keay, L., Jalbert, I., Sweeney, D. F. *et al.* (2001) Microcysts: clinical significance and differential diagnosis. *Optometry*, **72**, 452–460

Kiely, P. K., Carney, L. G. and Smith, G. (1982) Diurnal variations of corneal topography and thickness. *Am. J. Optom. Physiol. Opt.*, **59**, 976–982

King-Smith, P. E., Fink, B. A., Fogt, N. *et al.* (2000) The thickness of the human precorneal tear film: evidence from reflection spectra. *Invest. Ophthalmol. Vis. Sci.*, **41**, 3348–3359

Koers, D. (1982) Overnight corneal swelling. *Am. J. Optom. Physiol. Opt.*, **59**, 45

Koretz, J., Kaufman, P., Neider, M. *et al.* (1989) Accommodation and presbyopia in the human eye – aging of the anterior segment. *Vis. Res.*, **29**, 1685–1692

Ladage, P. M., Ren, D. H., Petroll, W. M. *et al.* (2003) Effects of eyelid closure and disposable and silicone hydrogel extended contact lens wear on rabbit corneal epithelial proliferation. *Invest. Ophthalmol. Vis. Sci.*, **44**, 1843–1849

La Hood, D. and Grant, T. (1990) Striae and folds as indicators of corneal edema. *Optom. Vis. Sci.*, **67**, 196

La Hood, D., Sweeney, D. and Holden, B. (1988) Overnight corneal edema with hydrogel, rigid gas-permeable and silicone elastomer contact lenses. *Int. Cont. Lens Clin.*, **15**, 149–152

Lambert, S. and Klyce, S. (1981) The origins of Sattler's veil. *Am. J. Ophthalmol.*, **91**, 51–56

Leach, R. M. and Treacher, D. F. (2002) The pulmonary physician in critical care 2: oxygen delivery and consumption in the critically ill. *Thorax*, **57**, 170–177

Lebow, K. and Plishka, K. (1980) Ocular changes associated with extended wear contact lenses. *Int. Cont. Lens Clin.*, **7**, 49–55

Lemp, M. A. and Gold, J. B. (1986) The effects of extended-wear hydrophilic contact lenses on the human corneal epithelium. *Am. J. Ophthalmol.*, **101**, 274–277

Li, H. F., Petroll, W. M., Moller, P. T. *et al.* (1997) Epithelial and corneal thickness measurements by *in vivo* confocal microscopy through focusing (CMTF). *Curr. Eye Res.*, **16**, 214–221

Lin, M. C., Graham, A. D., Polse, K. A. *et al.* (1999) Measurement of post-lens tear thickness. *Invest. Ophthalmol. Vis. Sci.*, **40**, 2833–2839

Liu, Z. and Pflugfelder, S. C. (1999) Corneal thickness is reduced in dry eye. *Cornea*, **18**, 403–407

Lowther, G. E. and Hill, R. M. (1973) Recovery of the corneal epithelium after a period of anoxia. *Am. J. Optom. Physiol. Opt.*, **50**, 234–241

Lowther, G. E. and Tomlinson, A. (1979) Clinical study of corneal response to the wear of low water content soft lenses. *Am. J. Optom. Physiol. Opt.*, **56**, 674–680

Makino, H., Cao, R., Svansson, K. *et al.* (2001) Association of CD40 ligand expression on HTLV-1-infected T cells and maturation of dendritic cells. *Scand. J. Immunol.*, **54**, 574–581

Maldonado, M. J., Ruiz-Oblitas, L., Munuera, J. M. *et al.* (2000) Optical coherence tomography evaluation of the corneal cap and stromal bed features after laser *in situ* keratomileusis for high myopia and astigmatism. *Ophthalmology*, **107**, 81–87

Mandell, R. B. and Polse, K. A. (1969) Keratoconus: spatial variation in thickness as a diagnostic test. *Arch. Ophthalmol.*, **82**, 182–188

Masters, B. R., Ghosh, A. K., Wilson, J. *et al.* (1989) Pyridine nucleotides and phosphorylation potential of rabbit corneal epithelium and endothelium. *Invest. Ophthalmol. Vis. Sci.*, **30**, 861–868

Mastropasqua, L., Ciancaglini, M., Di Tano, G. *et al.* (1998) Ultrastructural changes in rat cornea after prolonged hypobaric hypoxia. *J. Submicrosc. Cytol. Pathol.*, **30**, 285–293

Ménasche, M., Robert, L., Payrau, P., Hamada, R. and Pouliquen, Y. (1988) Comparative biochemical and morphometric studies on corneal wound healing. *Pathol. Biol.*, **36**, 781–789

Mertz, G. (1980) Overnight swelling of the living cornea. *J. Am. Optom. Assoc.*, **51**, 211–214

Miller, J. P., Coon, L. J. and Meier, R. F. (1980) Extended wear of Hydrocurve II soft contact lenses. *J. Am. Optom. Assoc.*, **51**, 225–230

Modis, L., Jr, Langenbucher, A. and Seitz, B. (2001) Corneal thickness measurements with contact and noncontact specular microscopic and ultrasonic pachymetry. *Am. J. Ophthalmol.*, **132**, 517–521

Mountford, J. (1997) An analysis of the changes in corneal shape and refractive error induced by accelerated orthokeratology. *Int. Cont. Lens Clin.*, **24**, 128–144

Mountford, J. (1998) Orthokeratology revisited. *Optician*, **215**, 28

Myrowitz, E. H., Melia, M. and O'Brien, T. P. (2002) The relationship between long-term contact lens wear and corneal thickness. *CLAO J.*, **28**, 217–220

Nichols, J. J. and King-Smith, P. E. (2003) Thickness of the pre- and post-contact lens tear film interferometry. *Invest. Ophthalmol. Vis. Sci.*, **44**, 68–77

Nichols, J. J., Marsich, M. M., Nguyen, M. *et al.* (2000) Overnight orthokeratology. *Optom. Vis. Sci.*, **77**, 252–259

Nissen, J., Hjortdal, J. O., Ehlers, N. *et al.* (1991) A clinical comparison of optical and ultrasonic pachometry. *Acta Ophthalmol. (Copenh.)*, **69**, 659–663

Nizam, A., Waring, G. O. 3rd, Lynn, M. J. and the PERK Study Group (1996) Stability of refraction during 11 years in eyes with simple myopia. *Invest. Ophthalmol. Vis. Sci.*, **37**, S1004

Odenthal, M. T., Nieuwendaal, C. P., Venema, H. W. *et al.* (1999) In vivo human corneal hydration control dynamics: a new model. *Invest. Ophthalmol. Vis. Sci.*, **40**, 312–319

O'Leary, D. J., Wilson, G. and Henson, D. B. (1981) The effect of anoxia on the human corneal epithelium. *Am. J. Optom. Physiol. Opt.*, **58**, 472–476

O'Neal, M. R. and Polse, K. A. (1985) In vivo assessment of mechanisms controlling corneal hydration. *Invest. Ophthalmol. Vis. Sci.*, **26**, 849–856

Papas, E. (1998) On the relationship between soft contact lens oxygen transmissibility and induced limbal hyperaemia. *Exp. Eye Res.*, **67**, 125–131

Papas, E. B., Vajdic, C. M., Austen, R. *et al.* (1997) High-oxygen-transmissibility soft contact lenses do not induce limbal hyperaemia. *Curr. Eye Res.*, **16**, 942–948

Patel, S. and Stevenson, R. W. (1994) Clinical evaluation of a portable ultrasonic and a standard optical pachometer. *Optom. Vis. Sci.*, **71**, 43–46

Perez, J. G., Meijome, J. M., Jalbert, I. *et al.* (2003) Corneal epithelial thinning profile induced by long-term wear of hydrogel lenses. *Cornea*, **22**, 304–307

Phillips, L. J., Cakanac, C. J., Eger, M. W. *et al.* (2003) Central corneal thickness and measured IOP: a clinical study. *Optometry*, **74**, 218–225

Polse, K. A., Brand, R. J., Vastine, D. W. *et al.* (1991) Clinical assessment of corneal hydration control in Fuchs' dystrophy. *Optom. Vis. Sci.*, **68**, 831–841

Pritchard, N. and Fonn, D. (1999) Myopia associated with extended wear of low-oxygen-transmissible hydrogel lenses. *Optom. Vis. Sci.*, **76**, S169

Rainer, G., Petternel, V., Findl, O. *et al.* (2002) Comparison of ultrasound pachymetry and partial coherence interferometry in the measurement of central corneal thickness. *J. Cat. Refract. Surg.*, **28**, 2142–2145

Rask, R. and Jensen, P. K. (1995) Corneal abrasion stimulates epithelial healing in the other eye. *Invest. Ophthalmol. Vis. Sci.*, **36**, S576

Reinstein, D. Z., Silverman, R. H., Rondeau, M. J. *et al.* (1994) Epithelial and corneal thickness measurements by high-frequency ultrasound digital signal processing. *Ophthalmology*, **101**, 140–146

Ribari, O. and Sziklai, I. (1995) Cochlear implantation improves hearing in the contralateral ear. *Acta Oto-Laryngol.*, **115**, 260–263

Riley, M. V. (1969) Glucose and oxygen utilization by the rabbit cornea. *Exp. Eye Res.*, **8**, 193–200

Riley, M. V. and Winkler, B. S. (1990) Strong Pasteur effect in rabbit corneal endothelium preserves fluid transport under anaerobic conditions. *J. Physiol.*, **426**, 81–93

Ripandelli, G., Coppe, A. M., Capaldo, A. and Stirpe, M. (1998) Optical coherence tomography. *Semin. Ophthalmol.*, **13**, 199–202

Sakamoto, R., Miyanaga, Y. and Hamano, H. (1991) Soft and RGP lens corneal swelling and deswelling with overnight wear. *Int. Cont. Lens Clin.*, **18**, 214–217

Sangwan, V. S. (2001) Limbal stem cells in health and disease. *Biosci. Rep.*, **21**, 385–405

Schoessler, J. and Barr, J. (1980) Corneal thickness changes with extended contact lens wear. *Am. J. Optom. Physiol. Opt.*, **57**, 729–733

Sloan, D. (1965) Another chapter in continuous contact lens wearing. *Contacto*, **9**, 19–22

Solomon, O. (1996) Corneal stress test for extended wear. *CLAO J.*, **22**, 75–78

Stapleton, F., Lakshmi, K. R., Kumar, S. *et al.* (1998) Overnight corneal swelling in symptomatic and asymptomatic contact lens wearers. *CLAO J.*, **24**, 169–174

Stone, J. (1976) The possible influence of contact lenses on myopia. *Br. J. Physiol. Opt.*, **31**, 89–114

Swarbrick, H., Wong, G. and O'Leary, D. (1998) Corneal response to orthokeratology. *Optom. Vis. Sci.*, **75**, 791–799

Sweeney, D. F. (1992) Corneal exhaustion syndrome with long-term wear of contact lenses *Optom. Vis. Sci.*, **69**, 601–608

Sweeney, D. F., Keay, L., Jalbert, I. *et al.* (2000) Clinical performance of silicone hydrogel lenses. In *Silicone Hydrogels: The Rebirth of Continuous Wear Contact Lenses* (ed. D. F. Sweeney). Oxford, Butterworth-Heinemann, pp. 90–149

Toth, C. A., Narayan, D. G., Boppart, S. A. *et al.* (1997) A comparison of retinal morphology viewed by optical coherence tomography and by light microscopy. *Arch. Ophthalmol.*, **115**, 1425–1428

Tsubota, K. and Yamada, M. (1992) Corneal epithelial alterations induced by disposable contact lens wear. *Ophthalmology*, **99**, 1193–1196

Tsubota, K., Hata, S., Toda, I. *et al.* (1996) Increase in corneal epithelial cell size with extended wear soft contact lenses depends on continuous wearing time. *Br. J. Ophthalmol.*, **80**, 144–147

Uniacke, C., Hill, R., Greenberg, M. *et al.* (1972) Physiological tests for new contact lens materials. 1. Quantitative effects of selected oxygen atmospheres on glycogen storage, LDH concentration and thickness of the corneal epithelium. *Am. J. Optom. Arch. Am. Acad. Optom.*, **49**, 329–336

Wang, J., Fonn, D., Simpson, T. L. and Jones, L. (2002a) The measurement of corneal epithelial thickness in response to hypoxia using optical coherence tomography. *Am. J. Ophthalmol.*, **133**, 315–319

Wang, J., Fonn, D. and Simpson, T. L. (2002b) Topographical thickness changes of the epithelium and total corneal after overnight lens wear of CRT™ rigid gas permeable lenses measured with OCT. *Optom. Vis. Sci.*, **79**, 2

Wang, J., Fonn, D., Simpson, T. L. *et al.* (2002c) Relation between optical coherence tomography and optical pachymetry measurements of corneal swelling induced by hypoxia. *Am. J. Ophthalmol.*, **134**, 93–98

Wang, J., Fonn, D. and Simpson, T. L. (2003a) Topographical thickness of the epithelium and total cornea after hydrogel and PMMA contact lens wear with eye closure. *Invest. Ophthalmol. Vis. Sci.*, **44**, 1070–1074

Wang, J., Fonn, D., Simpson, T. L. *et al.* (2003b) Precorneal and pre- and postlens tear film thickness measured indirectly with optical coherence tomography. *Invest. Ophthalmol. Vis. Sci.*, **44**, 2524–2528

Wilson, G. (1994) The effect of hypoxia on the shedding rate of the corneal epithelium. *Curr. Eye Res.*, **13**, 409–413

Wilson, G. and Fatt, I. (1980) Thickness of the corneal epithelium during anoxia. *Am. J. Optom. Physiol. Opt.*, **57**, 409–412

Wilson, G. S., Fatt, I. and Freeman, R. D. (1973) Thickness changes in the stroma of an excised cornea during anoxia. *Exp. Eye Res.*, **17**, 165–171

Wirbelauer, C., Scholz, C., Hoerauf, H. *et al.* (2002) Noncontact corneal pachymetry with slit lamp-adapted optical coherence tomography. *Am. J. Ophthalmol.*, **133**, 444–450

Wong, A. C., Wong, C. C., Yuen, N. S. *et al.* (2002) Correlational study of central corneal thickness measurements on Hong Kong Chinese using optical coherence tomography, Orbscan and ultrasound pachymetry. *Eye*, **16**, 715–721

Yaylali, V., Kaufman, S. C. and Thompson, H. W. (1997) Corneal thickness measurements with the Orbscan Topography System and ultrasonic pachymetry. *J. Cat. Refract. Surg.*, **23**, 1345–1350

You, X., Zheng, X., Bergmenson, J. *et al.* (1993) Corneal response and recovery to photorefractive keratectomy in rabbits. *Invest. Ophthalmol. Vis. Sci.*, **34**, 801

Chapter **6**

Clinical performance of silicone hydrogel lenses

Deborah F. Sweeney, Rènée du Toit, Lisa Keay,
Isabelle Jalbert, Padmaja R. Sankaridurg, Judith Stern,
Cheryl Skotnitsky, Andrew Stephensen, Michael Covey,
Brien A. Holden and Gullapalli N. Rao

INTRODUCTION

The global contact lens market is approaching US $6 billion at the supplier level, with close to 100 million wearers (Holden *et al.*, 2003). Nearly 35 million of these wearers are in the USA (Barr, 2003). Advances in material science, design, manufacturing, care systems and clinical research have made contact lenses safer, more comfortable and more convenient. The most recent advance has been the introduction of high-Dk rigid gas-permeable (RGP) materials, but there has also been development of multipurpose solutions, and advances in mass production and manufacturing technology, which have enabled low-cost production of disposable lenses.

As pointed out by Holden (1996), contact lenses must be more comfortable and more convenient than they are currently if they are to be attractive to the two billion wearers of spectacles worldwide. The ultimate contact lens will not only be superbly comfortable but also biocompatible, enabling it to be worn safely and effectively for an indefinite period. The first generation of a new range of continuous-wear (CW) products has been launched. These include silicone and fluorosilicone hydrogel lenses (see Chapter 1) and a RGP lens (Menicon Z), all of which have the potential to be worn continuously for up to 30 days and have overcome the first major barrier for CW lenses: hypoxia. Silicone hydrogel lenses also offer comfort that is comparable with current disposable soft contact lenses (DSCL), and have high oxygen permeability (Dk), allowing them to be used for daily wear (DW), extended wear (EW) or CW, with high patient acceptance.

THE CORNEA'S NEED: OXYGEN SUPPLY

As reviewed in Chapter 5, there is a direct correlation between the oxygen levels at the anterior surface of the cornea and the average corneal swelling response (Holden *et al.*, 1984). Corneal oedema can be avoided if the oxygen levels in the closed eye remain above at least 10–15 per cent (Mizutani *et al.*, 1983; Holden *et al.*, 1984).

EFFECTS OF CONTACT LENSES

Contact lenses almost invariably reduce the oxygen levels that are available to the anterior surface of the cornea. In the open-eye state the oxygen available is dependent primarily on the oxygen transmissibility (Dk/t) of the contact lens and is supplemented by oxygen in the tears behind the lens. The latter oxygen supply results from contact lens movement, which induces tear flow and tear replenishment. This supply, however, plays a relatively small role in the total oxygen available with hydrogel lenses (Polse, 1979; Polse *et al.*, 1997).

In the closed eye, oxygen is only available from under the lid and any contribution from the tears is reduced, if not abolished (Benjamin and Rasmussen, 1985). Therefore the Dk/t of the lens is of vital importance. The level of oxygen that is available to the cornea under closed-eye conditions can only be increased by either increasing the Dk of the contact lens material or by reducing the thickness of the lens.

Holden and Mertz (1984) determined that during overnight wear of lenses the minimum Dk/t that is required to reduce the level of closed-eye oedema to 4 per cent is 87×10^{-9} (cm/s) (mlO_2/ml·mmHg). However, to reduce the level of overnight oedema to 3.2 per cent (the mean level of overnight oedema with no lens recorded by La Hood *et al.*, 1988), the critical lens Dk/t calculated from the original Holden and Mertz criterion would need to be approximately 125×10^{-9} (cm/s) (mlO_2/ml·mmHg) (Figure 6.1).

The work of Harvitt and Bonanno (1998) supports this new criterion as they report that a Dk/t of 125×10^{-9} (cm/s) (mlO_2/ml·mmHg) is needed to avoid anoxia in the stroma. Smith *et al.* (1999) suggest that at least 10 per cent of the hypoxic stress of the average cornea remains with a lens Dk/t of 90×10^{-9} (cm/s) (mlO_2/ml·mmHg). To halve this residual hypoxia once again would require an estimated Dk/t of at least 175×10^{-9} (cm/s) (mlO_2/ml·mmHg).

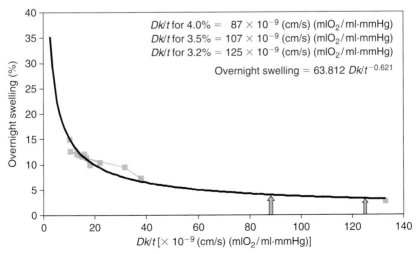

Figure 6.1   Revised criterion for avoiding oedema under EW conditions

Ideally, CW contact lenses should be available to correct a full range of refractive errors. Therefore, contact lens materials would need to have a Dk of at least 200×10^{-11} barrer, if lens thickness was limited to 0.16 mm.

SYSTEMS OF LENS WEAR

DAILY WEAR

Daily disposable lenses (DDs) represent the ultimate in convenience for daily lens wearers. These lenses are worn during waking hours and then discarded. No cleaning or other maintenance is required but the need and hassle of daily insertion and removal still remain. In the USA, approximately 4 per cent of lenses are now used in this way (Barr, 2003), while 28 per cent of new fits in the UK are DDs (Morgan and Efron, 2002a). However, many wearers of DDs still report symptoms of dryness and redness at the end of the day (Sweeney et al., 1997; Sankaridurg et al., 1999), and adverse responses continue to occur. Surveys of patients enrolled in studies with DDs at the Cornea and Contact Lens Research Unit (CCLRU) reveal that up to 15 per cent of patients sleep in their lenses (Jalbert et al., 1999a). Non-compliance with this modality may contribute to the occurrence of adverse events and complications. Hamano et al. (1994) reviewed the records of 893 eyes from patients wearing DDs and reported a 2.5 per cent rate of corneal 'complications'. Hingorani et al. (1995) described an event of contact lens-induced peripheral ulcer (CLPU) and one of microbial keratitis (MK) with DDs. Sweeney et al. (1997) reported incidents of infiltrates and corneal erosions with DDs, and CLPUs have been described in prospective clinical trials conducted at the L. V. Prasad Eye Institute (LVPEI) (Sankaridurg et al., 1999).

EXTENDED WEAR

The term 'extended wear' usually refers to wear of contact lenses for up to six nights and seven days continuously. Although EW of conventional hydrogels is still prescribed in the USA and to a far less extent in Europe and Australia, this modality is rarely used because of the hypoxic effects, adverse events and serious infections.

DSCLs that are discarded usually after one or possibly up to two weeks of wear were introduced in an attempt to avoid the adverse ocular effects associated with lens deposits and lens ageing. These lenses were made from low-Dk materials ($Dk/t = 18$–25 units) and research and clinical experience have shown that adverse effects continue to occur with the use of these products (Sankaridurg et al., 1999).

CONTINUOUS WEAR

Patients and practitioners still seek the 'Holy Grail' of contact lenses: a CW lens that can be worn safely and effectively for at least 30 days and nights.

PATIENT AND PRACTITIONER NEEDS

In surveys conducted by the CCLRU, patients have overwhelmingly indicated their desire for 'permanent' vision correction. In one survey, 97 per cent of 122 prospective patients expressed the desire to be able to wear their lenses continuously for at least six nights per week (Holden, 1989). In recent surveys of patients attending the CCLRU, the most important features in determining a patient's choice of a contact lens were initial comfort and quality of vision. We have found, however, that 85 per cent of patients believe that CW is also an essential feature in determining their choice of contact lens (Table 6.1). Nearly three-quarters of all myopic patients have indicated that they would try a high-*Dk* EW lens, especially if the lens was recommended to them for 30 days of CW (Barr, 1999).

While patients seek immediate comfort, excellent vision, convenience and safety from their contact lenses, practitioners seek a contact lens that can provide unaltered corneal physiology as well as patient comfort, safety and excellent vision.

PROBLEMS WITH HYDROGEL EW

EW materials that first became available during the 1970s posed a significant threat to corneal health and integrity. Changes in the corneal epithelium (epithelial microcysts, reduced epithelial adhesion), stroma (oedema) and endothelium (polymegethism) induced by chronic hypoxia and acidosis could be observed in all long-term hydrogel EW patients. Acute or chronic inflammatory adverse events affected a significant proportion of patients (up to 30 per cent over a 12-month period) (Vajdic and Holden, 1997) and serious infections associated with hydrogel EW were reported (Adams *et al.*, 1983; Weissman *et al.*, 1984; Chalupa *et al.*, 1987; Schein *et al.*, 1989; Nilsson and Montan, 1994). In addition, the media helped fuel public and practitioner scepticism regarding the safety of EW (Allegretti, 1985; Anon, 1986).

Table 6.1   Survey results of patients attending CCLRU clinics regarding their preferred option for lens wear schedule ($n = 1473$; 58% female; mean age = 31 years; range = 18–68 years)

CW (no overnight removals)	35%
EW full-time (6 nights weekly)	11%
EW occasional (2–5 nights weekly)	18%
EW/CW	**64%**
Full-time DW (all waking hours)	29%
Occasional DW (social occasions, sport, etc.)	6%
DW	**35%**
Other	1%

Frequent replacement of lenses every one to three months was introduced in an attempt to reduce complications with EW. This was soon followed by the concept of DSCLs with weekly or biweekly lens replacement. DSCLs were introduced with the claim that regular replacement of lenses would eliminate the contribution of handling, deposits and other contaminants to adverse responses and infection rates with hydrogel EW. While this system does reduce the risk of acute and inflammatory ocular responses, they are not eliminated. Kotow *et al.* (1987) reported that the annual incidence of contact lens-induced acute red eye (CLARE) was reduced from 15 per cent with non-replaced lenses to 2 per cent when lenses were replaced regularly. Grant (1991) reported a reduction in the number and severity of adverse responses, in particular CLARE and contact lens-induced papillary conjunctivitis (CLPC), with hydrogels that were replaced on a regular basis. While inflammatory problems are reduced, studies have shown that after three years of disposable hydrogel EW (Holden, 1992) only 6 per cent of patients are unaffected physiologically. Regular replacement also has little influence on corneal ulceration. An incidence of 2 per cent for CLPUs has been reported with both conventional EW and regularly replaced lenses (Grant, 1991; Grant *et al.*, 1998) and the rate of serious corneal infections is not reduced with disposable hydrogel lenses (Schein *et al.*, 1994). Complications that are either directly or indirectly attributable to chronic hypoxic stress and hypercapnic changes were not eliminated by frequent replacement because all of the lenses used were made from low-*Dk* materials. Therefore a new generation of soft materials providing significantly improved *Dk* was required to avoid the hypoxic side effects of EW.

HISTORY OF CW

CW is not a new concept. There are documented cases of patients wearing scleral or corneal lenses day and night for prolonged periods dating back to the 1940s (Dallos, 1946; Treissman and Plaice, 1946; Rengstorff, 1971; Mandell, 1974) and although few cases were reported, some patients could successfully wear low-water-content hydrophilic lenses for prolonged periods (Koetting, 1974). The early CW hydrogels were used for therapeutic reasons in corneal diseases such as bullous keratopathy and exposure keratitis (Gasset and Kaufman, 1970; Dohlman *et al.*, 1973; Ruben, 1976). However, de Carle (1972) is generally credited with the development of high-water-content hydrogel lenses for CW and for the fitting rationale and clinical guidelines for the general population.

Initial results reported with CW hydrogels were quite encouraging (Leibowitz *et al.*, 1973; Ezekiel, 1974; Hamano, 1974; Benson, 1975). de Carle (1972) reported he had achieved success with over 2000 patients in CW hydrogels. However, apart from Hodd (1975), who reported visual acuity (VA) problems related to lens fitting and spoilation, there is little objective information available on the ocular response to these first continuously worn contact lenses. Ruben (1977) was the first to report on all the frequent complications that occurred with CW hydrogel lenses in the late 1970s. Later Zantos (1981) and Zantos and Holden (1978) reported complication rates of over 35 per cent with CW of hydrogels. In his thesis,

Zantos (1981) evaluated the clinical performance of CW hydrogel contact lenses and determined some of the factors controlling the underlying ocular performance in such a regimen. He reported that only 29 per cent of his patients achieved successful wear (defined as four weeks or more) on their first attempt, with failure usually occurring in the first week of CW. The main adverse reactions observed were acute inflammatory conditions, in particular acute red eye (ARE) reactions, which at the time were thought to be associated with tight lens fitting. Nine per cent of the patients developed marginal ulcers and in one patient (3 per cent) a large central ulcer developed, leading to substantial loss of vision.

Silicone and high-*Dk* RGP lenses

The introduction of silicone elastomer lenses was promising for CW. Silicone lenses have a *Dk/t* well above the critical limits required for eliminating hypoxia with closed-eye wear (approximately 300×10^{-9} (cm/s) (mlO$_2$/ml·mmHg)). Overnight oedema levels with these lenses were actually significantly less than those observed during eye closure with no lens wear (Sweeney and Holden, 1987) as the lens provides a reservoir of oxygen to the cornea. The high oxygen levels also resulted in no increase in endothelial polymegethism (Schoessler *et al.*, 1984), a marker of corneal hypoxic stress. In addition, these lenses demonstrated therapeutic potential as they promoted epithelial wound healing (Sweeney and Holden, 1988). Despite these positive signs, silicone lens wear was fraught with problems. Manufacturing difficulties resulted in poor edge shape, which was associated with discomfort. The material proved to be prone to excessive lipid deposition and, because of their time-dependent mechanical properties, lenses tended to bind to the cornea. The greatest limits to the success of silicone lenses were reports of adverse events, including ulcers, which were mainly attributable to the effects of lens binding (Gurland, 1976; Ruben and Guillon, 1979; Blackhurst, 1985; Mannarino *et al.*, 1985; Nelson *et al.*, 1985).

High-*Dk* RGP materials were also developed in the 1980s. Several articles were published reporting 'superpermeable' GP lenses with *Dk* values in the 100–200 range (Hill *et al.*, 1985; Brezinski and Hill, 1986; Hill and Brezinski, 1987). Long-term clinical trials at the CCLRU involving more than 300 patients for over 10 years with some of these high-*Dk* materials ($Dk/t > 85 \times 10^{-9}$ (cm/s) (mlO$_2$/ml·mmHg)) demonstrated that, when RGP lenses were adequately fitted, their high *Dk/t* afforded an excellent physiological response. These lenses also offered both excellent vision and convenience. Various authors have reported that 70–95 per cent of their patients were successful with CW of high-*Dk* RGP lenses (Kastl and Johnson, 1989; Kreis-Gosselin and Lumbruso, 1990). In these studies patients were able to wear lenses without removal for periods ranging from nine days to approximately five weeks and, in some cases, several months or a year at a time (Kastl and Johnson, 1989; CCLRU unpublished data, 1990). The only long-term effects of concern noted in the CCLRU clinical trials were the development of papillary lid changes (which could be managed by yearly lens replacement) and a very low 'chronic' microcyst response, averaging around 10 microcysts. Other problems related to poor wettability and deposit formation contributed to the dropout rate.

The experience gained with these high-*Dk* RGP materials demonstrates that CW can be safe and convenient. Nevertheless, this modality has had no significant impact on either the market or wearing trends. This is because of two main factors. First is the inherent initial discomfort related to mechanical characteristics of RGP materials. Nearly one-third of patients in CCLRU studies ceased wear for comfort-related reasons, with most discontinuations occurring during the first month of wear. The second problem is the need for practitioners to be skilled in the art of fitting the lenses and their reluctance to fit them.

In 2002 Menicon Z (*Dk* 163 barrer) received USA Food and Drug Administration (FDA) approval for 30-day RGP CW. The FDA clinical trials, with over 660 patients at 24 clinical sites for 12 months, reported excellent physiological results with increases in 3 and 9 o'clock staining. For the most part, adverse responses with Menicon Z are caused by foreign body abrasions whereas those associated with Acuvue are caused by bacterial infection (Gleason and Albright, 2003).

Experience with both silicone elastomer lenses and high-*Dk* RGPs has shown that, to meet our patients' needs, new-generation lenses need to provide more than oxygen. Lenses must also satisfy the patients' desire for immediate comfort and be able to perform at least as well as currently marketed hydrogel products in terms of fitting and lens surface characteristics.

WHY HIGH-*Dk* SOFT LENSES?

High-*Dk* soft contact lenses (SCLs) promise to meet the needs of both the practitioner and patient. The silicone hydrogel and fluorosilicone hydrogel materials offer practitioners and patients the first significant breakthrough in the past 30 years. Silicone hydrogel lenses promise immediate comfort and performance similar to current DSCLs in terms of fitting and surface characteristics. They have the additional benefit that they alleviate hypoxia and prevent the changes in corneal function and structure associated with conventional hydrogels.

It is generally accepted that corneal hypoxia during sleep with low-*Dk/t* contact lenses brings about corneal changes that predispose the cornea to infection (Baum and Barza, 1990; Donshik, 1994). Chronic hypoxic stress reduces corneal sensitivity (Millodot, 1974; Millodot and O'Leary, 1980), increases epithelial fragility (O'Leary and Millodot, 1981) and compromises epithelial adhesion (Madigan *et al.*, 1987; Madigan and Holden, 1992). Also, Ren *et al.* (1999) have shown a relationship between *Dk/t* and binding of *Pseudomonas aeruginosa* to exfoliated epithelial cells. Solomon *et al.* (1994) have shown in their work with animals that the greater the degree of corneal hypoxia, the greater the likelihood of MK. More subtle effects on the epithelium, the primary barrier to invasion of pathogens, may also result from the continuous presence of the lens and the absence of blink-activated cleansing of the ocular surface. Now that silicone hydrogel lenses are available on the market, large-scale clinical trials can be conducted to determine the effects of the elimination of hypoxia on the rates of corneal infection.

This chapter will discuss and detail our clinical findings in physiological performance, fitting performance and patient subjective responses with silicone hydrogel lenses. These lenses have been worn on both a six-night EW and 30-night CW basis. The long-term clinical performance of silicone hydrogel lenses will be contrasted with that observed for six-night EW DSCLs and, where applicable, with DW or no-lens-wear findings.

SILICONE HYDROGEL MATERIALS

LENSES AVAILABLE

The major contact lens corporations are currently developing silicone hydrogel lenses.

Bausch & Lomb has brought to market PureVision (balafilcon A), which has a water content of 35 per cent and a Dk/t of 110×10^{-9} (cm/s) (mlO$_2$/ml·mmHg) at -3.00 D, and CIBA Vision has introduced Focus Night & Day (lotrafilcon A), which is made from a fluorosiloxane hydrogel material and has a water content of 24 per cent and a Dk/t of 175×10^{-9} (cm/s) (mlO$_2$/ml·mmHg) at -3.00 D (for further details of these materials and their properties, refer to Chapter 1). Both products have received FDA approval to be worn for up to 30 nights continuously with monthly replacement.

THE STUDIES

The clinics at the CCLRU, School of Optometry and Vision Science, the University of New South Wales in Sydney, Australia and the Brien A. Holden Research Centre at LVPEI in Hyderabad, India, have conducted numerous short-term, overnight and long-term dispensing trials of a range of prototype and commercially available silicone hydrogel contact lenses, and have conducted trials with spectacles, conventional DW, DD and EW of DSCLs (Table 6.2).

Although many observers were involved in the collection of the data discussed here, steps were taken to ensure that their judgements were concordant (Terry et al., 1995). The majority of the biomicroscopy findings were graded using a previously established 0–4 scale (CCLRU, 1996), where 1 = very slight, 2 = slight, 3 = moderate and 4 = severe (Figure 6.2) and the observers used decimalized scale divisions to enhance sensitivity (Bailey et al., 1991). Where a different scale was used, e.g. for lens wettability, a description of the scale and the

Table 6.2 Patients involved in the clinical trials at the CCLRU and LVPEI

	Number of patients	Eye years
Spectacles	147	240
DW (DD)	146	200
EW (6 nights, 13 nights)	1132	2287
CW (6 nights, 30 nights)	964	1518

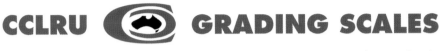

CCLRU GRADING SCALES

Cornea and Contact Lens Research Unit, School of Optometry and Vision Science, University of New South Wales

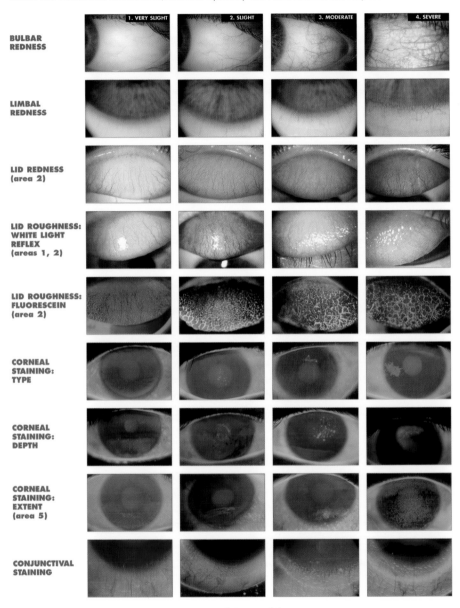

Sponsored by an Educational Grant from *Johnson & Johnson* VISION CARE, INC.

Figure 6.2   CCLRU grading scales

CCLRU GRADING SCALES

APPLICATION OF GRADING SCALES

- Patient management is based on how much the normal ocular appearance has changed.
- In general, a rating of slight (grade 2) or less is considered within normal limits (except staining).
- A change of one grade or more at follow up visits is considered clinically significant.

PALPREBRAL CONJUNCTIVAL GRADES

- The palprebal conjunctiva is divided into five areas to grade redness and roughness.
- Areas 1, 2 and 3 are most relevant in contact lens wear.

ADVERSE EFFECTS WITH CONTACT LENSES

CLPC CONTACT LENS PAPILLARY CONJUNCTIVITIS

Inflammation of the upper palprebal conjunctiva

Signs
- Redness
- Enlarged papillae
- Excess mucus

Symptoms
- Itchiness
- Mucus strands
- Lens mislocation
- Intolerance to lenses

INFILTRATES

Accumulation of inflammatory cells in corneal sub-epithelial stroma. Inset: high magnification view

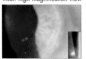

Signs
- Whitish opacity (focal) or grey haze (diffuse)
- Usually confined to 2-3mm from limbus
- Localized redness

Symptoms
- Asymptomatic or scratchy, foreign body sensation
- Redness, tearing and photophobia possible

CLARE CONTACT LENS REDUCED RED EYE

An acute corneal inflammatory episode associated with sleeping in soft contact lenses

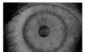

Signs
- Unilateral
- Intense redness
- Infiltrates
- No epithelial break

Symptoms
- Wakes with irritation or pain
- Photophobia
- Lacrimation

POLYMEGETHISM

CORNEAL STAINING GRADES

- Staining assessed immediately after single instillation of fluorescein using cobalt blue light and written 12 (yellow) filter over the slit lamp objective.
- The cornea is divided into five areas. The type, extent and depth of staining are graded in each area.

Type
1. Micropunctate
2. Macropunctate
3. Coalescent macropunctate
4. Patch

Extent: Surface area
1	1 – 15%
2	16 – 30%
3	31 – 45%
4	> 45%

Depth*
1. Superficial epithelium
2. Deep epithelium, delayed stromal glow
3. Immediate localized stromal glow
4. Immediate diffuse stromal glow

*Based on penetration of fluoroscein and slit lamp optic section

EROSION

Full thickness epithelial loss over a discrete area

Signs
- No stromal inflammation
- Immediate spread of fluoroscein into stroma

Symptoms
- Can be painful
- Photophobia
- Lacrimation

CLPU CONTACT LENS PERIPHERAL ULCER

Round, full thickness epithelial loss with inflamed base, typically in the corneal periphery which results in a scar. Insets: with fluorescein, scar

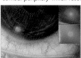

Signs
- Unilateral, "white spot"
- Localized redness
- Infiltrates
- Post healing scar

Symptoms
- Varies from foreign body sensation to pain
- Lacrimation and photophobia may occur

INFECTED ULCER

Full thickness epithelial loss with stromal necrosis and inflammation, typically central or paracentral

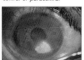

Signs
- Intense redness
- "White patch" (raised edges)
- Infiltrates
- Epithelial and stromal loss
- Anterior chamber flare
- Conjunctival and lid edema

Symptoms
- Pain, photophobia
- Redness, mucoid discharge
- VA (if over pupil)

 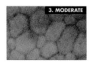

1. VERY SLIGHT   2. SLIGHT   3. MODERATE   4. SEVERE

VASCULARIZATION

Vessel extension beyond translucent limbal zone is recorded (mm)

STROMAL STRIAE and FOLDS

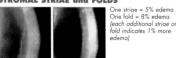

One striae = 5% edema
One fold = 8% edema
(each additional striae or fold indicates 1% more edema)

Record number observed

MICROCYSTS and VACUOLES

Located in epithelium. Identified by side showing brightness.

reversed
Microcysts
Vacuoles
unreversed

Record number observed

Sponsored by an Educational Grant from Johnson & Johnson VISION CARE, INC.

Figure 6.2   *Continued*

evaluation technique is included in the relevant section. For some findings, such as striae, microcysts and mucin balls, the number of features were counted rather than graded. Patient ratings of symptoms, as well as information pertaining to their satisfaction and attitudes to 30-night CW compared to laser refractive surgery, are also presented and discussed. Where no differences in the performance of balafilcon A and lotrafilcon A have been found, results are presented as a response to silicone hydrogels.

CORNEAL SWELLING WITH SILICONE HYDROGEL MATERIALS

Several studies (MacDonald *et al.*, 1995; Fonn *et al.*, 1998, 1999; Comstock *et al.*, 1999; Mueller *et al.*, 2001; Bullimore *et al.*, 2002) have been conducted using the protocol described by La Hood *et al.* (1988) to determine the level of overnight oedema with silicone hydrogel lenses compared with no lens wear and commercially available DSCLs. These studies have confirmed that induced overnight oedema is significantly lower relative to the oedema observed with conventional products and is indeed similar to no lens wear (Table 6.3). However, some patients with higher than average corneal demands will still experience oedema, even with lenses of high Dk/t. As Comstock *et al.* (1999) have shown, 11 per cent of patients can be expected to show greater than 7.7 per cent corneal oedema with overnight wear of balafilcon A. Holden *et al.* (1983) demonstrated that the cornea is able to eliminate about 8 per cent of oedema during the open-eye phase of EW with hydrogels. Therefore, for some patients low-grade oedema is still expected.

Striae and folds

Hypoxic oedema commonly results in the development of corneal striae and folds (Sarver, 1971) (Figure 6.3). The presence of striae indicates that corneal swelling is at least 6 per cent (Kerns, 1974; La Hood and Grant, 1990), whereas the observation of folds indicates swelling of 10–15 per cent or greater (Kame, 1976; La Hood and Grant, 1990). La Hood and Grant (1990) have demonstrated a link between the percentage of corneal swelling and the number of striae and folds observed in the cornea. In their study the presence of one stria represented a mean corneal swelling of 5 per cent, five striae were equivalent to 8 per cent swelling and 10 striae to 11 per cent swelling. The presence of one fold indicated a mean oedema response of 8 per cent, five folds 11 per cent oedema and 10 folds 14 per cent oedema. This approach provides the practitioner with a clinical method of evaluating the oedema response by simply counting the number of striae and folds present. If striae are observed 1 hour after eye opening, then corneal swelling is still at least 5–6 per cent.

The number of corneal striae, as an indicator of hypoxic stress to the cornea, is monitored in our clinical trials. As would be expected from the reported levels of overnight corneal swelling, striae are evident less frequently in silicone hydrogel lens-wearing groups compared with DSCL lens-wearing groups. Low levels

Table 6.3   Overnight corneal oedema responses (mean ± SD) with SCLs, rigid gas-permeables (RGPs), silicone hydrogel and silicone elastomer lenses

Lens type[a]	Material	Tc (mm)[b]	n[c]	Overnight oedema response (%)
SCLs				
Permalens	Perfilcon A	204	31	12.3 ± 2.1
Hydrocurve II	Bufilcon A	56	15	11.8 ± 3.4
03/04 (SeeQuence)	Polymacon	37	14	11.7 ± 2.7
B&L 70	Lidofilcon A	149	12	11.5 ± 1.8
Durasoft 3	Phemfilcon A	47	10	10.9 ± 3.3
Permaflex Natural	Surfilcon A	144	44	10.5 ± 2.4
Acuvue	Etafilcon A	69	24	10.4 ± 3.2
NewVues	Vifilcon A	81	10	10.3 ± 3.0
Cibathin	Tefilcon	35	5	10.2 ± 2.1
RGPs				
Boston IV	Pasifocon A	145	16	12.9 ± 3.5
Equalens	Itafluorofocon A	158	20	10.2 ± 2.8
Quantum	Fluorosilicone acrylate	154	16	10.1 ± 2.5
Fluoroperm 92	Fluorosilicone acrylate	146	8	7.6 ± 2.5
Advent	Fluorofocon A	203	22	6.0 ± 2.7
Menicon SF-P	Melafocon A	160	10	5.0 ± 2.8
Silicone hydrogels				
Prototype A	Silicone hydrogels	72	10	3.8 ± 1.8
Prototype B	Silicone hydrogels	75	9	3.9 ± 1.3
Prototype C	Silicone hydrogels	90	7	3.6 ± 2.3
Silicone elastomer				
Silsoft	Elastofilcon A	110	11	2.0 ± 1.9
No lens	–	–	41	3.2 ± 16

[a]All lenses were −3.00 D back vertex power.
[b]Measured lens centre thickness (mean).
[c]Number of subjects.
Data from La Hood *et al.* (1988) and unpublished CCLRU studies.

of overnight oedema followed by rapid deswelling on eye opening for the majority of patients suggest that practitioners are unlikely to observe striae unless aftercare visits are early in the morning.

As hyperopic and toric and bifocal silicone hydrogel lenses become available, areas of regional lens thickness may result in more frequent observations of striae in some patients.

Bulbar hyperaemia

According to Terry *et al.* (1993) the standard for EW should be no more than a one-grade increase in persistent redness of the bulbar conjunctiva. Judgements of bulbar redness are made in the nasal, temporal, superior and inferior quadrants.

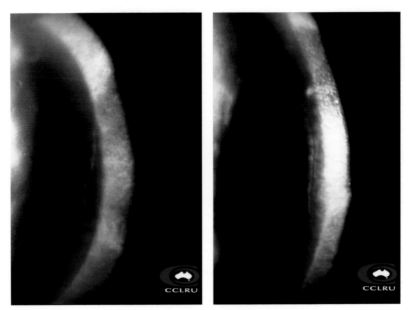

Figure 6.3   Typical appearance of striae and folds (from CCLRU)

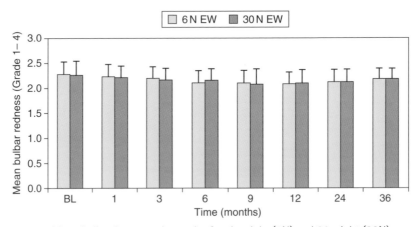

Figure 6.4   Mean bulbar hyperaemia results for six-night (6N) and 30-night (30N) silicone hydrogel lens wear across time

Figure 6.4 shows the bulbar hyperaemia response to silicone hydrogels worn on a six- or 30-night schedule. While DSCL wearers have an increase in bulbar redness with increasing length of wear, silicone hydrogel wearers have a reduction in redness, though this is less consistent than the response that is observed with limbal hyperaemia. Dumbleton *et al.* (1998, 2001) and Fonn *et al.* (2002) have also reported reduced bulbar hyperaemia with high-Dk/t lenses.

Limbal hyperaemia

According to standards suggested by Terry *et al.* (1993), for successful hydrogel EW, a lens must cause no change in the appearance of a patient's eyes which is unacceptable to either the patient or practitioner. There should be no more than a one-grade increase in persistent redness with lens wear. Limbal hyperaemia is represented by the filling and engorgement of the limbal capillaries and is a well-documented change accompanying both DW (Larke *et al.*, 1981; McMonnies *et al.*, 1982) and EW (Holden *et al.*, 1986) with hydrogels. In a study of long-term wearers of hydrogels and RGPs with a group of spectacle-wearing control patients, the hydrogel wearers could be correctly identified in 85 per cent of cases based on their levels of limbal hyperaemia (Sweeney *et al.*, 1992). In fact, Efron (1987) has suggested that an increased level of hyperaemia in hydrogel wearers represents the norm.

As clinicians we are well aware of and concerned for our patients' desire for white eyes as opposed to the circumlimbal flush seen with conventional and disposable hydrogels in the majority of our wearers. In the study by Vajdic *et al.* (1999) redness is reported as occurring often or constantly in 16 per cent of SCL wearers. However, limbal hyperaemia is also a clinical concern as there is evidence that it is a necessary precursor to corneal vascularization (Cogan, 1948; Collin, 1973).

Several aetiologies for lens-induced limbal hyperaemia have been suggested. Tomlinson and Haas (1980) suggested that the hyperaemia is a result of central corneal oedema, while McMonnies *et al.* (1982), using the clinical finding that the level of hyperaemia with RGPs is similar to that of spectacle wearers, has associated hyperaemia with the overlying presence or pressure of the hydrogel lens on the limbal capillaries.

Papas (1998) and Papas *et al.* (1997) have demonstrated that there is a relationship between induced limbal hyperaemia and lens Dk/t. Time series studies over 16 hours, including 8 hours of eye closure, show that silicone hydrogel lenses produce fluctuations in limbal hyperaemia similar to those seen in non-lens wearers, i.e. a significant increase is seen only after eye closure. In contrast, there are marked increases in limbal hyperaemia in DSCL wearers after as little as 4 hours of lens wear which are significantly greater than the increase seen with either no lens wear or silicone hydrogel lens wear after 8 hours of eye closure (Figure 6.5). This work confirms earlier reports of reduced limbal hyperaemia with such lenses (Papas *et al.*, 1994; Covey *et al.*, 1995; MacDonald *et al.*, 1995) and further reports substantiating these findings have been published (Dumbleton *et al.*, 1998, 2001; du Toit *et al.*, 1998; Morgan and Efron, 2002b). Work by Papas (1998) also demonstrates a strong link between Dk/t in the lens periphery and increased limbal hyperaemia. Papas suggests, based on a logarithmic model, that the peripheral Dk/t required to avoid limbal hyperaemia is in the range of $56-274 \times 10^{-9}$ (cm/s) (mlO$_2$/ml·mmHg) and averages 125×10^{-9} (cm/s) (mlO$_2$/ml·mmHg) (Figure 6.6). This provides further support that the critical lens Dk/t for EW/CW should be greater than the original 87×10^{-9} (cm/s) (mlO$_2$/ml·mmHg) of the Holden–Mertz criterion.

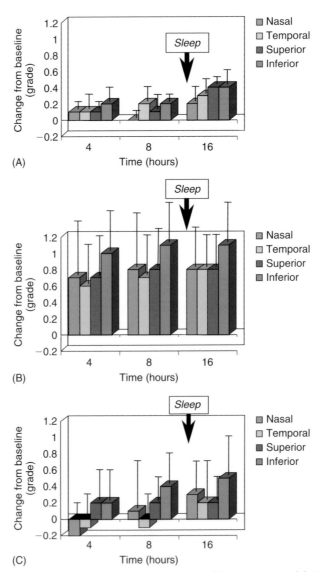

Figure 6.5 Limbal hyperaemia across a 16-hour period: (A) no lens wear; (B) 38 per cent hydroxyethyl methacrylate (HEMA); (C) silicone hydrogel

In our clinical trials limbal hyperaemia is quantified by observing the change in redness caused by vascular activity at the limbus and, as for bulbar redness, judgements are made in the nasal, temporal, superior and inferior quadrants. Our longer-term clinical studies have confirmed the findings of Papas and others. Although the levels of redness in our silicone hydrogel and DSCL groups are similar at baseline, reduced limbal hyperaemia is observed with silicone hydrogels. Dumbleton *et al.* (1998, 2001) have also reported a lower vascular response

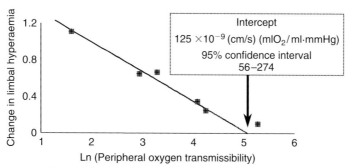

Figure 6.6 Predicted Dk/t to avoid increased limbal hyperaemia

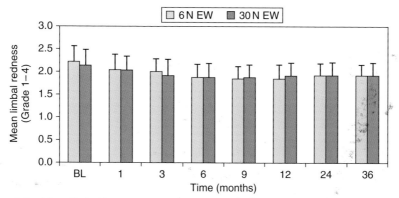

Figure 6.7 Mean limbal hyperaemia with six-night (6N) and 30-night (30N) silicone hydrogel lens wear across time

at both the limbal surface and in the deeper neovascular stromal vessels with silicone hydrogel lenses worn on a CW basis over nine months compared to conventional hydrogel lenses worn on an EW basis. Studies show that this reduction is stable in the long term (over three years) and occurs in both six-night and 30-night wear groups (Figure 6.7).

Limbal vascularization

Duke-Elder (1963) indicated that vascularization is a response to a 'call for help' by tissue in difficulty. Limbal vascularization is the vessel penetration into the cornea beyond the translucent zone. These vessels may empty but will refill with the return of hypoxic stress (McMonnies, 1983). McMonnies *et al.* (1982) and Holden *et al.* (1986) have shown that more limbal vessel penetration occurs with hydrogel EW than with DW.

In our studies we measure the amount of superficial corneal vascularization using a 16× graticule. There is less vascularization in silicone hydrogel lens-wearing patients than in DSCL wearers (Figure 6.8). The amount of vascularization

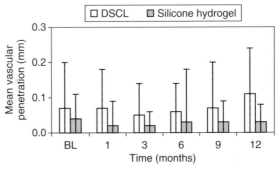

Figure 6.8   Levels of vascularization observed with DSCL and silicone hydrogel lenses across time. The silicone hydrogel levels represent emptying of limbal vessels

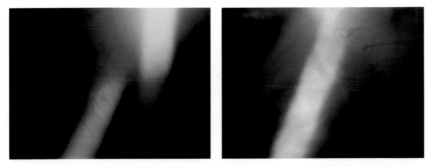

Figure 6.9   Limbal vascularization in a patient after 15 years of DSCL wear (left). After six months of silicone hydrogel lens wear a significant reduction in the filling of the limbal vessels was observed (right)

increases over time with DSCLs but remains at a constant and low amount with silicone hydrogel lenses. Dumbleton *et al.* (2001) also report that there is no corneal neovascularization with silicone hydrogel lenses after nine months of wear and that moderate neovascularization develops in conventional hydrogel lens wearers after two to three months of EW. A study that assessed the amount of vascularization in a group of patients who had previously worn DSCLs and who were refitted with silicone hydrogel lenses showed that silicone hydrogel lens wear results in the emptying of limbal blood vessels over time (Figure 6.9).

These results strongly suggest the use of silicone hydrogels for those patients with high refractive corrections where peripheral lens thickness is greater. These patients are prone, as a result of reduced Dk/t in the periphery, to develop neovascularization.

Epithelial microcysts

Epithelial microcysts are small (15–50 µm), irregular-shaped inclusions usually found in the paracentral to mid-peripheral zones of the cornea in an annular

Figure 6.10   Appearance of microcysts

pattern (Zantos and Holden, 1978; Humphreys *et al.*, 1980; Zantos, 1983; Holden *et al.*, 1987; Holden and Sweeney, 1991). Microcysts are best observed with retro-illumination. They show reversed illumination and thus are believed to have a higher refractive index than the surrounding tissue. Microcysts have been described as accumulated cellular debris (Zantos, 1983), degenerated epithelial cells (Humphreys *et al.*, 1980; Bergmanson, 1987) or apoptotic cells (Madigan, 1989) (Figure 6.10).

Holden *et al.* (1987) have shown that the overnight corneal oedema during EW is closely related to development of epithelial microcysts. That is, the lower the Dk/t of the lens, the higher the overnight oedema and the greater the number of microcysts (Figure 6.11).

A mechanism has been proposed for development of microcysts involving a reduction in the rate of epithelial cell mitosis and an increase in the regeneration time of the epithelium (Holden *et al.*, 1985). Impaired cellular synthesis and waste removal are features related to altered metabolism. With cessation of lens wear the number of microcysts increases within two to three months before it decreases significantly. The increase in microcyst numbers after discontinuation of lens wear (Figure 6.12), a 'rebound effect', may be related to the return to normal epithelial metabolism and mitotic rate and subsequent accelerated removal of encapsulated cellular matter (Holden *et al.*, 1985).

In clinical trials microcysts are used as the classic marker of hypoxia. They can occur in low numbers with DW of DSCLs (Epstein and Donnenfeld, 1989;

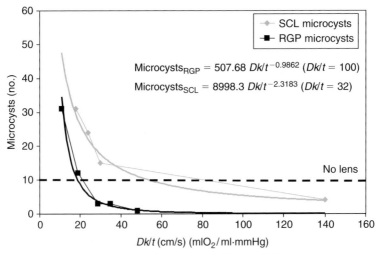

Figure 6.11   Relationship between microcysts and Dk/t for RGP and soft lenses

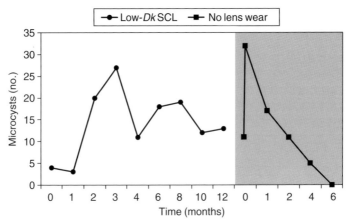

Figure 6.12   Time course for the induction of microcysts and their elimination after cessation of SCL EW

Grant, 1991; Holden and Sweeney, 1991; Efron and Veys, 1992) and even with spectacles (Ruben, 1976; Hickson and Papas, 1997) but are usually observed in significant numbers after two to three months of EW lens wear. Typically, patients with epithelial microcysts are asymptomatic and the microcysts have no effect on vision. No relationships between the number of microcysts and adverse inflammatory or infectious responses during hydrogel EW have been reported (Holden and Sweeney, 1991).

In CCLRU clinical trials microcysts are observed using 16× magnification with an optic section that is swept across the cornea. Significantly lower numbers of microcysts are seen in silicone hydrogel lens wearers compared with the numbers

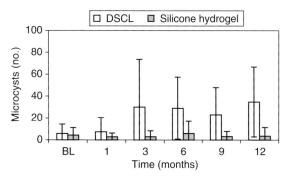

Figure 6.13   Microcyst numbers with DSCL and silicone hydrogel materials across a 12-month period

observed with DSCLs. In our long-term study we have found that the number of microcysts observed with silicone hydrogels remains at the levels observed with spectacle wearers for over three years and that there are no differences in the numbers of microcysts observed in subjects on six- or 30-night wear schedules. In comparison, the number of microcysts significantly increases with time in EW with DSCLs (Figure 6.13).

When the number of microcysts is followed in patients who have been refitted with CW silicone hydrogel lenses following long-term wear of DSCLs on an EW basis, there is a spike in the number of microcysts within the first weeks of wear of silicone hydrogels. The number of microcysts then reduces to the levels seen with spectacle wearers over about three months (Keay *et al.*, 2000) (Figure 6.14). These findings confirm that wearers of low Dk/t lenses who are exposed to a significant increase in oxygen (either by no contact lens wear or by wearing high-Dk/t lenses) can experience a 'rebound' effect characterized by an increase in the number of microcysts for a month or so, during which epithelial metabolism presumably returns to a more normal level. This 'rebound' effect is observed in 50 per cent of patients (Keay *et al.*, 2000).

Corneal staining

Corneal epithelial staining occurs when fluorescein penetrates damaged cell membranes or when it fills gaps in the epithelial cell surface that are created when cells are damaged or displaced. A break in the protective epithelial layer presumably increases the possibility of corneal infection, particularly during EW/CW. The integrity of the epithelium should therefore be assessed carefully at each contact lens aftercare visit.

In CCLRU trials biomicroscopic examination and assessment of the type, depth and extent of staining of the cornea are performed after a single instillation of fluorescein. The cobalt blue light source is used in conjunction with a Wratten 12 filter over the objective lens.

In the CCLRU grading system for corneal staining (Table 6.4), the corneal surface is divided into five zones of approximately equal area. Grade 2 or more in any

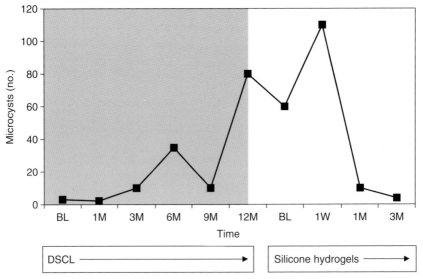

Figure 6.14   Rebound effect in microcyst response observed when a patient is refitted with silicone hydrogel lenses after 12 months' wear of low-Dk/t DSCLs

area is considered unacceptable staining. To assess the depth of staining, the time since first instillation of fluorescein should be noted. Depth of staining should be assessed using a fine optic section and high magnification under white light.

It should be noted that 20 per cent of asymptomatic non-lens wearers will exhibit corneal staining (Norn, 1972). Contact lens wear results in mechanical and biochemical disruption of the anterior epithelium, which is evidenced clinically as corneal staining. A number of causes of corneal staining have been reported during lens wear: hypoxia, deposits, care products, lens fit, lens surface or edge irregularities, foreign bodies and tear film disruption, to name but a few. Hamano *et al.* (1994) conducted an extensive review of complications, including corneal staining with conventional and DSCLs, and reported a frequency between 0.2 and 3.5 per cent of eyes examined. Jalbert *et al.* (1996) found the levels of staining with DSCLs used on either a DW or EW basis to be low.

The levels of corneal staining in our DSCL group and in our six- and 30-night CW silicone hydrogel groups are low. However, in any of these groups there are occasions when severe corneal staining (patch staining with stromal glow or very occasional full-thickness corneal erosions) occurs.

Inferior corneal staining (Figure 6.15) is usually attributed to lens dehydration and typically appears as 'snowflakes' on the cornea with either punctate or coalescent punctate staining as a result of localized areas of dehydration on the corneal surface. This type of staining is often exacerbated by mid-water-content DSCLs and is lower with silicone hydrogels, possibly because of their lower water content (Figure 6.16). The lower levels of inferior staining with silicone hydrogels may be related to the better end-of-day comfort that is reported with these lenses compared with DSCLs.

Table 6.4   CCLRU grading system for corneal staining

Grade	Description
Extent	
0	Absent
1	1–15% surface involvement
2	16–30% surface involvement
3	31–45% surface involvement
4	46% or greater surface involvement
Depth	
0	Absent
1	Superficial epithelial involvement
2	Stromal glow present
3	Immediate localized stromal glow
4	Immediate diffuse stromal glow
Type	
0	Absent
1	Micropunctate
2	Macropunctate
3	Coalescent macropunctate
4	Patch

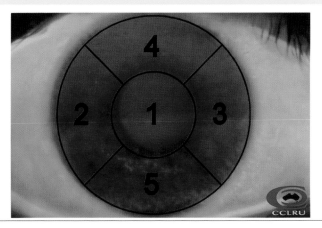

In contrast, Morgan and Efron (2002b) report high levels of corneal staining with silicone hydrogels and suggest that these levels are higher than the staining observed in their patients who wear conventional DW hydrogels. They attribute the higher degree of corneal staining that they find with silicone hydrogels to the potentially greater impact of these lenses on the eye. The evidence put forward for the greater impact is the relatively stiffer modulus of silicone hydrogel materials and the epithelial 'depressions' or microtrauma (Pritchard *et al.*, 2000) associated with mucin balls (see Figure 6.30). Another phenomenon that results in staining and that is attributed to the potentially greater impact of silicone hydrogel lenses on the corneal surface is superior epithelial arcuate lesions (SEALs: Chapter 7).

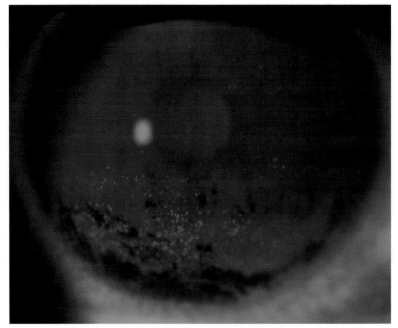

Figure 6.15   Typical inferior corneal staining observed with DSCLs

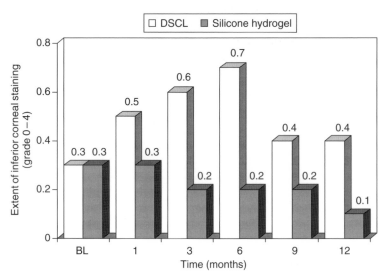

Figure 6.16   Levels of inferior corneal staining observed with DSCL and silicone hydrogel wearers

A recent study has also suggested that incompatibility of the silicone hydrogel lens materials with care solutions may result in increased levels of corneal staining with DW of silicone hydrogels. Jones *et al.* (2002) report that certain multi-purpose care systems that contain polyaminopropyl biguanide can potentially

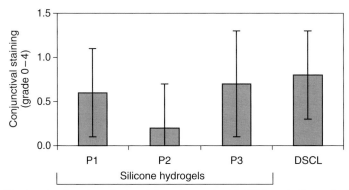

Figure 6.17   Levels of conjunctival staining observed with DSCL and silicone hydrogels

cause significant levels of corneal staining when they are used in conjunction with balafilcon lenses. However, the use of hydrogen peroxide or polyquad systems eliminates these staining problems.

Conjunctival staining

During clinical trials at the CCLRU, conjunctival staining is recorded on the standard 0–4 scale. It is assessed under cobalt blue light with a Wratten filter following the instillation of fluorescein.

There have been isolated reports in which bulbar conjunctival staining is proposed as a basis for comparison of contact lenses or as an indicator of contact lens compatibility with the eye (Seger and Mutti, 1988; Devries *et al.*, 1989; Robboy and Cox, 1991). In general, however, little attention is paid to conjunctival staining. Lakkis and Brennan (1996) reported that 48 out of 50 control non-lens-wearing patients had some degree of conjunctival staining and suggested that fine punctate conjunctival staining is physiological rather than pathological. They further proposed that only staining with a grading of three or above be regarded as clinically significant, since their control patients had staining equivalent to Grade 1 or 2. The higher levels of staining they observed with contact lens wearers was attributed to increased lens dryness during wear and the mechanical effect of the lens itself. Robboy and Cox (1991) suggested that reduced tear film quality predisposed lens wearers to conjunctival staining. Furthermore, the considerably greater conjunctival damage seen with RGP lens wear also appears to be of little consequence.

CCLRU studies indicate that the level of conjunctival staining with silicone hydrogels is low and occurs at levels similar to DSCLs (Figure 6.17). Conjunctival staining with silicone hydrogels primarily appears to be edge-induced (Figure 6.18) and does not worsen over time.

Palpebral conjunctiva

The level of redness and roughness of the upper palpebral conjunctiva is assessed at every aftercare visit at the CCLRU. The eyelids are everted and viewed at

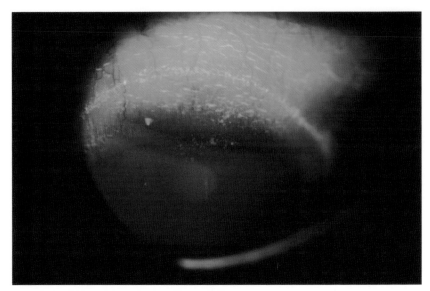

Figure 6.18   Edge-induced conjunctival staining

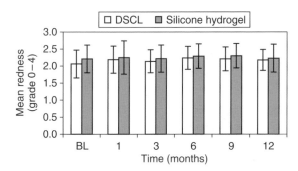

Figure 6.19   Levels of palpebral redness observed with DSCLs and silicone hydrogels

low to moderate magnification. Instillation of fluorescein aids in the assessment of palpebral roughness. With lens wear, levels of both redness and roughness increase to slight or moderate levels. Similar increases are observed across time for both silicone hydrogels and DSCLs in our studies (Figures 6.19 and 6.20).

Although both general and local events of CLPC have been observed with silicone hydrogels, these lenses are associated with greater numbers of localized events (Skotnitsky *et al.*, 2002). The aetiology of CLPC is unclear, but preliminary evidence indicates that the initial steps leading to local CLPC are primarily driven by mechanical factors. In contrast, general CLPC appears to be associated with surface deposits that potentially expose the conjunctival membrane to antigen and initiate a hypersensitivity reaction (Molinari, 1983).

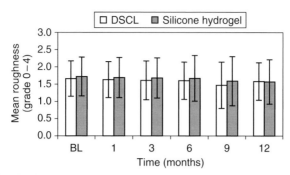

Figure 6.20   Levels of palpebral roughness observed with DSCLs and silicone hydrogels

OVERALL PHYSIOLOGICAL PERFORMANCE

The results from CCLRU and other studies all confirm that many of the short- or long-term hypoxic effects seen with EW in the past have been overcome with silicone hydrogel lenses.

We conducted a prospective, masked assessment of two groups of age- and sex-matched patients; 16 had worn silicone hydrogels for an average of nine months on a 30-night wear schedule and 16 were non-lens wearers (Covey *et al.*, 2001). No significant differences could be found in the classic markers of hypoxic stress – epithelial microcysts, endothelial polymegethism or limbal hyperaemia – for these two groups. As expected, levels of corneal and, in particular, conjunctival staining were greater in the silicone hydrogel lens-wearing group.

LENS PERFORMANCE

FITTING PERFORMANCE

Assessment of silicone hydrogel lens fit is conducted with the same standard protocol used for DSCLs (Table 6.5). Corneal coverage in primary and lateral gaze, movement in the primary gaze position and behaviour with the push-up test (Young *et al.*, 1993) are assessed with diffuse white light and a 16× graticule. The fit assessment of silicone hydrogel lenses can be performed as soon as five minutes or so after insertion, as long as there is no lacrimation or reflex tearing. These materials are less susceptible to tear-induced change than has been reported with ionic materials because of their low water content.

In CCLRU studies we reviewed the number of patients who were unable to be fitted with DSCLs and silicone hydrogel contact lens prototypes. With the DSCLs, the main reasons for failure were insufficient limbal coverage and instability. More subtle fitting issues such as edge lifting or fluting were observed with the silicone hydrogel lenses (Figure 6.21). Edge lift or fluting may be intermittent and is best observed by watching the lens edge move over the inferior limbal area. Fluorexon may help with the detection of these phenomena. Edge lift does not

Table 6.5   CCLRU lens fit grading system

Grade	Description
Corneal coverage	
2	Full corneal coverage
1	Corneal coverage but lens decentres to limbus
0	Incomplete corneal coverage
Tightness (push–up)	
0%	Falls from cornea without lid support
100%	No movement
50%	Optimum
Acceptance rating	
0	Should not be worn
1	Should not be dispensed although no immediate danger
2	May be dispensed but should be reviewed the following day
3	Not perfect but would be adequate to dispense
4	Perfect

After Young *et al.* (1993).

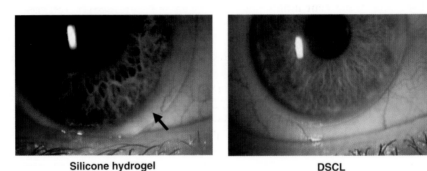

Silicone hydrogel   **DSCL**

Figure 6.21   Edge buckling commonly observed in an unsuccessful fit of silicone hydrogels. Poor corneal coverage is generally the reason for an unsuccessful fit with DSCLs

reduce or settle with wear and will result in reduced comfort. If lens fluting is observed the patient should not be fitted with lenses. As well as aiding the assessment of edge lift, fluorexon will allow the practitioner to observe any transition zones with silicone hydrogels. Hard transition zones may result in problems such as SEALs (see Chapter 7) and should be avoided. Our data suggest that a similar percentage of the population will achieve a successful fit with silicone hydrogel lenses as with DSCLs.

Dumbleton *et al.* (2002) have reported that 98 per cent of 95 subjects obtain a satisfactory initial fit (less edge fluting) and initial subjective comfort response with the two base curves that are available for lotrafilcon A. The study suggests that a lens with a steeper base curve might be the first choice for patients with steep keratometry readings over 45.50 D. However, for CW especially, maximizing movement and potential tear exchange without a detrimental effect on comfort should be the objective.

Primary gaze movement

The amount of post-blink lens movement is measured in primary gaze. Measurements are made by observing the inferior lens edge and gently moving the lower lid to aid viewing if necessary.

Owing to the higher rigidity of silicone-based materials, lenses exhibit approximately 0.3 mm of movement in primary gaze whereas DSCLs exhibit approximately 0.2 mm. This increase in lens movement may facilitate or increase tear exchange. However, whether significant clinical consequences, as a result of this increase, will be observed with silicone hydrogel lenses is not yet known (Chapter 3).

Lens tightness

The push-up test provides a means of gauging lens tightness in terms of the ease of upward displacement when the lower lid is moved against the lens edge. Tightness is rated on a continuous scale from 0 to 100 per cent. Fifty per cent is considered optimum, 100 per cent indicates a lens that is almost impossible to dislodge and 0 per cent indicates a lens that is so loose that it slides from the cornea when the lids retract. Martin *et al.* (1989) have shown this subjective measurement to be fairly reproducible. The overall acceptability of fit is subjectively assessed on a 0–4 scale. Lenses graded between three or four are regarded as being optimal fits.

A lens that is rated as slightly loose, i.e. one that maintains corneal coverage but has a tightness rating of slightly less than 50 per cent, is seen as desirable for both EW and CW. The distribution of lens fits according to percentage tightness ratings observed in the 12-month clinical trials for silicone hydrogel and DSCLs is presented in Figure 6.22. There are no differences between the groups and over half of the fits have a tightness rating between 40 and 50 per cent.

Lens adherence

The binding of lenses to the cornea has been observed with both RGP (Gasson, 1977; Lippman, 1978; Levy, 1985; Zantos and Zantos, 1985; Swarbrick and Holden, 1987) and silicone elastomer lenses (Blackhurst, 1985), and is a major factor that has limited the clinical acceptance of silicone elastomer lenses. The binding of silicone lenses has been reported in relation to complications including corneal ulceration as well as acute inflammatory reactions. Closed-eye hydrogel lens wear frequently leads to lens binding and may be associated with stipple or punctate fluorescein staining (Kenyon *et al.*, 1988; Lin and Mandell, 1991). In a study where subjects wore a hydrogel lens in one eye and a RGP lens in the other, Kenyon *et al.* (1988) reported that either lens type adhered to 48 per cent of eyes on eye opening. Normal movement patterns are gradually established after eye opening so that binding is not usually observed clinically. Patients may only

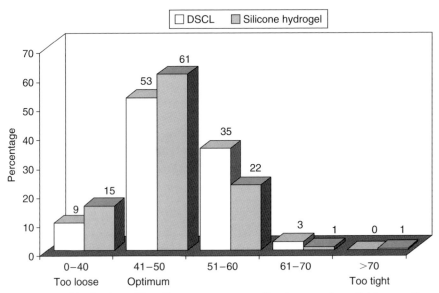

Figure 6.22 Distribution of lens fit assessment according to percentage tightness ratings

become aware of the condition if they need to remove their lenses soon after eye opening. Bruce and Brennan (1992) have suggested that binding occurs when there is a decrease in aqueous content of the post-lens tear film, rendering it viscous and adhesive. Persistent adherence of hydrogel lenses can trap debris behind the lens and potentially provoke a CLARE reaction (Mertz and Holden, 1981).

During the initial assessment of experimental silicone hydrogel lenses, binding was observed and was associated with significant peripheral corneal staining (Austen *et al.*, 1996). However, we did not find any occurrence of lenses adhering to patients' eyes during our long-term clinical trials with silicone hydrogels. CCLRU overnight studies show that the new silicone-based hydrogels typically resume movement 5–10 minutes after eye opening, which is very similar behaviour to that of DSCLs.

Routine instillation of two to three drops of sterile, unpreserved saline after overnight lens wear is recommended to all our patients in clinical trials. We believe this acts to initiate lens movement and flush debris from behind the lens. Approximately 50 per cent of our patients find this saline rinse beneficial. A saline rinse is also recommended in the evening, before sleep, to aid the flushing of back surface debris from beneath the lens.

OVERALL LENS FIT

CW should not be considered unless a comfortable lens fit can be achieved. With an optimum fitting there is 0.2–0.3 mm of primary gaze lens movement with good corneal coverage in all directions of gaze. The lens should be slightly loose (i.e. 45–50 per cent) on push-up and no edge lift should be observed. In our experience, lens fit does not alter with time and so a lens that does not fit well or is not comfortable after initial settling should not be dispensed. Unlike RGPs, lens adaptation does not occur and the fit will remain unsuccessful.

SURFACE PERFORMANCE

LENS WETTABILITY

The CCLRU scale for assessing lens wettability is a subjective assessment made after observations at the slit-lamp. It takes into account the pattern in which tears break over the contact lens, the speed of break-up, the stability of the tear film, the lipid layer appearance and the non-invasive break-up time (NIBUT). The grading scale (Table 6.6) was designed around two benchmarks. The first is the wettability of the healthy corneal epithelium (Grade 5) which typically has a NIBUT greater than 30 seconds and has a stable, even lipid layer. The second is the wettability of hydroxyethyl methacrylate (HEMA) lenses which typically have a NIBUT of 5–7 seconds (Guillon and Guillon, 1993) and is Grade 2 on our scale. Our clinical observers review video footage of tear film stability to establish concordance and standardization of this scale.

The silicone hydrogel prototypes all display very similar surface wettability to that observed with DSCLs. The wettabilities observed across a 12-month period for silicone hydrogels and DSCLs are shown in Figure 6.23.

DEPOSITS

Front and back surface deposits

Both front and back surface deposition are generally low after one week of DSCL wear. The levels observed with the silicone hydrogel lenses are also low regardless of a six- or 30-night wear schedule (Figures 6.24 and 6.25).

Biochemical analyses have shown that silicone hydrogel lenses have significantly lower levels of protein deposition compared to disposable hydrogels (McKenney et al., 1998; Jones et al., 2003) and higher levels of lipid. Interestingly it has been shown that the degree of lysozyme denaturation on silicone hydrogel lenses is higher compared to ionic lenses (Jones et al., 2003). This may have an impact on the development of CLPC with silicone hydrogel lenses.

Table 6.6   CCLRU front surface wettability grading scale

Grade	Description
0	Totally hydrophilic (non-wetting)
1	Non-wetting patches immediately after blinking
2	Appearance equivalent to the HEMA surface
3	More wettable than the HEMA surface
4	Appearance approaching that of normal healthy corneas
5	Appearance equivalent to normal healthy corneas

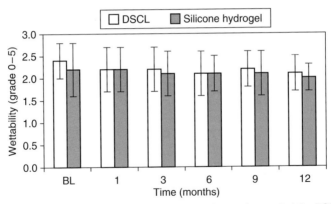

Figure 6.23 Front surface wettability across 12-month wearing period for DSCLs and silicone hydrogels. The low-*Dk* lenses are approximately six nights old, while the silicone hydrogel lenses are approximately 30 nights old

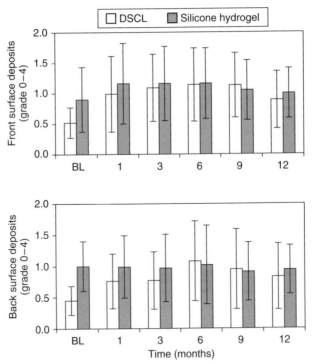

Figure 6.24 Front surface and back surface deposit levels observed with DSCL and silicone hydrogels

Film and globules

The greater interaction of silicone hydrogels with both the tear film and the anterior ocular surface is in part due to the composition of the lens materials. A manifestation

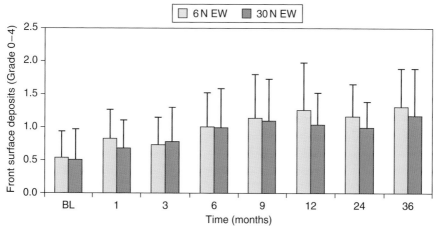

Figure 6.25   Front surface deposit levels observed with six-night (6N) and 30-night (30N) silicone hydrogel lens wear across time

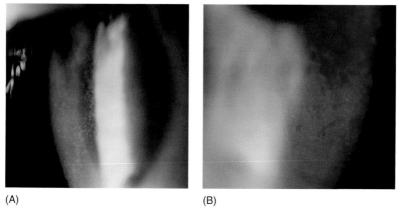

(A)   (B)

Figure 6.26   Appearance of haze and globule-type deposits on (A) a DSCL and (B) a silicone hydrogel lens

of the interaction between silicone hydrogels and the cornea is the appearance of characteristic deposits which we have termed 'haze' and 'globules'. These deposits are whitish in colour and either form a haze or film on the lens surface or appear as discrete globules (Figure 6.26). Both front and back surfaces may be affected and biochemical analyses in our laboratory suggest that the deposits are primarily lipid in composition.

These deposits, however, are not limited to silicone hydrogels, as similar deposits have also been observed with DSCLs. In CCLRU studies, a greater percentage of patients wearing silicone hydrogel lenses display these types of deposits than those wearing disposable lenses and generally there is no difference in the levels of film or globule deposition between DSCL and silicone hydrogel

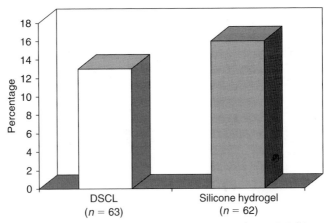

Figure 6.27 Percentage of lenses with greater than Grade 1 (very slight) haze or globule deposition

lenses. The percentage of lenses seen with greater than Grade 1 film/haze and globules on either surface for both lens groups is shown in Figure 6.27.

These deposits may interfere with vision but the build-up usually takes several days before becoming noticeable to the patient. Occasionally, however, more rapid accumulation may occur, requiring intervention after only several hours of lens wear. Cleaning with a surfactant is sufficient to remove the deposits and restore vision.

In our experience some patients are more susceptible to the development of this type of deposit. Such patients are advised to remove and clean their lenses as frequently as required. Wear schedule does not appear to impact the occurrence of these deposits significantly.

Mucin balls

Mucin balls, pre-corneal deposits or lipid plugs have been described with both hydrogel and RGP lens materials (Fleming *et al.*, 1994). It has been suggested that because hydrogel lenses drape the cornea and allow little post-lens tear exchange (Polse, 1979) they entrap by-products of corneal metabolism, exfoliated epithelial cells and debris in the post-lens tear film. Mucin balls are round and vary in size and clarity. The smaller 'deposits' are generally 10–20 μm in diameter and are typically translucent. Larger mucin balls, 20–50 μm in diameter, tend to appear opalescent (Figure 6.28). The 'deposits' may be either scattered or clumped and are generally observed in the superior quadrant of the cornea beneath the resting position of the upper eyelid.

Mucin balls can be observed within minutes of lens insertion (Figure 6.29). They increase in number and size in the initial stages of lens wear. Mucin balls appear to be trapped against the corneal surface because they do not move as the lens moves. Lens removal and/or subsequent blinking causes them to dislodge and

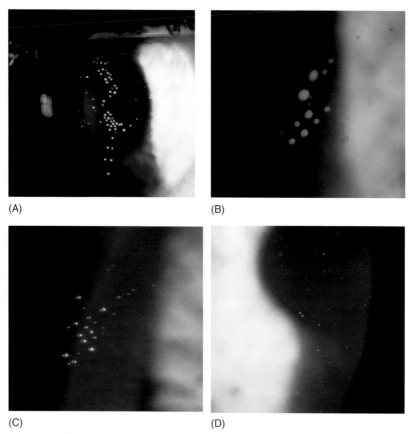

Figure 6.28   (A) Scattered translucent mucin balls; (B) clumped translucent mucin balls; (C) clumped opalescent mucin balls; (D) opalescent mucin balls

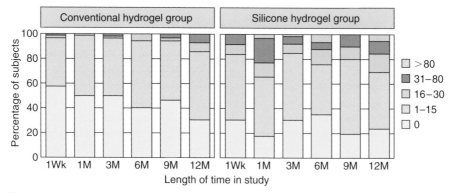

Figure 6.29   Frequency of subjects with mucin balls after one year of EW in the conventional and silicone hydrogel groups

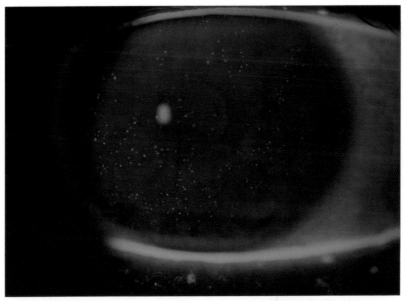

Figure 6.30   Indentations in the corneal surface as a result of mucin balls beneath a silicone hydrogel lens

leaves an indentation in the corneal surface which resolves rapidly (Figure 6.30). Confocal microscopy examination shows that mucin balls appear to indent both the overlying contact lens and the underlying cornea well below the level of the surrounding Bowman's layer (Jalbert *et al.*, 2003).

Mucin balls tend to be patient-specific and have been observed in both adapted and non-adapted patients. Patients with mucin balls are totally asymptomatic. Although it is suggested that mucin balls may need to be managed by changing the lens type or by introducing more frequent overnight lens removals during EW/CW (Fleming *et al.*, 1994), our clinical trial experience with silicone hydrogels suggests that there is no link between the appearance of mucin balls and adverse responses of any nature. Pritchard *et al.* (2000) have reported one case where mucin balls were found embedded within the epithelium of a patient without further consequence. Similar numbers of mucin balls occur in patients on both six- and 30-night wear schedules with silicone hydrogels (Figure 6.31).

Mucin balls are different from corneal staining and other contact lens-related features at the corneal surface such as 'corneal blotting' (Lin and Mandell, 1991), micro-deposits (Bourassa and Benjamin, 1988) and dimple veiling. They should not be confused with either epithelial microcysts or epithelial vacuoles. Vacuoles described by Zantos (1983) are fluid-filled vesicles which vary in size from 20 to 50 μm. They are almost circular, intra-epithelial inclusions that show unreversed illumination, which indicates that they are of a lower refractive index than the surrounding tissue (Figure 6.32). Zantos (1981) reported an incidence of 32 per cent of vacuoles in his CW patients.

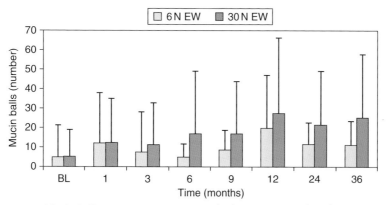

Figure 6.31   Mucin ball numbers with six-night (6N) and 30-night (30N) silicone hydrogel lens wear across time

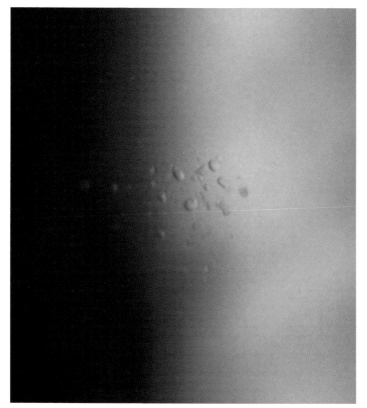

Figure 6.32   Epithelial vacuoles

Biochemical analyses of mucin balls that have been collected by corneal washing indicate that the deposits are composed mainly of mucin and tear proteins and have little lipid content (Fleming *et al.*, 1994). These results prompted the renaming of this phenomenon, which was classically termed 'lipid plugs'. Mucin balls absorb fluorescein but do not stain with rose bengal, which suggests that there is no coexisting disturbance of the integrity of the corneal surface (Feenstra and Tseng, 1992).

Studies by Dumbleton *et al.* (2000) and Tan *et al.* (2003) indicate that a higher incidence of mucin balls can be observed in patients with steep corneas. This suggests that together with the stiffness of the silicone hydrogels, the mismatch in fit between the lens and cornea contributes to the formation of mucin balls.

Mucin balls have been hypothesized to result from interactions between the lens surface and the corneal epithelium and occur in a variety of distributions and densities with both DSCLs and silicone hydrogels. Generally, higher numbers are observed with silicone hydrogels although, as stated, certain individuals tend to be predisposed, regardless of lens type. Reports have suggested that higher numbers are observed with lotrafilcon A than with balafilcon A lenses (Dumbleton *et al.*, 2000; Morgan and Efron, 2002b). We have noted that altering the composition of a surface treatment can affect the number of mucin balls observed with a particular material substrate, indicating that it is not the modulus of the lens material alone that accounts for the interaction with the lens and anterior ocular surface.

OTHER DEPOSITS AND SURFACE DURABILITY

Jelly bumps and calcium deposits have been reported to occur with silicone hydrogels (Fonn *et al.*, 2000).

Our clinical experience indicates that there are no concerns with the durability of coatings when lenses are replaced according to manufacturers' guidelines (i.e. monthly).

For example, a 19-year-old patient in a clinical trial who was non-compliant with instructions reported for a follow-up visit where the right lens had been worn for 90 days and the left for 40 days without replacement. The front surface ratings for deposits were very low (0.8, 0.5 respectively, 0–4 CCLRU gradings), while comfort was excellent (95) and there were no clinically significant ocular signs.

Back surface debris

Back surface debris is observed routinely in patients on an EW regime (Pritchard and Fonn, 1998), particularly at early-morning visits. Mertz and Holden (1981) suggest that entrapped debris may be responsible for inflammatory reactions observed with EW and this debris has also been implicated in corneal infections. Increased levels of microflora during EW (Willcox *et al.*, 1995; Holden *et al.*, 1996), reduced tear film thickness and the increased susceptibility of the epithelium to bind to bacteria when under chronic hypoxic stress (Imayasu *et al.*, 1994) may also contribute to these reactions.

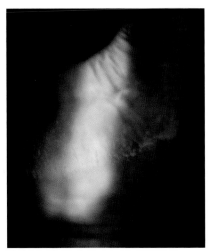

Figure 6.33   Typical appearance of back surface debris with contact lens wear

Back surface debris appears as greyish-white amorphous material (Figure 6.33). The material will move as the lens moves but if substantial amounts are accumulated it can result in corneal staining.

The levels of back surface debris observed with silicone hydrogels worn for either six or 30 nights consecutively are similar to those observed with the low-*Dk* materials worn for six nights and in both cases the levels are low.

ADVERSE RESPONSES

Adverse responses, their clinical manifestation and management are presented in Chapter 7. Inflammatory events have been observed with silicone hydrogels and include the infiltrative events such as CLPU, CLARE, infiltrative keratitis (IK) and asymptomatic infiltrates (AI).

Mechanically mediated ocular complications such as SEALs, erosions and CLPC occur with a greater frequency with silicone hydrogels compared to conventional hydrogels. These differences in mechanically induced events between lens types are likely to be caused by the differences in the way the lenses interact with the cornea. Silicone hydrogel materials are slightly more rigid than conventional polymers and it is anticipated that lenses made from these different types of materials will have different pressure profiles.

Solomon *et al.* (1994) demonstrated a link between the level of oedema and rates of infection in an animal model. Whether reducing oedema translates to a reduction in the rate of corneal infection for human contact lens wearers will not be known until the post-marketing surveillance studies have been conducted with silicone hydrogel lenses. To date, preliminary information suggests that the risk of MK with EW/CW is lower with silicone hydrogels compared to conventional hydrogels (Holden *et al.*, 2003).

SUBJECTIVE RESPONSES, REFRACTIVE ERROR AND COMPLIANCE

COMFORT

At aftercare visits at the CCLRU, patients rate lens comfort on a scale from 1 to 100, where 1 indicates that the lens causes pain and 100 indicates that the lens cannot be felt at all. Patients are asked to rate their comfort overall, on waking, during the day and at the end of the day.

Ocular discomfort is the chief cause of dissatisfaction and patient dropout from contact lens wear (du Toit *et al.*, 2003). According to the standards suggested by Terry *et al.* (1993), a successful patient must consistently experience comfort equivalent to a rating of 60 or better both immediately on insertion and throughout the period of wear. The patient must report only occasional lens awareness that abates without the need for lens removal.

Overall, both silicone hydrogel and DSCL lenses are very comfortable when worn on their respective schedules. Although comfort in both groups reduces towards the end of the day, end-of-day comfort is significantly higher with silicone hydrogel lenses. We have postulated that this is associated with reduced levels of dehydration with silicone hydrogel materials and is evidenced by the lower levels of inferior corneal staining during wear.

Comfort is lower on awakening for both silicone hydrogel and hydrogel groups relative to average daytime levels. This may be associated with early-morning dryness. Early-morning dryness is believed to be associated with lens dehydration and the reduction in aqueous tears during sleep, which creates a relatively dry environment (Baum and Barza, 1990) or may be associated with changes in tear composition.

SYMPTOMATOLOGY

The aetiologies and mechanisms of the symptoms reported as 'dryness' by contact lens wearers are not well understood. Dryness is a persistent complaint of symptomatic contact lens wearers. Brennan and Efron (1989) reported that only 25 per cent of wearers never experience the symptom.

Vajdic *et al.* (1999) conducted a survey of prospective volunteers for contact lens clinic trials at the CCLRU. Questions pertaining to lens wear experience and ocular symptoms were answered by 883 untrained individuals without active ocular disease. The group included 48 current RGP wearers, 171 current soft lens wearers and 664 spectacle wearers. The frequencies of 10 ocular symptoms (dryness, redness, grittiness, itchiness, aching, tiredness, watering, burning, pain and excessive blinking) were compared for each group. Contact lens wearers experienced the same type and severity of symptoms as non-contact lens wearers. This is puzzling since ocular discomfort is the primary reason for discontinuation of lens wear. SCL and RGP wearers reported significantly more ocular redness and dryness than spectacle wearers.

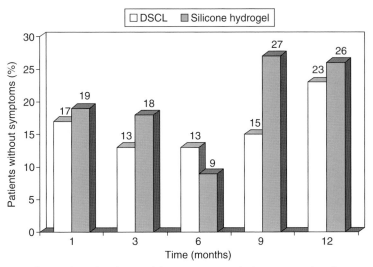

Figure 6.34 Proportion of patients with no symptoms during 12 months of lens wear

During the course of all our clinical trials, patients are surveyed at each visit for symptoms, in particular blurred vision, halos/flare, photophobia, burning/sting-ing, itching, dryness, lens awareness, tearing, unusual secretions, redness and other miscellaneous complaints. Patients are required to provide details of when the symp-tom occurred, its frequency, severity, duration and possible cause.

Approximately 20 per cent of patients in CCLRU DSCL and silicone hydro-gel lens trials report no symptoms with their lens wear (Figure 6.34). The types of symptoms that are experienced by patients are similar for both lens types and wear schedules, although silicone hydrogel wearers report fewer symptoms of lens dryness.

VISION

Quality of vision is evaluated by obtaining a rating (1–100) from each patient at all aftercare visits. As a guide, 100 would be taken as 'perfect' or comparable with the best corrected spectacle performance. Similar to comfort, vision is rated at the end of the day, in the morning and overall.

Obviously, visual satisfaction is a high priority for contact lens wearers. Terry *et al.* (1993) suggest that this should be maintained at least to a rating of 60, with no significant blur, visual fluctuation, halos or flare.

Both silicone hydrogel and DSCL lenses give excellent overall vision through-out the day when worn on their respective schedules. When problems are encoun-tered by certain individuals, these are most often associated with lens deposits (in particular with haze and globule-type deposition).

REFRACTIVE ERROR CHANGES

The influences of polymethyl methacrylate (PMMA) (Rengstorff, 1979; Hovding, 1983), RGP (Briceno-Garbi, 1984; Sevigny, 1986) and hydrogel (Grosvenor, 1975; Hovding, 1983) lens wear on corneal curvature are well documented. RGP lenses typically induce slight overall corneal flattening and a reduction in corneal toricity (sphericalization) as a result of more pronounced flattening of the steeper (usually vertical) meridian. The term 'myopic creep' has been used to refer to the need for increased minus power in subjects wearing DW or EW hydrogel contact lenses (Caroline and Campbell, 1991; Edmonds, 1993). Corneal changes during hydrogel lens wear include an initial flattening followed by gradual steepening as lens wear continues. Both mechanical moulding of the cornea toward the back surface of the lens and lens-induced oedema have been suggested as causes (Rengstorff, 1979).

According to Terry *et al.* (1993), contact lens-induced refractive changes should not exceed ±0.50 D sphere and ±0.75 D cyl.

In CCLRU studies, monocular subjective refractions are performed to achieve the minimum negative power consistent with best VA. Binocular adjustments are not made. All refractions are done in the spectacle plane and adjusted for vertex distance where necessary. Baseline refractions are performed after a minimum of 12 hours without lens wear, while follow-up refractions occur shortly after lens removal.

EW of disposable low-*Dk* hydrogel lenses induces a myopic shift of about −0.25 D after 12 months of wear in new contact lens wearers. By comparison, 30-night CW of silicone hydrogel contact lenses does not appear to affect refraction in neophytes significantly. Long-term wearers of DSCLs who are refitted with silicone hydrogel contact lenses experience a reduction in myopia in the order of −0.25 D after 12 months of silicone hydrogel wear. Jalbert *et al.* (1999b) have shown the decrease in myopia is associated with corneal flattening, while the increase in myopia is associated with corneal steepening. Similar results for myopic creep have been reported by both Dumbleton *et al.* (1999) and McNally and McKenney (2002). These findings suggest that hypoxia may play a role in any topographical shifts induced by contact lens wear.

COMPLIANCE ISSUES

Wearing time is defined as the number of consecutive days and nights that a patient is able to wear lenses before either a scheduled or unscheduled removal. The length of time that a contact lens can be worn comfortably will be affected by factors such as the build-up of surface deposits, any decrease in lens comfort and the level of overnight oedema. One test of the success of the 30-night modality of lens wear is how successful the patients are in complying with the proposed wear schedule. This is also important because of its impact on lens care and maintenance regimes. Compliance with care and maintenance schedules plays an important role in minimizing complications related to lens wear. With

CW an important issue is how frequently patients must break the 30-night cycle, either just to rub, rinse and immediately reinsert their lenses or to remove lenses for longer periods, possibly involving an overnight break, which means that lenses must be disinfected.

For CCLRU studies, DSCL wearers are instructed to leave their lenses in place for six consecutive nights and silicone hydrogel wearers are instructed to leave their lenses in place for six or 30 nights depending on the trial. Overriding this is the general advice that lenses may be removed at any time should there be a perceived need. This allows the wearer to manage minor episodes of discomfort, dryness or blurred vision as they occur.

More serious problems, such as a red eye, persistent blurred vision or persistent discomfort, may demand prolonged removal and require appropriate lens care strategies. All patients are instructed in these strategies.

In addition, all patients in EW/CW are advised to avoid overnight lens wear if they are unwell or in poor general health. Routine scrutiny of the eyes before sleep and upon awakening is also encouraged to ensure that they:

LOOK GOOD, FEEL GOOD and SEE WELL!

This was first proposed by Yamane and Kuwabara (1987) as part of their patient education programme for ensuring compliance in patients wearing EW contact lenses.

Patients in our clinical studies are asked at each visit if they had to remove their lenses overnight outside their scheduled routine. The majority of patients are able to adhere to their prescribed wear schedule. For all visits combined over a 12-month period, 86 per cent of DSCL wearers and 79 per cent of 30-night silicone hydrogel lens wearers could wear lenses as prescribed with no unscheduled overnight removals, and over 90 per cent of silicone hydrogel patients removed their lenses only once or twice for an overnight break during the 30-night period (Figure 6.35).

Patients are also asked if they had ever needed to remove their lenses temporarily to rinse and/or clean as opposed to overnight removal. The percentage of patients who had removed their lenses at any time outside the schedule is shown in Figure 6.36. Approximately 50 per cent of patients needed to remove their lenses temporarily during their assigned wear schedule.

PATIENT SATISFACTION

We surveyed 74 patients who had worn silicone hydrogel lenses on a CW basis for 12 months or longer. Approximately one-quarter of these patients had not worn contact lenses previously, 45 per cent had previously used DW lenses and the remainder had worn either six-night EW or had used EW lenses intermittently. These patients were asked about their satisfaction with the wear regimens, the best and worst features of the wear system and to suggest any improvements. In addition, they were questioned with regard to their attitudes towards refractive surgery before and after experience with CW contact lenses.

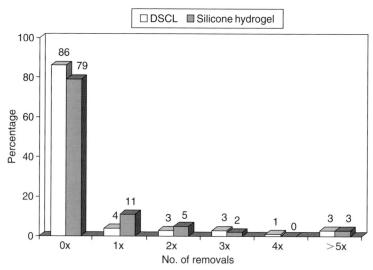

Figure 6.35   Number of overnight removals required by DSCL and silicone hydrogel patients, all visits combined over a 12-month period

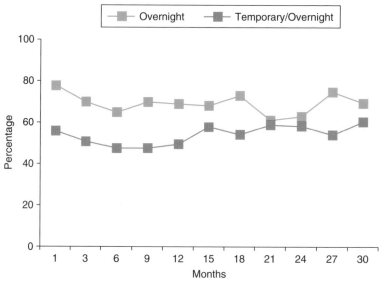

Figure 6.36   Percentage of patients who removed their lenses outside the scheduled routine (overnight and temporary removals)

Patients in the survey were overwhelmingly satisfied with the concept of CW. Ninety-three per cent of patients rated their lens system as excellent. The main reason for their satisfaction with the CW system was its convenience. Factors such as no lens care and maintenance or lens handling (88 per cent), being able to see

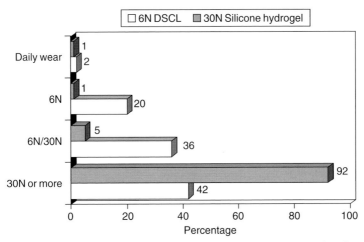

Figure 6.37 Preferred wear option for six-night (6N) DSCL and 30-night (30N) silicone hydrogel EW wearers

in the morning (7 per cent) and excellent comfort (5 per cent) were reported. Ten per cent of patients reported that they forgot that they were wearing lenses at all.

The disadvantages of the lenses were also rated by CW patients. Problems with discomfort (8 per cent) and dryness (38 per cent) persisted even with the lower-water-content materials and 18 per cent of patients wanted to be able to wear their lenses for even longer than one month. Approximately 10 per cent of the group surveyed listed deposits as a disadvantage of their current lenses and 30-night schedule. Problems with deposits which can interfere with the quality of vision and require lenses to be removed and cleaned need to be overcome or reduced. These results indicate the need for further development in the area of true biocompatibility with the ocular environment.

Having worn lenses on a 30-night CW schedule, 50 per cent of these patients indicated that they wished to continue with their 30-night schedule, while 42 per cent indicated that they wanted to be able to wear contact lenses for longer than 30 nights at a time. In comparison, patients on a six-night schedule indicated that they wanted to be able to wear lenses for 30 nights (27 per cent), while fewer sought lens wear for longer than 30 nights (only 16 per cent). This difference (Figure 6.37) in preferred option clearly demonstrates that once the 30-night modality is experienced, patients will demand lenses that can sustain CW.

Before trying CW, 66 per cent of these patients had considered refractive or laser surgery to correct their vision permanently. Following their experience with CW, only a third of these patients still considered refractive surgery and 68 per cent preferred the use of CW contact lenses to provide their vision correction. This again indicates a strong preference for the modality once it has been tried and the patients' need for a convenient form of 'permanent' vision correction are met. Fitting appropriate patients using CW lenses could, therefore, contribute positively to building and maintaining a contact lens practice as well as offering a safer vision alternative for patients.

PERMANENT DISCONTINUATIONS

Jalbert *et al.* (1998) reported a discontinuation rate of 0.8 per cent per patient year with DW, and 19 per cent and 16 per cent respectively for neophytes and experienced patients in EW. In a prospective clinical trial of DSCLs, Sankaridurg *et al.* (1998) showed that non-lens-related discontinuations such as patient relocation and non-compliance occur twice as frequently as lens-related discontinuations such as discomfort, lens deposits and adverse events. Twelve-month CCLRU clinical trials indicate that there are no significant differences in the number of permanent discontinuations between DSCL and silicone hydrogel contact lens wearers. When the classification of discontinuations is broken down further into lens-related versus non-lens-related reasons for permanent discontinuation, we also find no differences in the number of discontinuations between DSCL and silicone hydrogel wearers.

Furthermore, there are no differences in the rates of discontinuation between patients wearing silicone hydrogels on a six- or 30-night wear schedule. After three years, and excluding non-lens-related discontinuations, 80 per cent of patients in both groups were able to continue with their assigned wear schedule.

SUMMARY

The development of silicone hydrogel lenses marks the beginning of a new era for both practitioners and patients. These lenses offer vision and comfort comparable with current DSCLs but have overcome the significant hurdle of hypoxia, so that lenses can be worn for up to 30 days continuously. Our studies have shown that the side effects caused by hypoxia when lenses are worn on a CW basis, such as microcysts, limbal hyperaemia and vascularization, are eliminated regardless of whether a six- or 30-night wear schedule is used. The patient response to lenses and especially to the convenience offered by the flexible wear schedule has been extremely enthusiastic. Unless there is a patient-specific contradiction, performance of silicone hydrogels on a 30-night wear schedule offers patients convenience without deleterious hypoxia-associated effects.

Now that silicone hydrogel lenses have been released on the marketplace, we can begin to test the hypothesis that a healthy epithelium, as a result of the alleviation of hypoxia, will reduce the rates of infection traditionally observed with EW/CW of hydrogel lenses.

FURTHER STEPS REQUIRED

Further developments are needed and manufacturers are still striving to develop the ultimate contact lens. Future strategies may include producing lenses with enhanced designs that are truly biocompatible so that improved comfort, reduced deposition and reduced inflammatory and mechanical events can be offered to the wearer. Antibacterial treatments and solutions may help minimize infections as well as bacterial-driven inflammatory events. This 'Holy Grail' lens will promote a healthy, resistant epithelium. Ideally, the truly safe high-Dk/t biocompatible SCL will allow months of CW before disposal. It should also be durable enough to use for long-term DW in regions such as Asia, where millions of potential wearers would find a reusable contact lens more economically feasible (Swarbrick and Holden, 1999). This lens should truly challenge spectacles and refractive surgery as a means of vision correction.

ACKNOWLEDGEMENT

We would like to acknowledge Eric Papas and Serina Stretton for their helpful comments during the preparation of this chapter.

REFERENCES

Adams, C. P., Cohen, E. J., Laibson, P. R. *et al.* (1983) Corneal ulcers in patients with cosmetic extended-wear contact lenses. *Am. J. Ophthalmol.*, **96**, 705–709

Allegretti, D. (1985) Extended wear lens: blessing or public peril? *Capital Times* (Madison, WI), 3 October

Anon. (1986). A sceptic eye on contacts. *Time*, 27 January, 57

Austen, R., Papas, E., Evans, V. *et al.* (1996) The cat as a model to predict on eye performance of contact lenses in the human. *Invest. Ophthalmol. Vis. Sci.*, **37**, s71

Bailey, I. L., Bullimore, M. A., Raash, T. W. and Taylor, H. R. (1991) Clinical grading and the effects of scaling. *Invest. Ophthalmol. Vis. Sci.*, **32**, 422–432

Barr, J. (1999) The 1998 annual report on contact lenses. *Cont. Lens Spectrum*, January, 25–28

Barr, J. (2003) Contact lenses 2002: annual report. *Cont. Lens Spectrum*, January, 24–31

Baum, J. and Barza, M. (1990) *Pseudomonas* keratitis and extended-wear soft contact lenses. *Arch. Ophthalmol.*, **108**, 663–664

Benjamin, W. J. and Rasmussen, M. A. (1985) The closed lid tear pump: oxygenation? *Int. Eyecare*, **1**, 251–257

Benson, C. (1975) Continuous use of contact lenses. *Aust. J. Ophthalmol.*, **4**, 99

Bergmanson, J. P. G. (1987) Histopathological analysis of the corneal epithelium after contact lens wear. *J. Am. Optom. Assoc.*, **58**, 812–818

Blackhurst, R. T. (1985) Personal experience with hydrogel and silicone extended wear lenses. *J. Cont. Lens Assoc. Ophthalmol.*, **11**, 136–137

Bourassa, S. and Benjamin, W. J. (1988) Transient corneal surface 'micro-deposits' and associated epithelial surface pits occurring with gel contact lens extended wear. *Int. Cont. Lens Clin.*, **15**, 338–340

Brennan, N. A. and Efron, N. (1989) Symptomatology of HEMA contact lens wear. *Optom. Vis. Sci.*, **66**, 834–838

Brezinski, S. D. and Hill, R. M. (1986) The new superpermeables. *Cont. Lens Forum*, November, 22–23

Briceno-Garbi, E. A. (1984) Variations in corneal curvature and refractive error in CAB gas-permeable contact lens wearers. *J. Am. Optom. Assoc.*, **55**, 217–219

Bruce, A. S. and Brennan, N. A. (1992) Hydrogel lens binding and the post-lens tear film. *Clin. Eye Vis. Care*, **4**, 111–116

Bullimore, M. A., Nguyen, M., Bozic, J. and Mitchell, G. L. (2002) Overnight swelling with 7-day continuous wear of soft contact lenses. *Invest. Ophthalmol. Vis. Sci.*, 43, abstract 3100

Caroline, P. and Campbell, R. (1991) Long term effects of hydrophilic contact lenses on myopia. *Cont. Lens Spectrum*, June, 68

Chalupa, E., Swarbrick, H. A., Holden, B. A. and Sjostrand, J. (1987) Severe corneal infections associated with contact lens wear. *Ophthalmology*, **94**, 17–22

Cogan, D. G. (1948) Vascularisation of the cornea: its experimental induction by small lesions and a new theory of its pathogenesis. *Trans. Am. Ophthalmol. Soc.*, **46**, 457–471

Collin, H. B. (1973) Limbal vascular response prior to corneal vascularisation. *Exp. Eye Res.*, **16**, 443–455

Comstock, T., Robboy, M., Cox, I. *et al.* (1999). In *British Contact Lens Association Conference*, Birmingham, May poster available at: http://www.siliconehydrogels.com/, accessed February 2003

Covey, M. A., Papas, E., Austen, R. *et al.* (1995) Limbal vascular response during daily wear of conventional and high *Dk* soft lenses. *Optom. Vis. Sci.*, **72**, 12 (suppl.), 171

Covey, M. A., Sweeney, D. F., Terry, R. L. *et al.* (2001) Hypoxic effects on the anterior eye of high *Dk* soft contact lens wearers are negligible. *Optom Vis. Sci.*, **18**, 95–99

Dallos, J. (1946) Sattler's veil. *Br. J. Ophthalmol.*, **30**, 607

de Carle, J. (1972) Developing hydrophilic lenses for continuous wearing. *Aust. J. Optom.*, **55**, 343–346

Devries, D. K., Lingel, N. J., Patrick, T. C. *et al.* (1989) A clinical evaluation of edge induced conjunctival staining with Acuvue SeeQuence disposable lenses. *Optom. Vis. Sci.*, **66**(suppl.), 115

Dohlman, C. H., Boruchoff, A. and Mobilia, E. F. (1973) Complications in use of soft contact lenses in corneal disease. *Arch. Ophthalmol.*, **90**, 367–371

Donshik, P. C. (1994) Corneal ulceration revisited. *J. Cont. Lens Assoc. Ophthalmol.*, **20**, 86–87

du Toit, R., Simpson, T. and Fonn, D. (1998) Recovery from hyperemia after overnight wear of hydrogel lenses. *Invest. Ophthalmol. Vis. Sci.*, **39**, s336

du Toit, R., Papas, E., Stahl, U. and Sweeney, D. F. (2003) Initial comfort ratings of soft contact lenses. *Invest. Ophthalmol. Vis. Sci.*, **44**, 3696

Duke-Elder, S. (1963) Corneal vascularization. In *System of Ophthalmology*, 2nd edn, vol. VIII. Henry Kimpton, London, pp. 676–691

Dumbleton, K., Richter, D., Simpson, T. and Fonn, D. (1998) A comparison of the vascular response to extended wear of conventional lower *Dk* and experimental high *Dk* hydrogel contact lenses. *Optom. Vis. Sci.*, **75** (suppl.), 170

Dumbleton, K. A., Chalmers, R. L., Richter, D. B. and Fonn, D. (1999) Changes in myopic refractive error in nine months' extended wear of hydrogel lenses with high and low oxygen permeability. *Optom. Vis. Sci.*, **76**, 845–849

Dumbleton, K., Jones, L., Chalmers, R. *et al.* (2000) Clinical characterization of spherical post-lens debris associated with lotrafilcon high-*Dk* silicone lenses. *CLAO J.*, **26**, 186–192

Dumbleton, K., Chalmers, R. L., Richter, D. B. and Fonn, D. (2001) Vascular response to extended wear of hydrogel lenses with high and low oxygen permeability. *Optom. Vis. Sci.*, **78**, 147–151

Dumbleton, K. A., Chalmers, R. L., McNally, J., Bayer, S. and Fonn, D. (2002) Effect of lens basecurve on subjective comfort and assessment of fit with silicone hydrogel continuous wear contact lenses. *Optom. Vis. Sci.*, **79**, 633–637

Edmonds, C. R. (1993) Myopia reduction with frequent replacement of Acuvue lenses. *Int. Cont. Lens Clin.*, **20**, 195–199

Efron, N. (1987) Vascular response of the cornea to contact lens wear. *J. Am. Optom. Assoc.*, **58**, 836–846

Efron, N. and Veys, J. (1992) Defects in disposable contact lenses can compromise ocular integrity. *Int. Cont. Lens Clin.*, **19**, 8–18

Epstein, A. B. and Donnenfeld, E. D. (1989) Epithelial microcysts associated with the Acuvue disposable CL. *Cont. Lens Forum*, **14**, 35

Ezekiel, D. F. (1974) High water content hydrophilic contact lenses. *Aust. J. Optom.*, **57**, 317–324

Feenstra, R. P. G. and Tseng, S. C. G. (1992) Comparison of fluorescein and rose bengal staining. *Ophthalmology*, **99**, 605–617

Fleming, C., Austen, R., Davies, S. *et al.* (1994) Pre-corneal deposits during soft contact lens wear. *Optom. Vis. Sci.*, **71** (suppl.), 152–153

Fonn, D., du Toit, R., Situ, P. *et al.* (1998) Apparent sympathetic response of contralateral non-lens wearing eyes after overnight lens wear in the fellow eye. *Invest. Ophthalmol. Vis. Sci.*, **39**, s336

Fonn, D., du Toit, R., Simpson, T. *et al.* (1999) Sympathetic swelling response of the control eye to soft lenses in the other eye. *Invest Ophthalmol. Vis. Sci.*, **40**, 3116–3121

Fonn, D., Pritchard, N. and Dumbleton, K. (2000) Factors affecting the success of silicone hydrogels. In *Silicone Hydrogels: The Rebirth of Continuous Wear Contact Lenses*, 1st edn (ed. D. F. Sweeney). Butterworth-Heinemann, Oxford, pp. 214–234

Fonn, D., MacDonald, K., Richter, D. *et al.* (2002) The ocular response to extended wear of a high *Dk* silicone hydrogel contact lens. *Clin. Exp. Optom.*, **85**, 176–182

Gasset, A. R. and Kaufman, H. E. (1970) Therapeutic uses of hydrophilic contact lenses. *Am. J. Ophthalmol.*, **69**, 252–259

Gasson, A. (1977) Preliminary observations in fitting Silflex silicone contact lenses. *Optician*, **174** (4509), 7–12

Gleason, W. and Albright, R. A. (2003) Menicon Z 30-day continuous wear lenses: a clinical comparison to Acuvue 7-day extended wear lenses. *Eye Cont. Lens*, **29**, s149–s152

Grant, T. (1991) Clinical aspects of planned replacement and disposable lenses. In *The Contact Lens Year Book* (ed. C. Kerr). Medical and Scientific Publishing, Hythe, UK, p. 7

Grant, T., Chong, M. S., Vajdic, C. *et al.* (1998) Contact lens induced peripheral ulcers (CLPUs) during hydrogel contact lens wear. *J. Cont. Lens Assoc. Ophthalmol.*, **24**, 145–151

Grosvenor, T. (1975) Changes in corneal curvature and subjective refraction of soft contact lens wearers. *Am. J. Optom. Physiol. Opt.*, **52**, 405–413

Guillon, J. P. and Guillon, M. (1993) Tear film examination of the contact lens patient. *Optician*, **206**, 21–29

Gurland, J. E. (1976) Use of silicone lenses in infants and children. *Ophthalmology*, **86**, 1599–1604

Hamano, H. (1974) Continual wearing of soft contact lenses. In *Proceedings of the 1st International Conference on Contact Lenses*, Toyo, Nagoya, October

Hamano, H., Watanabe, K., Hamano, T. *et al.* (1994) A study of the complications induced by conventional and disposable contact lenses. *J. Cont. Lens Assoc. Ophthalmol.*, **20**, 103–108

Harvitt, D. M. and Bonanno, J. A. (1998) Minimum contact lens transmissibility values for daily and extended wear contact lenses. *Optom. Vis. Sci.*, **75**, 12s, 189

Hickson, S. and Papas, E. (1997) Prevalence of idiopathic corneal anomalies in a non-contact lens wearing population. *Optom. Vis. Sci.*, **74**, 293–297

Hill, R. M. and Brezinski, S. D. (1987) The super permeables: an examination of the Bes-Con V, Equalens I, and Optacryl Z. *Cont. Lens Spectrum*, January, 60–61

Hill, R. M., Brezinski, S. and Flynn, W. J. (1985) The rigid 'super-permeables'. *Cont. Lens Forum*, January, 35–39

Hingorani, M., Christie, C. and Buckley, R. J. (1995) Ulcerative keratitis in a person wearing daily disposable contact lenses. *Br. J. Ophthalmol.*, **79**, 1138

Hodd, N. F. B. (1975) Some observations on 62 permanent wear soft lens cases. *Ophthalmic Optician*, **15**, 2–8

Holden, B. A. (1989) The Glenn A. Fry award lecture 1988: the ocular response to contact lens wear. *Optom. Vis. Sci.*, **66**, 717–733

Holden, B. A. (1992) Factors affecting the corneal response to contact lenses. In *Current Perspectives in Vision Care* (eds R. P. Franz, A. J. Hanks and R. E. Weisbarth). No. 1, CIBA Vision Monograph Series, CIBA Vision, Bulach/Zurich, p. 9

Holden, B. A. (1996) Creating the 'spectacle killer' contact lens. *Cont. Lens Spectrum*, January, 31–34

Holden, B. A. and Mertz, G. W. (1984) Critical oxygen level to avoid corneal edema for daily and extended wear contact lenses. *Invest. Ophthalmol. Vis. Sci.*, **25**, 1161–1167

Holden, B. A. and Sweeney, D. F. (1991) The significance of the microcyst response: a review. *Optom. Vis. Sci.*, **68**, 703–707

Holden, B. A., Mertz, G. W. and McNally, J. J. (1983) Corneal swelling response to contact lenses worn under extended wear conditions. *Invest. Ophthalmol. Vis. Sci.*, **24**, 218–226

Holden, B. A., Sweeney, D. F. and Sanderson, G. (1984) The minimum precorneal oxygen tension to avoid corneal edema. *Invest. Ophthalmol. Vis. Sci.*, **25**, 476–480

Holden, B. A., Sweeney, D. F, Vannas, A. *et al.* (1985) Effects of long-term extended contact lens wear on the human cornea. *Invest. Ophthalmol. Vis. Sci.*, **26**, 1489–1501

Holden, B. A., Sweeney, D. F., Swarbrick, H. *et al.* (1986) The vascular response to long term extended contact lens wear. *Clin. Exp. Optom.*, **69**, 112–119

Holden, B. A., La Hood, D. and Sweeney, D. F. (1987) Prediction of extended wear microcyst response on the basis of the mean overnight corneal response in an unrelated sample of non-wearers. *Am. J. Optom. Physiol. Opt.*, **64**, 83

Holden, B. A., La Hood, D., Grant, T. *et al.* (1996) Gram-negative bacteria can induce contact lens related acute red eye (CLARE) responses. *J. Cont. Lens Assoc. Ophthalmol.*, **22**, 47–52

Holden, B. A., Sweeney, D. F. and Sankaridurg, P. R. (2003) Microbial keratitis and vision loss with contact lenses. *Eye Cont. Lens*, **29**, s131–134

Hovding, G. (1983) Variations of central corneal curvature during the first year of contact lens wear. *Acta Ophthalmol. (Kbh.)*, **61**, 117–128

Humphreys, J. A., Larke, J. R. and Parrish, S. T. (1980) Microepithelial cysts observed in extended contact-lens wearing subjects. *Br. J. Ophthalmol.*, **64**, 888–889

Imayasu, M., Petroll, W. M., Jester, J. V. *et al.* (1994) The relation between contact lens oxygen transmissibility and binding of *Pseudomonas aeruginosa* to the cornea after overnight wear. *Ophthalmology*, **101**, 371–388

Jalbert, I., Sweeney, D. F. and Holden, B. A. (1996) Corneal staining in daily wearers and extended wearers of hydrogel contact lenses. *Optom. Vis. Sci.*, **73**, 103

Jalbert, I., Sweeney, D. F., Sankaridurg, P. R. and Holden, B. A. (1998) Measuring success in daily wearers and extended wearers of disposable hydrogel lenses: discontinuation rates and unscheduled removals. *Optom. Vis. Sci.*, **75**, 41

Jalbert, I., Sweeney, D. F. and Holden, B. A. (1999a) Patient satisfaction with daily disposable contact lens wear. *Optom. Vis. Sci.*, **12s**, 164

Jalbert, I., Holden, B. A., Keay, L. and Sweeney, D. (1999b) Refractive and corneal power changes associated with overnight lens wear differences between low *Dk/t* hydrogel and high *Dk/t* silicone hydrogel lenses. *Optom. Vis. Sci.*, **76**, S234

Jalbert, I., Stapleton, F., Papas, E. *et al.* (2003) *In vivo* confocal microscopy of the human cornea. *Br. J. Ophthalmol.*, **87**, 225–236

Jones, L., MacDougall, N., Sorbara, G. (2002) Asymptomatic corneal staining associated with the use of balafilcon silicone-hydrogel contact lenses disinfected with a polyaminopropyl biguanide-preserved care regimen. *Optom. Vis. Sci.*, **79**, 753–761

Jones, L., Senchyna, M., Glasier, M. A. *et al.* (2003) Lysozyme and lipid deposition on silicone hydrogel contact lens materials. *Eye Cont. Lens*, **29**, 575–579

Kame, R. T. (1976) Clinical management of hydrogel-induced edema. *Am. J. Optom. Physiol. Opt.*, **53**, 468–473

Kastl, P. R. and Johnson, W. C. (1989) Fluoroperm 7 extended wear RGP contact lenses for myopia, hyperopia, aphakia, astigmatism and keratoconus. *J. Cont. Lens Assoc. Ophthalmol.*, **15**, 61–63

Keay, L., Sweeney, D. F., Jalbert, I., Skotnitsky, C. and Holden, B. A. (2000) Microcyst response to high *Dk/t* silicone hydrogel contact lenses. *Optom. Vis. Sci.*, **77**, 582–585

Kenyon, E., Polse, K. A. and Mandell, R. B. (1988) Rigid contact lens adherence: incidence, severity and recovery. *J. Am. Optom. Assoc.*, **59**, 168–174

Kerns, R. L. (1974) A study of striae observed in the cornea from contact lens wear. *Am. J. Optom. Physiol. Opt.*, **51**, 998–1004

Koetting, R. A. (1974) Soflens J contact lens worn continuously for more than one year: a report on three patients. *Am. J. Optom. Arch. Am. Acad. Optom.*, **51**, 583–586

Kotow, M., Holden, B. A. and Grant, T. (1987) The value of regular replacement of low water content contact lenses for extended wear. *J. Am. Optom. Assoc.*, **58**, 461–464

Kreis-Gosselin, F. and Lumbroso, P. (1990) Extended wear of rigid gas permeable, high *Dk* contact lenses in myopia. *Contactologia*, **12E**, 158–162

La Hood, D. and Grant, T. (1990) Striae and folds as indicators of corneal edema. *Optom. Vis. Sci.*, **67** (suppl.), 196

La Hood, D., Sweeney, D. F. and Holden, B. A. (1988) Overnight corneal edema with hydrogel, rigid gas-permeable and silicone elastomer contact lenses. *Int. Cont. Lens Clin.*, **15**, 149–154

Lakkis, C. and Brennan, N. A. (1996) Bulbar conjunctival fluorescein staining in hydrogel contact lens wearers. *J. Cont. Lens Assoc. Ophthalmol.*, **22**, 189–194

Larke, J. R., Humphreys, J. A. and Holmes, R. (1981) Apparent corneal vascularisation in soft lens wearers. *J. Br. Cont. Lens Assoc.*, **4**, 105–106

Leibowitz, H. M, Laing, R. A. and Sandstrom, M. (1973) Continuous wear of hydrophilic contact lenses. *Arch. Ophthalmol.*, **89**, 306–310

Levy, B. (1985) Rigid gas-permeable lenses for extended wear: a 1-year clinical evaluation. *Am. J. Optom. Physiol. Optics*, **62**, 889–894

Lin, S. T. and Mandell, R. B. (1991) Corneal trauma from overnight wear of rigid or soft contact lenses. *J. Am. Optom. Assoc.*, **62**, 224–227

Lippman, J. I. (1978) Silicone lenses in aphakia: fact vs fancy. *Cont. Intraoc. Lens Med. J.*, **4**, 58–62

MacDonald, K. E., Fonn, D., Richter, D. B. and Robboy, M. (1995) Comparison of the physiological response to extended wear of an experimental high *Dk* soft lens versus a 38 per cent HEMA lens. *Invest. Ophthalmol. Vis. Sci.*, **36**, s310

Madigan, M. C. (1989) Cat and monkey as models for extended hydrogel contact lens wear in humans. PhD thesis, University of New South Wales, Sydney, Australia

Madigan, M. C. and Holden, B. A. (1992) Reduced epithelial adhesion after extended contact lens wear correlates with reduced hemidesmosome density in cat cornea. *Invest. Ophthalmol. Vis. Sci.*, **33**, 314–323

Madigan, M. C., Holden, B. A. and Kwok, L. S. (1987) Extended wear of contact lenses can compromise corneal epithelial adhesion. *Curr. Eye Res.*, **6**, 1257–1259

Mandell, R. B. (1974) *Contact Lens Practice: Hard and Flexible Lenses*, 2nd edn. C. Thomas, Springfield, IL

Mannarino, A. P., Belin, M. W. and Weiner, B. M. (1985) Clinical fitting characteristics of extended wear silicone (Silsight) lenses. *J. Cont. Lens Assoc. Ophthalmol.*, **11**, 339–342

Martin, D. K., Boulos, J., Gan, J. *et al.* (1989) A unifying parameter to describe the clinical mechanics of hydrogel contact lenses. *Optom. Vis. Sci.*, **66**, 87–91

McKenney, C., Becker, N., Thomas, S. *et al.* (1998) Lens deposits with a high *Dk* hydrophilic soft lens. *Optom. Vis. Sci.*, **75**, 276

McMonnies, C. W. (1983) Contact lens-induced corneal vascularization. *Int. Cont. Lens Clin.*, **10**, 12–15

McMonnies, C. W., Chapman-Davies, A. and Holden, B. A. (1982) The vascular response to contact lens wear. *Am. J. Optom. Physiol. Optics*, **59**, 795–799

McNally, J. and McKenney, C. (2002) A clinical look at a silicone hydrogel extended wear lens. *Cont. Lens Spectrum*, January, 38–41

Mertz, G. W. and Holden, B. A. (1981) Clinical implications of extended wear research. *Can. J. Optom.*, **43**, 203–205

Millodot, M. (1974) Effect of soft lenses on corneal sensitivity. *Acta. Ophthalmol.*, **52**, 603–608

Millodot, M. and O'Leary, D. J. (1980) Effect of oxygen deprivation on corneal sensitivity. *Acta Ophthalmol.*, **58**, 434–439

Mizutani, Y, Matsunaka, H., Takemoto, N. and Mizutani, Y. (1983) The effect of anoxia on the human cornea. *Jpn Ophthalmol. Soc. Acta*, **87**, 644–649

Molinari, J. F. (1983) Review, giant papillary conjunctivitis. *Aust. J. Optom.*, **66**, 59

Morgan, P. B. and Efron, N. (2002a) Trends in UK contact lens prescribing 2002. *Optician*, **5849** (223), 28–29

Morgan, P. B. and Efron, N. (2002b) Comparative performance of two silicone hydrogel contact lenses for continuous wear. *Clin. Exp. Optom.*, **85**, 183–192

Mueller, N., Caroline, P., Smythe, J., Mai-Le, K. and Bergenske, P. (2001) A comparison of overnight swelling response with two high *Dk* silicone hydrogels (AAO Abstract). *Optom. Vis. Sci.*, **78**, S199

Nelson, L. B., Cutler, S. I., Calhoun, J. H. *et al.* (1985) Silsoft extended wear contact lenses in pediatric aphakia. *Ophthalmology*, **92**, 1529–1531

Nilsson, S. E. G. and Montan, P. G. (1994) The hospitalized cases of contact lens induced keratitis in Sweden and their relation to lens type and wear schedule: results of a three year retrospective study. *J. Cont. Lens Assoc. Ophthalmol.*, **20**, 97–101

Norn, M. S. (1972) Vital staining of cornea and conjunctiva. *Cont. Lens J.*, **3**, 19–22

O'Leary, D. J. and Millodot, M. (1981) Abnormal epithelial fragility in diabetes and in contact lens wear. *Acta Ophthalmol.*, **59**, 827

Papas, E. (1998) On the relationship between soft contact lens oxygen transmissibility and induced limbal hyperemia. *Exp. Eye Res.*, **67**, 125–131

Papas, E., Fleming, C., Austen, R. and Holden, B. A. (1994) High *Dk* soft contact lenses reduce the limbal vascular response. *Optom. Vis. Sci.*, **71** (suppl.), 14

Papas, E. B., Vajdic, C. M., Austen, R. and Holden, B. A. (1997) High-oxygen-transmissibility soft contact lenses do not induce limbal hyperaemia. *Curr. Eye. Res.*, **16**, 942–948

Polse, K. A. (1979) Tear flow under hydrogel contact lenses. *Invest. Ophthalmol. Vis. Sci.*, **18**, 409–413

Polse, K. A., McNamara, N. A. and Brand, R. J. (1997) Bulk tear flow under a soft contact lens. *Invest Ophthalmol. Vis. Sci.*, **38**, s201

Pritchard, N. and Fonn, D. (1998) Post-lens tear debris during extended wear of hydrogels. *Can. J. Optom.*, **60**, 87–91

Pritchard, N., Jones, L., Dumbleton, K. and Fonn, D. (2000) Epithelial inclusions in association with mucin ball development in high oxygen permeability hydrogel lenses. *Optom. Vis. Sci.*, **77**, 68–72

Ren, D. H., Petroll, W. M., Jester, J. V., *et al.* (1999) The relationship between contact lens oxygen permeability and binding of *Pseudomonas aeruginosa* to human corneal epithelial cells after overnight and extended wear. *J. Cont. Lens Assoc. Ophthalmol.*, **25**, 80–100

Rengstorff, R. H. (1971) Wearing contact lenses during sleep: corneal curvature changes. *Am. J. Optom. Arch. Am. Acad. Optom.*, **48**, 1034–1037

Rengstorff, R. H. (1979) Changes in corneal curvature associated with contact lens wear. *J. Am. Optom. Assoc.*, **50**, 375–377

Robboy, M. W. and Cox, I. G. (1991) Patient factors influencing conjunctival staining with soft contact lens wearers. *Optom. Vis. Sci.*, **68**, 163

Ruben, M. (1976) Acute eye disease secondary to contact lens wear. *Lancet*, **i**, 138

Ruben, M. (1977) Constant wear vs daily wear. *Optician*, August, 5, 7, 9, 11–14

Ruben, M. and Guillon, M. (1979) Silicone rubber lenses in aphakia. *Br. J. Ophthalmol.*, **63**, 471–474

Sankaridurg, P., Sweeney, D. F., Gora, R. *et al.* (1998) Rates and trends of corneal infiltrative responses observed during extended wear with disposable hydrogels. *Invest. Ophthalmol. Vis. Sci.*, **39s**, poster 2506

Sankaridurg, P. R., Sweeney, D. F., Sharma, J. *et al.* (1999) Adverse events with extended wear of disposable hydrogels: results for the first thirteen months of lens wear. *Ophthalmology*, **106**, 1671–1680

Sarver, M. D. (1971) Striate corneal lines among patients wearing hydrophilic contact lenses. *Am. J. Optom. Arch. Am. Acad. Optom.*, **48**, 762–763

Schein, O. D., Glynn, R. K., Poggio, E. C. *et al.* (1989) The relative risk of ulcerative keratitis among users of daily-wear and extended-wear soft contact lenses: a case-control study. *N. Engl. J. Med.*, **321**, 773–778

Schein, O. D., Buehler, P. O., Stamler, J. F. *et al.* (1994) The impact of overnight wear on the risk of contact lens-associated ulcerative keratitis. *Arch. Ophthalmol.*, **112**, 186–190

Schoessler, J. P., Barr, J. T. and Freson, D. R. (1984) Corneal endothelial observations of silicone elastomer contact lens wearers. *Int. Cont. Lens. Clin.*, **11**, 337–340

Seger, R. G. and Mutti, D. O. (1988) Conjunctival staining and single-use CLs with unpolished edges. *Cont. Lens Spectrum*, **3**, 36–37

Sevigny, J. (1986) Clinical comparison of the Boston IV contact lens under extended wear vs the Boston II lens under daily wear. *Int. Eyecare*, **2**, 260–264

Skotnitsky, C., Sankaridurg, P. R., Sweeney, D. F. and Holden, B. A. (2002) General and local contact lens induced papillary conjunctivitis (CLPC). *Clin. Exp. Optom.*, **85**, 193

Smith, B. J., Fink, B. A. and Hill, R. M. (1999) *Dk/L*: Into the ultra-high zone. *Cont. Lens Spectrum*, January, 31–34

Solomon, O. D., Loff, H., Perla, B. *et al.* (1994) Testing hypotheses for risk factors for contact lens-associated infectious keratitis in an animal model. *J. Cont. Lens Assoc. Ophthalmol.*, **20**, 109–113

Swarbrick, H. A. and Holden, B. A. (1987) Rigid gas permeable lens binding: significance and contributing factors. *Am. J. Optom. Physiol. Optics*, **64**, 815–823

Swarbrick, H. A. and Holden, B. A. (1999) Extended wear lenses. In *Contact Lenses*, 5th edn (eds A. J. Phillips and L. Speedwell). Butterworth-Heinemann, Oxford, Ch. 15, pp. 494–539

Sweeney, D. F. and Holden, B. A. (1987) Silicone elastomer lens wear induces less overnight corneal edema than sleep without lens wear. *Curr. Eye Res.*, **6**, 1391–1394

Sweeney, D. F. and Holden, B. A. (1988) Silicone elastomers enhance corneal physiology. In *Transactions of the World Congress on the Cornea III* (ed. H. D. Cavanagh). Raven Press, New York, pp. 293–296

Sweeney, D. F., Gauthier, C., Terry, R. *et al.* (1992) The effects of long-term contact lens wear on the anterior eye. *Invest. Ophthalmol. Vis. Sci.*, **33s**, 1293

Sweeney, D. F., Sankaridurg, P. R., Covey, M. A. *et al.* (1997) Masked assessment of the ocular responses of daily disposable lens wearers and extended wear hydrogel lens wearers compared to a non-lens wearing population. *Optom. Vis. Sci.*, **74** (suppl.), 75

Tan, J., Keay, L., Jalbert, I. *et al.* (2003) Mucin balls with wear of conventional and silicone hydrogel contact lenses. *Optom. Vis. Sci.*, **80**, 291–297

Terry, R. L., Schnider, C. M., Holden, B. A. *et al.* (1993) CCLRU standards for success of daily and extended wear contact lenses. *Optom. Vis. Sci.*, **70**, 234–243

Terry, R., Sweeney, D. F., Wong, R. and Papas, E. (1995) Variability of clinical investigators in contact lens research. *Optom. Vis. Sci.*, **72** (suppl.), 16

Tomlinson, A. and Haas, D. D. (1980) Changes in corneal thickness and circumcorneal vascularisation with contact lens wear. *Int. Cont. Lens Clin.*, **7**, 45–56

Treissman, H. and Plaice, E. A. (1946) *Principles of the Contact Lens.* Henry Kimpton, London, pp. 82–83

Vajdic, C. M. and Holden, B. A. (1997) Extended wear contact lenses. In *Corneal Physiology and Disposable Contact Lenses* (eds H. Hamano and H. Kaufman). Churchill Livingstone, Edinburgh

Vajdic, C., Holden, B. A., Sweeney, D. F. and Cornish, R. (1999) The frequency of ocular symptoms during spectacle and daily soft and rigid contact lens wear. *Optom. Vis. Sci.*, **76**, 705–711

Weissman, B. A., Mondino, B. J., Pettit, T. H. and Hofbauer, J. D. (1984) Corneal ulcers associated with extended-wear soft contact lenses. *Am. J. Ophthalmol.*, **97**, 476–481

Willcox, M. D. P., Sweeney, D. F., Sharma, S. *et al.* (1995) Culture negative peripheral ulcers are associated with bacterial contamination of contact lenses. *Invest. Ophthalmol. Vis. Sci.*, **36**, s152

Yamane, S. J. and Kuwabara, D. M. (1987) Ensuring compliance in patients wearing contact lenses on an extended-wear basis. *Int. Cont. Lens Clin.*, **14**, 108–112

Young, G., Holden, B. and Cooke, G. (1993) Influence of soft contact lens design on clinical performance. *Optom. Vis. Sci.*, **70**, 394–403

Zantos, S. G. (1981) The ocular response to continuous wear of contact lenses. PhD thesis, School of Optometry, University of New South Wales, Sydney

Zantos, S. G. (1983) Cystic formations in the corneal epithelium during extended wear of contact lenses. *Int. Cont. Lens Clin.*, **10**, 128–146

Zantos, S. G. and Holden, B. A. (1978) Ocular changes associated with continuous wear of contact lenses. *Aust. J. Optom.*, **61**, 418–426

Zantos, S. G. and Zantos, P. O. (1985) Extended wear feasibility of gas-permeable hard lenses for myopes. *Int. Eyecare*, **1**, 66–75

Chapter 7

Adverse events and infections: which ones and how many?

Padmaja R. Sankaridurg, Brien A. Holden and
Isabelle Jalbert

INTRODUCTION

The use of contact lenses has increased considerably in recent years and current estimates suggest that at the beginning of 2003 there were approximately 110 million lens wearers worldwide (IACLE, 2003). In comparison, spectacles are used by over two billion (USA scale) people. Silicone hydrogel lenses were approved for up to 30 days of continuous wear (CW) in Australia and Europe in 1999 and in the USA in 2001 and since then have seen a steady market growth. In the UK, 3 per cent of all refits with soft lens materials in 2000 were with silicone hydrogel lenses, which increased to 12 per cent in 2001 (Morgan and Efron, 2000, 2001). In 2002 more than 95 per cent of all extended-wear (EW) fits in Australia, Norway and the UK were with silicone hydrogel lenses (Morgan et al., 2002). In Australia, in 2002, 18 per cent of refits and 7 per cent of new fits were with silicone hydrogel lenses (Morgan et al., 2002).

While this trend is promising for silicone hydrogels, scepticism towards EW still remains (Cheung et al., 2002; Jones et al., 2002), as both its safety and the inconvenience of possible adverse events are of concern. The wariness stems from the previous publicity surrounding the use of EW and the risk of microbial keratitis (MK). EW of conventional low-Dk hydrogel lenses, introduced in the early 1970s, was shown to increase the risk of developing potentially blinding MK (Ruben, 1976; Cooper and Constable, 1977; Spoor et al., 1984; Patrinely et al., 1985; Alfonso et al., 1986; Chalupa et al., 1987). 'Disposable' contact lenses, introduced in the late 1980s, neither increased nor decreased the risk of MK (Dunn et al., 1989; Kent et al., 1989; Killingsworth and Stern, 1989; Maguen et al., 1991; Poggio and Abelson, 1993; Chatterjee et al., 1995; Cohen et al., 1996). The incidence of some significant adverse events, e.g. contact lens-induced papillary conjunctivitis (CLPC) and contact lens-induced acute red eye (CLARE), seems to have been reduced by regular lens replacement (Grant et al., 1987).

In the face of these challenges, the key to successful contact lens practice lies in educating practitioners and helping them promptly detect, diagnose and appropriately manage any adverse reactions to lens wear.

In this chapter we discuss the symptoms, signs, diagnosis, management and treatment of the complications seen in a contact lens practice, especially with EW of hydrogels. We also report and discuss the impact the silicone hydrogel lenses has had on the incidence of these complications.

The Cornea and Contact Lens Research Unit (CCLRU) and the L. V. Prasad Eye Institute (LVPEI) have developed a categorization and management system entitled 'The CCLRU/LVPEI Guide to Infiltrative Conditions seen in Contact Lens Practice' (The CLIC Guide). Excerpts from the guide are used in this chapter to provide a clearer definition of these conditions and help the practitioner correctly identify and manage adverse events.

In the first section, definitions of the terms 'serious adverse reactions, adverse reactions and adverse events' are provided as an introduction and the later sections deal with specific adverse events.

WHAT IS A SERIOUS ADVERSE REACTION?

The definition of a serious adverse reaction or event as per the International Conference on Harmonization (Food and Drug Administration (FDA) Federal Register, 1995) is given in Table 7.1. Also, Spilker (1991) defines a *serious adverse reaction* as one that 'produces a significant impairment of functioning or incapacitation, is a definite hazard to the patient's health and warrants counteractive treatment or alteration of therapy'.

WHAT IS AN ADVERSE REACTION OR EVENT?

An adverse reaction is 'any noxious and unintended response(s) to a product related to any dose'. The phrase 'responses to a product' means that a causal relationship between a product and an adverse event is at least a reasonable possibility, i.e. the relationship cannot be ruled out (FDA Federal Register, 1995). Other definitions for an adverse reaction include an 'unwanted effect(s) (i.e. physical and/or psychological symptoms and signs) resulting from treatment', or 'any undesirable effect or problem that is present during the period of treatment' (Spilker, 1991).

The mildest of the noteworthy occurrences is defined as an *adverse event*, which is 'an unwanted effect(s) that occurs and is detected in populations'. The term is used whether or not there is any attribution to a medicine or other cause. Similarly, International Conference on Harmonisation guidelines (FDA Federal Register,

Table 7.1   Serious adverse reaction

A serious adverse reaction is any untoward medical occurrence that at any dose:
● results in death
● is life-threatening
● requires inpatient hospitalization or prolongation of existing hospitalization
● results in persistent or significant disability/incapacity

1995) define an adverse event to be 'any untoward medical occurrence in a patient administered a pharmaceutical product and which does not necessarily have to have a causal relationship with this treatment'. Again the suggestion is that the condition may or may not be related to the use of the product.

CATEGORIZATION OF ADVERSE REACTIONS

Categorization of adverse reaction(s) or event(s) into distinct groups helps formulate a systematic approach to managing and treating the condition.

Currently, widespread confusion exists in the literature and in clinical practice, with either the same adverse reaction(s) being categorized differently or different reactions being labelled as the same type of event. A typical example is the use of the term 'corneal infiltrate', which can be used to describe either a large infected ulcer or a few cells in the cornea. Corneal ulcers, whether infected or not, are variously referred to as 'keratitis' (Matthews et al., 1992; Nilsson and Montan, 1994), 'corneal ulcer' (Cohen et al., 1987, 1996; Dunn et al., 1989; Macrae et al., 1991), 'MK' (Ormerod and Smith, 1986; Dart, 1988), 'ulcerative keratitis' (Alfonso et al., 1986; Schein et al., 1989; Schein and Poggio, 1990; Matthews et al., 1992), 'presumed MK' (Stapleton et al., 1993), 'infiltrative keratitis' (Josephson and Caffery, 1979), 'peripheral corneal infiltrative keratopathy' (Levy et al., 1997), 'suppurative keratitis' (Stapleton et al., 1993) and 'corneal infiltrates' (Stein et al., 1988). In the absence of clear guidelines, interpretation of the nature of the adverse events with regard to potential damage to the eye becomes difficult, as does making advances in prevention or management strat-egies. The FDA of the USA recognized the need for a categorization system and conducted a review of the definition of the terms 'adverse reactions' and 'corneal infiltrates' in 1998, with the focus on conditions seen with contact lens wear.

The CCLRU, at the School of Optometry and Vision Science, the University of New South Wales, Australia, and the LVPEI, Hyderabad, India, have conducted numerous prospective clinical trials in the past decade involving spectacles, daily disposable hydrogel lenses, daily wear (DW) and EW of rigid gas-permeable (RGP) lenses, disposable hydrogel lenses and silicone hydrogel materials. Clinical and laboratory researchers discussed in detail the signs, symptoms, appearance, laboratory findings, treatment and management of a range of adverse conditions seen during spectacle and hydrogel contact lens wear in order to develop the CLIC Guide. The outcome was presented for discussion by the Adverse Event Panel of the International Society for Contact Lens Research and then presented to the FDA. Using the criteria laid down by the ICH guidelines, the conditions were categorized as 'Serious', 'Significant' and 'Non-Significant' events, based on the severity of the condition, the level of clinical concern and the patient/event outcome and action criteria associated with the event. The clinical features for each of the event types and the treatment and management options were detailed.

Table 7.2 provides a description for the categories Serious, Significant and Non-Significant adverse reaction(s) and event(s) commonly seen in a contact lens practice.

Table 7.2 Adverse reactions/events in contact lens practice

Classification	Serious (symptomatic)	Significant (mostly symptomatic)	Non–significant (asymptomatic)	
Description	Adverse reaction • of sufficient clinical concern to warrant permanently discontinuing lens wear • that produces or has the potential to produce significant visual impairment	Adverse reaction of sufficient clinical concern to warrant temporary or permanent discontinuation of lens wear	Adverse event not of sufficient clinical concern. May not warrant discontinuation of the patient from lens wear	An observation of no clinical concern
Conditions	Microbial keratitis	• Contact lens-induced acute red eye • Contact lens-induced peripheral ulcer • Infiltrative keratitis • Viral keratoconjunctivitis • Superior epithelial arcuate lesion • Corneal erosion • Corneal wrinkling • Contact lens papillary conjunctivitis	• Asymptomatic infiltrative keratitis • Corneal vascularization • Corneal striae	Asymptomatic infiltrates

SERIOUS ADVERSE REACTIONS (SYMPTOMATIC)

The only serious adverse reaction seen with contact lens wear is MK.

Microbial keratitis

MK is a serious ocular condition because it is potentially sight-threatening. The major risk factors for development of MK include hypoxia, trauma, ocular surface disease, certain systemic conditions and contact lens wear (Dart, 1988; Dart *et al.*, 1991; Solomon *et al.*, 1994; Cheung and Slomovic, 1995; Bennett *et al.*, 1998). In developed countries where the use of contact lenses is substantial, contact lens wear has emerged as the major risk factor for MK (Liesegang and Forster, 1980; McClellan *et al.*, 1989; Cheung and Slomovic, 1995; Bennett *et al.*, 1998; Lam *et al.*, 2002). Reports since the 1980s from these countries suggest that 30–60 per cent of all MK events in the younger age group are associated with contact lens wear (Liesegang and Forster, 1980; Dart, 1988; Cohen *et al.*, 1996; Bennett *et al.*, 1998; Schaefer *et al.*, 2001; Lam *et al.*, 2002). In contrast, in developing countries where contact lens wear has not yet achieved the popularity it enjoys in developed countries, trauma and ocular surface diseases remain the major risk factors for MK (Upadhyay *et al.*, 1982; Ormerod, 1987).

Events of MK with contact lens wear were reported as early as the 1960s with polymethyl methacrylate (PMMA) lens wear (Dixon *et al.*, 1966). In subsequent years MK was seen with all lens types, i.e. hard or PMMA, RGPs, conventional soft, disposable soft and also with all modes of lens wear, i.e. DW, EW, therapeutic wear and CW (Brown *et al.*, 1974; Ruben, 1976; Cooper and Constable, 1977; Donnenfeld *et al.*, 1986; Ormerod and Smith, 1986; Wilhelmus, 1987; Dart, 1988; Cohen *et al.*, 1996; Sharma *et al.*, 2003). However, it was the increased incidence seen with CW or EW of low-oxygen-permeable hydrogel materials in the late 1970s and the 1980s that led to public prominence of this complication. Since then it has been clearly established that the risk of MK is significantly greater with EW of hydrogel lenses in comparison to other types and modes of lens wear (Donnenfeld *et al.*, 1986; Ormerod and Smith, 1986; Chalupa *et al.*, 1987; Wilhelmus, 1987; Cohen *et al.*, 1996, Cheng *et al.*, 1999). More recently, events of MK have been reported with CW of silicone hydrogel lenses (Lim *et al.*, 2002).

Incidence with contact lens wear

Several difficulties exist in trying to determine the incidence of MK with contact lens wear. First, the lack of a standardized descriptive terminology makes it difficult to gather information on the real incidence of this condition. For this review we have chosen reports from the literature which presume the condition to be microbial in nature.

Second, while there have been many case series and case reports in the literature of MK with all types and modes of contact lens wear, epidemiological information on the incidence of MK in lens wearers is limited. Interestingly, information on the incidence of MK in non-lens wearers is even more limited. This is largely due to the fact that, while the condition is serious with potentially blinding consequences, the incidence of all cases of MK (lens and non-lens wearers) is limited in developed countries to a few individuals per 100 000 wearers. For example, the annual incidence for all cases of MK (lens plus non-lens wearers) from a population-based cohort study in Scotland was 0.26 per 10 000 persons (Seal *et al.*, 1999). Due to the relatively low rate of occurrence of the condition one would be required to sample hundreds of thousands of people or conduct a large-scale clinical trial to arrive at reasonable estimates of the incidence of the condition. Conducting such large-scale population studies poses practical difficulties. In addition, extrapolating information from small-scale clinical studies to project the annual incidence carries the risk of overestimating or underestimating the condition.

Estimates of the incidence of MK with contact lens wear have been derived from clinical surveys (Dixon *et al.*, 1966), reviews of pre-market clinical trial data (Macrae *et al.*, 1991), population surveys (Poggio *et al.*, 1989) and retrospective studies (Maguen *et al.*, 1991, 1992, 1994; Boswall *et al.*, 1993). Each of these

Table 7.3   Annualized incidence of microbial keratitis across studies

Lens type	Mode of wear	Terminology used	Incidence (%)	Eyes/ people	Authors
PMMA	–	Ulcerative keratitis	0.02	People	Poggio et al. (1989)
RGP	–	Ulcerative keratitis	0.040	People	Poggio et al. (1989)
RGP	DW	Corneal ulcer	0.00068	People	Macrae et al. (1991)
RGP	DW	Contact lens-induced keratitis	0.012	People	Nilsson and Montan (1994)
RGP	DW	Microbial keratitis	0.011	People	Cheng et al. (1999)
RGP	EW	Corneal ulcer	0.00239	People	Macrae et al. (1991)
Soft	DW	Corneal ulcer	0.00052	People	Macrae et al. (1991)
Soft	DW	Ulcerative keratitis	0.041	People	Poggio et al. (1989)
Soft	DW	Contact lens-induced keratitis	0.005	People	Nilsson and Montan (1994)
Soft	DW	Microbial keratitis	0.035	People	Cheng et al. (1999)
Conventional soft	EW	Keratitis (year 1)	3.7	People	Boswall et al. (1993)
Conventional soft	EW	Keratitis (year 2)	2.3	People	Boswall et al. (1993)
Conventional soft	EW	Keratitis (year 3)	9.1	People	Boswall et al. (1993)
Conventional soft	EW	Corneal ulcer	0.31	Eyes	Poggio and Abelson (1993)
Conventional soft	EW	Corneal ulcer	0.00182	People	Macrae et al. (1991)
Conventional soft	EW	Ulcerative keratitis	0.209	People	Poggio et al. (1989)
Conventional soft	EW	Contact lens-induced keratitis	0.031	People	Nilsson and Montan (1994)
Conventional soft	EW	Microbial keratitis	0.20	People	Cheng et al. (1999)
Disposable soft	DW	Contact lens-induced keratitis	0.002	People	Nilsson and Montan (1994)
Disposable soft	EW	Contact lens-induced keratitis	0.042	People	Nilsson and Montan (1994)
Disposable soft	EW	Corneal ulcers (year 1)	1.6	People	Maguen et al. (1991)
Disposable soft	EW	Corneal ulcers (year 3)	2.0	People	Maguen et al. (1994)
Disposable soft	EW	Corneal ulcer	0.38	Eyes	Poggio and Abelson (1993)
Disposable soft	EW	Microbial keratitis	0.27	Eyes	CCLRU/LVPEI database
Silicone hydrogel	CW	Microbial keratitis	0.14	Eyes	CCLRU/LVPEI database

methods has its own limitations. Also, continual changes in lens materials, lens care regimens and lens wear patterns influence the incidence.

The earliest record of the incidence of infectious corneal ulcers was from a national survey (USA) of ophthalmologists conducted by Dixon et al. (1966). The incidence of lost eyes or blinding ulcers was recorded to be 0.3 per cent of the entire lens-wearing population. Table 7.3 gives the incidence of MK reported in a number of recent studies of contact lens wear.

Table 7.4 Relative risk of developing microbial keratitis

Lens type					Authors
Hard (PMMA)	Rigid	DW soft	EW soft	EW disposable soft	
1.0 (referent)	–	1.13	4.08	17.36	Matthews et al. (1992)
–	0.90	1.66	1.87	14.34	Buehler et al. (1992)
–	1.0 (referent)	2.64	23.29	–	Stapleton et al. (1993)
0.5	1.0 (referent)	1.0	5.15	–	Poggio et al. (1989)
1.3	1.0 (referent)	3.6	20.8	–	Dart et al. (1991)
–	1.0 (referent)	3.3	18.9	–	Cheng et al. (1999)

Whatever the nature of the study, it is clear that the incidence of MK is usually greater with EW of both disposable and conventional hydrogel lenses in comparison to other lens types and modes. This is further illustrated by case-control studies which established the relative risk of developing MK with different lens types and modes of wear (Table 7.4).

Silicone hydrogel lenses and MK

As mentioned before, MK has been observed with CW of silicone hydrogel lenses (Lim *et al.*, 2002). Also to date, in the CCLRU/LVPEI studies, three events of MK have been seen in approximately 2073 patient eye years (incidence of 0.14 per cent) of silicone hydrogel CW experience compared with an MK rate of six per 2226 patient eye years (incidence of 0.27 per cent) with six-night hydrogel lens EW studies (Table 7.3). In addition, the CCLRU has attempted to collate all the known cases of MK that have occurred with silicone hydrogel lenses worldwide by actively contacting members of the ophthalmic community through international meetings, and directly from practitioners. The list, while not comprehensive, offers a first approximation of what the incidence of MK with these lenses may be. There have been 21 cases (excluding CCLRU/LVPEI studies) and if we consider that there are currently 850 000 wearers of silicone hydrogel lenses (lens sales data, assuming 20 lenses per patient per year), this equates to approximately 640 000 patient years and an estimated annualized incidence of 0.33 per 10 000 wearers per year (0.003 per cent). While this figure is low, clearly further experience and controlled clinical studies are needed to estimate reliably the incidence of MK with silicone hydrogel lenses.

Clinical features of MK

The clinical features of MK vary depending on the type and virulence of microorganism infecting the cornea, the stage at which the patient presented, i.e. an early or an advanced stage of infection, use of prior medication, if any, and the inflammatory response mounted by the host cornea associated with the condition.

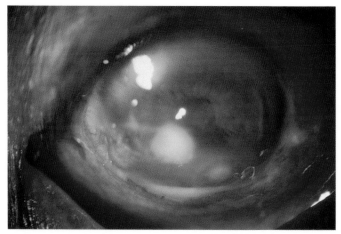

Figure 7.1   MK caused by *Pseudomonas* sp. Note the large, dense, yellowish–white infiltrate close to the pupil and a smaller infiltrate on the inferior cornea. Hypopyon is also observed (courtesy LVPEI, India)

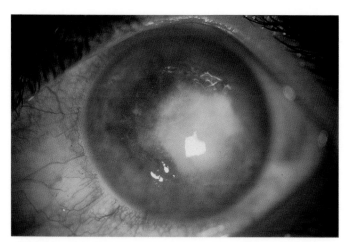

Figure 7.2   Fungal keratitis. Note the large, dense, white infiltrate and the branching figures extending from the infiltrate (courtesy LVPEI, India)

For example, *Pseudomonas* keratitis is characterized by a rapid, suppurative stromal infiltrate with necrosis and excessive mucopurulent discharge (Figure 7.1). A ring infiltrate may be seen in the surrounding paracentral cornea. Fungal keratitis is characterized by an infiltrate with 'fluffy' or branching margins and satellite lesions (Figure 7.2). Oedema of the surrounding cornea is common and endothelial plaques may be seen. *Acanthamoeba* keratitis can present with dendritic involvement or patchy stromal infiltrates (Figure 7.3). Such wide-ranging clinical features make it difficult to describe each of the specific clinical patterns in this section and therefore we have attempted to define the frequently observed clinical symptoms and signs that would alert the clinician to a possible MK event

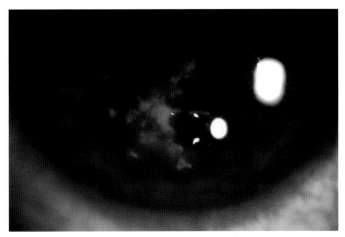

Figure 7.3   *Acanthamoeba* keratitis (courtesy LVPEI, India)

Table 7.5   Symptoms associated with microbial keratitis

Symptoms
- Moderate to severe pain of rapid onset
- Severe redness ('meaty' appearance)
- Blurred or hazy vision; decreased visual acuity if the lesion is on the visual axis
- Discharge (purulent), tearing
- Photophobia
- Puffiness of lids

(Tables 7.5 and 7.6). Figure 7.4 shows the photograph of an event of *Pseudomonas* keratitis in a contact lens wearer.

Many micro-organisms have been implicated in contact lens-related MK, with bacteria, fungi and protozoa found (Table 7.7). However, for the past two decades, the predominant organism isolated from contact lens-related MK has been *Pseudomonas aeruginosa* (Alfonso *et al.*, 1986; Donnenfeld *et al.*, 1986; Ormerod and Smith, 1986; Cohen *et al.*, 1987; Dart, 1988; Chatterjee *et al.*, 1995; Sharma *et al.*, 2003). Other frequently reported organisms include *Staphylococcus* sp. and *Acanthamoeba* (Donnenfeld *et al.*, 1986; Mondino *et al.*, 1986; Ormerod and Smith, 1986; Wilhelmus, 1987; Cohen *et al.*, 1987, 1996), although *Acanthamoeba* appears almost exclusively as a DW contaminated lens storage problem.

Risk factors and pathogenesis

A normal, healthy cornea is rarely infected. Conditions that breach or affect the corneal epithelium are the major risk factors for an event of MK and include trauma (Upadhyay *et al.*, 1982; Ormerod, 1987; Dart, 1988; Cruz *et al.*, 1993; Gebauer *et al.*, 1996; Bennett *et al.*, 1998), contact lens wear (Dart, 1988;

Table 7.6   Clinical signs of microbial keratitis

Feature	Signs
Corneal infiltrate	
– Location	Mainly central or paracentral, sometimes peripheral
– Type	Large, dense, irregular infiltrate (>1 mm); possibly multiple focal
– Depth	Anterior to mid-stroma, may involve entire depth; ulceration and necrosis of infiltrate with severe disease
Surrounding cornea	Involved, ranges from oedema, diffuse infiltrates to satellite lesions or ring infiltrate
Overlying epithelium	Commonly full-thickness loss (when active)
Endothelium	Ranges from none to endothelial dusting with cells, keratic precipitates/plaques
Anterior chamber reaction	Common, ranging from flare to hypopyon
Lid oedema	Usual; blepharospasm may be present
Bulbar/limbal redness	Severe; conjunctival chemosis may be present
Unilateral/bilateral	Typically unilateral

Schematic representation

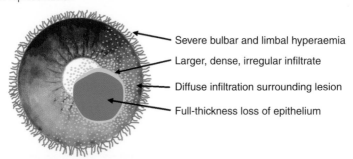

Severe bulbar and limbal hyperaemia

Larger, dense, irregular infiltrate

Diffuse infiltration surrounding lesion

Full-thickness loss of epithelium

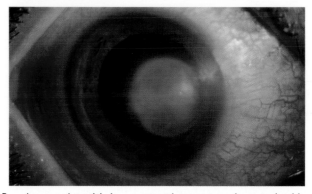

Figure 7.4   *Pseudomonas* keratitis in a contact lens wearer characterized by severe ocular redness and a large, dense paracentral infiltrate (courtesy LVPEI, India)

Table 7.7 Microbes isolated from corneal scrapes of events with lens-related microbial keratitis

Micro-organism reported	Authors
Bacteria (Gram-negative)	
Pseudomonas aeruginosa	Alfonso *et al.* (1986)
	Bennett *et al.* (1998)
	Chalupa *et al.* (1987)
	Chatterjee *et al.* (1995)
	Cheng *et al.* (1999)
	Cooper and Constable (1977)
	Dart (1988)
	Kent *et al.* (1989)
	Killingsworth and Stern (1989)
	Mondino *et al.* (1986)
	Nilsson and Montan (1994)
	Ormerod and Smith (1986)
	Patrinely *et al.* (1985)
	Sharma *et al.* (2003)
	Weissman *et al.* (1984)
Pseudomonas fluorescens	Dunn *et al.* (1989)
Pseudomonas cepacia	Patrinely *et al.* (1985)
Stenotrophomonas maltophila	Cheng *et al.* (1999)
	Lemp *et al.* (1984)
Pseudomonas spp.	Adams *et al.* (1983)
	Alfonso *et al.* (1986)
	Cohen *et al.* (1987)
	Cohen *et al.* (1996)
	Donnenfeld *et al.* (1986)
	Sharma *et al.* (2003)
	Stapleton *et al.* (1993)
Moraxella lacunata	Dart (1988)
Moraxella spp.	Stapleton *et al.* (1993)
Serratia liquefaciens	Cooper and Constable (1977)
Serratia marcescens	Alfonso *et al.* (1986)
	Cheng *et al.* (1999)
	Cohen *et al.* (1987)
	Dart (1988)
	Donnenfeld *et al.* (1986)
	Lemp *et al.* (1984)
Serratia spp.	Adams *et al.* (1983)
	Ormerod and Smith (1986)
Klebsiella oxytoca	Dart (1988)
	Lemp *et al.* (1984)
Klebsiella pneumoniae	Lemp *et al.* (1984)
Klebsiella spp.	Cheng *et al.* (1999)
	Donnenfeld *et al.* (1986)
Acinetobacter calcoaceticus	Cheng *et al.* (1999)
	Lemp *et al.* (1984)

Table 7.7 *Continued*

Acinetobacter spp.	Bennett *et al.* (1998)
	Ormerod and Smith (1986)
Haemophilus influenzae	Mondino *et al.* (1986)
Morganella morganii	Mondino *et al.* (1986)
Proteus mirabilis	Alfonso *et al.* (1986)
	Lemp *et al.* (1984)
	Spoor *et al.* (1984)
Proteus morganii	Alfonso *et al.* (1986)
Proteus vulgaris	Lemp *et al.* (1984)
Escherichia coli	Cooper and Constable (1977)
	Lemp *et al.* (1984)
	Weissman *et al.* (1984)
Enterobacter aerogenes	Cooper and Constable (1977)
Enterobacter spp.	Cheng *et al.* (1999)
Unidentified Gram-negative bacilli	Alfonso *et al.* (1986)
	Ormerod and Smith (1986)

Bacteria (Gram-positive)

Staphylococcus epidermidis	Cohen *et al.* (1987)
	Dart (1988)
	Maguen *et al.* (1991)
	Mondino *et al.* (1986)
	Nilsson and Montan (1994)
	Ormerod and Smith (1986)
	Patrinely *et al.* (1985)
	Sharma *et al.* (2003)
	Spoor *et al.* (1984)
Staphylococcus spp.	Cheng *et al.* (1999)
	Cohen *et al.* (1996)
	Donnenfeld *et al.* (1986)
	Stapleton *et al.* (1993)
Staphylococcus aureus	Alfonso *et al.* (1986)
	Bennett *et al.* (1998)
	Chalupa *et al.* (1987)
	Cohen *et al.* (1987)
	Cooper and Constable (1977)
	Mondino *et al.* (1986)
	Nilsson and Montan (1994)
	Ormerod and Smith (1986)
	Patrinely *et al.* (1985)
	Sharma *et al.* (2003)
	Spoor *et al.* (1984)
	Weissman *et al.* (1984)
Alpha-haemolytic streptococci	Bennett *et al.* (1998)
	Dart (1988)
	Ormerod and Smith (1986)
	Sharma *et al.* (2003)

Table 7.7   *Continued*

Streptococcus pneumoniae	Bennett *et al.* (1998)
	Dart (1988)
Streptococcus viridans	Bennett *et al.* (1998)
	Dart (1988)
Streptococcus spp.	Alfonso *et al.* (1986)
	Cheng *et al.* (1999)
	Donnenfeld *et al.* (1986)
	Sharma *et al.* (2003)
Diphtheroids	Cohen *et al.* (1987)
	Dunn *et al.* (1989)
Propionibacterium acnes	Dunn *et al.* (1989)
	Mondino *et al.* (1986)
	Weissman *et al.* (1984)
Coagulase-negative *Staphylococcus*	Bennett *et al.* (1998)
Nocardia spp.	Weissman *et al.* (1984)
Bacillus cereus	Patrinely *et al.* (1985)
Bacillus spp.	Ormerod and Smith (1986)
Micrococcus spp.	Ormerod and Smith (1986)
Corynebacterium diphtheriae	Cheng *et al.* (1999)
Aerobic spore-forming bacilli	Cheng *et al.* (1999)
Protozoa	
Acanthamoeba spp.	Bennett *et al.* (1998)
	Cohen *et al.* (1996)
	Ficker *et al.* (1989)
	Nilsson and Montan (1994)
	Sharma *et al.* (2003)
	Stapleton *et al.* (1993)
Vahlkampfia	Bennett *et al.* (1998)
Fungi	
Fusarium solani	Wilhelmus *et al.* (1988)
Fusarium spp.	Alfonso *et al.* (1986)
Cephalosporium spp.	Wilhelmus *et al.* (1988)
Paecilomyces spp.	Wilhelmus *et al.* (1988)
Aspergillus wentii	Wilhelmus *et al.* (1988)
Candida spp.	Wilhelmus *et al.* (1988)
Candida parapsilosis	Wilhelmus *et al.* (1988)
Candida tropicalis	Wilhelmus *et al.* (1988)
Arthographis kalrae	Perlman and Binns (1997)
Penicillium spp.	Ormerod and Smith (1986)

McClellan *et al.*, 1989; Cruz *et al.*, 1993; Cheung and Slomovic, 1995; Gebauer *et al.*, 1996; Bennett *et al.*, 1998), pre-existing ocular surface disease such as dry eye or corneal erosions (Dart, 1988; McClellan *et al.*, 1989; Cruz *et al.*, 1993; Gebauer *et al.*, 1996; Bennett *et al.*, 1998), systemic conditions such as diabetes

(Cruz *et al.*, 1993), and previous ocular surgery (Cruz *et al.*, 1993; Cheung and Slomovic, 1995).

Contact lens wear

Various factors have been found to encourage the risk of developing an event of MK with contact lens wear. These include EW of both conventional and disposable hydrogels (Weissman *et al.*, 1984; Donnenfeld *et al.*, 1986; Ormerod and Smith, 1986; Cohen *et al.*, 1987; Dart, 1988; Dunn *et al.*, 1989; Schein *et al.*, 1989; Schein and Poggio, 1990; Macrae *et al.*, 1991; Buehler *et al.*, 1992; Matthews *et al.*, 1992; Cohen *et al.*, 1996), use of contaminated lens care solutions and products (Cooper and Constable, 1977; Patrinely *et al.*, 1985; Mondino *et al.*, 1986; Dart, 1988; Wilhelmus *et al.*, 1988), therapeutic lens wear in the presence of a compromised ocular surface (Ormerod and Smith, 1986), concomitant usage of corticosteroids and contact lens wear (Chalupa *et al.*, 1987), diabetes (Eichenbaum *et al.*, 1982), and smoking (Schein and Poggio, 1990).

In DW the overwhelming factor appears to be lens contamination through inadequate care, storage and disinfection. For EW it appears to be the oxygen transmissibility of the lens. Holden *et al.* (1985) reported that EW of low-*Dk* hydrogel lenses induced significant structural and functional changes in all layers of the cornea. Importantly, lens wear was found to suppress the aerobic epithelial metabolism. This compromises the epithelial barrier to infection as evidenced by epithelial thinning and the accumulation of microcysts (Holden *et al.*, 1985) and a decrease in mitosis (Hamano *et al.*, 1983). Madigan (1990) reported significant changes in the epithelium of cat and monkey animal models induced by EW of hydrogels, including decreased numbers of cells and misshapen cells. Madigan *et al.* (1987) reported a significant loss of corneal epithelial adhesion in the model eyes wearing EW hydrogel lenses in comparison to the control non-lens-wearing eyes due to defective epithelial basement membrane attachment caused by a decrease in the density of the hemidesmosomes (Madigan and Holden, 1988, 1992). It was said that these effects could be minimized by fitting lenses that have greater oxygen transmissibility. Solomon *et al.* (1994) demonstrated that corneal hypoxia, with a contact lens in place, was the major risk factor for the development of *Pseudomonas* corneal ulcers in studies. Remarkably, they reported that a contaminated contact lens and closed-eye rabbit model was more effective in inducing corneal infection than corneal incision, inoculation with the bacteria and closed eye. The authors proposed that a swollen cornea may lead to abrasion of the corneal epithelium and thus provide an entry point for the infectious agent. All these reports indicate that a break in the continuity of the epithelium or a compromised epithelium is an important risk factor for the development of an event of MK, but that a contaminated contact lens–closed-eye wear combination presented the greatest hazard.

Fleiszig *et al.* (1998) suggested that certain cytotoxic bacteria can damage the epithelium on an uninjured corneal surface, provided there is prolonged bacterial contact. It would appear, however, that such a mechanism is rarely, if ever, operative without a contact lens in place. As discussed in Chapter 4, the external

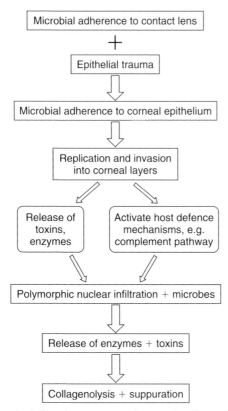

Figure 7.5   Flow chart depicting the sequence of events leading to MK

ocular surface has highly organized defence mechanisms which are able to eliminate pathogens in contact with the ocular surface and therefore microbes would
not be expected to be infective in a normal non-lens-wearing situation. However,
a contact lens can act both as a trap and as a substratum for the microbes (Miller
and Ahearn, 1987) and, in EW, is able to promote contact of the microbes with
the ocular surface for prolonged periods.

Possible mechanisms involved in the pathogenesis of an event of MK are complex and are dealt with elsewhere. We present, however, a simple flow chart depicting the possible sequence of events leading to MK (Figure 7.5). The initial step
in the pathogenesis of MK with hydrogel EW involves colonization of the contact lens by the microbes. Studies have demonstrated the ability of microbes such
as *Acanthamoeba* and *Pseudomonas* to adhere to hydrogel lenses (Miller and
Ahearn, 1987; Gorlin *et al.*, 1995; Sharma *et al.*, 1995). Given suitable conditions
these organisms can then adhere to, damage and/or invade the epithelium (Stern
et al., 1982, 1985; Fleiszig *et al.*, 1998). Without antibiotics or other modu-
lating factors, bacteria then invade, survive and replicate in the corneal stroma
(Wilhelmus, 1996), leading to a cascade of events culminating in tissue inflammation, destruction and a dense corneal infiltrate.

Severity as an eye disease

The CLIC Guide rates severity of each condition as an eye disease where 1 = very slight, 2 = slight, 3 = moderate and 4 = severe, e.g. a sight-threatening eye disease such as a centrally located MK. As the rating is based on direct observation of the patient, ratings will obviously vary with both the severity of the condition and the stage of the condition. The event ratings for five events of MK seen in these studies were 2.8 ± 0.3 with conventional soft lenses and 2.8 ± 0.8 with silicone hydrogel lenses.

Management

Prompt attention and aggressive treatment are essential for suspected corneal infection as infections associated with virulent organisms or many bacterial ulcers can progress rapidly to involve the entire cornea.

A corneal scrape and culture is the most *predictive* of the tests that will help determine the type of microbe infecting the cornea and will need to be conducted prior to instillation of any topical antibiotic. Other tests that can be helpful in making a tentative diagnosis include Gram stains of the corneal scrapes, and lid and conjunctival cultures. In addition, if the patient presents with a contact lens on the eye, it should be removed using sterile gloves and submitted for microbial culture. The lens care solutions and lens case that the patient may have been using at the time of the event should also be processed, as they could provide valuable information on the involved pathogen.

Aggressive antibiotic therapy delivered topically at frequent intervals is the usual practice; however, treatment could vary depending on the stage and severity of the condition. The common practice is to start empirical therapy with broad-spectrum antibiotic(s) drops delivered topically at frequent intervals. This therapy may then be modified based on the results of the corneal smears.

For suspected bacterial infections, the empirical therapy should include an antibiotic to cover Gram-positive organisms and a fluoroquinolone or an aminoglycoside to cover Gram-negative organisms. However, a single agent like ciprofloxacin 0.3 per cent is widely used as the antibiotic of choice for its activity against a range of Gram-positive and Gram-negative organisms. However, a second-line agent is needed where resistance is demonstrated, especially with Gram-positive organisms such as *Streptococcus* spp. as recent studies suggest that, while ciprofloxacin is effective against 94 per cent of Gram-negative isolates that were tested, only 61 per cent of Gram-positive isolates were susceptible to ciprofloxacin (Graves *et al.*, 2001).

Wherever a fungal infection is suspected, treatment will need to include an antifungal agent (5 per cent natamycin) and with a protozoal infection, an aminoglycoside (e.g. neomycin) or a diamidine (dibromopropamidine 0.3 per cent) needs to be used. The patient should be closely monitored. If the condition is potentially sight-threatening or severe, hospitalization is necessary. Adjunctive medications (e.g. cycloplegics) or other routes of drug delivery (e.g. subconjunctival injections, collagen shields) may be indicated depending on the presenting clinical features.

Severe and large events threatening the integrity of the globe may require more radical therapy such as application of cyanoacrylate tissue adhesive or therapeutic keratoplasty; however, a discussion of these procedures is beyond the scope of this chapter.

MK resolves in a scar which may impair vision if it is in the visual axis or if it induces astigmatism due to the cicatrization process. Secondary corneal changes such as corneal vascularization or calcific degeneration can occur with severe events.

The outcome of the disease in terms of vision and corneal changes will determine whether the patient can continue in contact lens wear. Many patients will not wish to resume contact lens wear and the practitioners may be unwilling to prescribe lenses. However, if the patient wishes to continue with lenses, the practitioner will need to discuss the likelihood of a repeat infection.

If there is induced astigmatism or an irregular corneal surface due to corneal scarring, the practitioner may want to consider RGP lenses. These lenses are also an option if there is any vascularization as a result of the disease. If soft lenses can be prescribed and if the patient is willing to be refitted, they need to be prescribed on a DW schedule. Importantly, all lens wearers need to be educated to recognize and minimize risk factors through precautions such as:

- using protective eye wear in places where they are exposed to contaminants;
- not swimming in their lenses without swimming goggles;
- rigorous cleaning of hands before lens handling;
- rigorous cleaning of lens cases;
- care to ensure that lens care solutions remain sterile (capping the lens care solution bottle tightly, keeping the bottle nozzle clean and not using old solutions);
- if lenses are discontinued and stored for any period of time, proper cleaning and disinfection of lenses prior to reinserting on eye;
- discontinuing lens wear during periods of acute illness which may expose the eyes to pathogens; and
- checking eyes regularly and discontinuing lens wear in response to any potential warning signs such as increased redness or discomfort.

For any suspected corneal infection, the single most important factor determining the outcome is the immediate removal of the lens and the speed at which appropriate treatment is initiated. Clinical practice demonstrates that if the lens is removed immediately and appropriate treatment vigorously commenced, the prognosis is usually good. Delay in removal and treatment can be disastrous. Practitioners prescribing EW lenses need to provide a 24-hour service, e.g. using a pager or a mobile telephone.

SIGNIFICANT ADVERSE EVENTS (COMMONLY SYMPTOMATIC)

Six types of significant adverse events will be reviewed in this chapter: CLARE, contact lens peripheral ulcer (CLPU), infiltrative keratitis (IK), CLPC, superior epithelial arcuate lesion (SEAL) and corneal erosion.

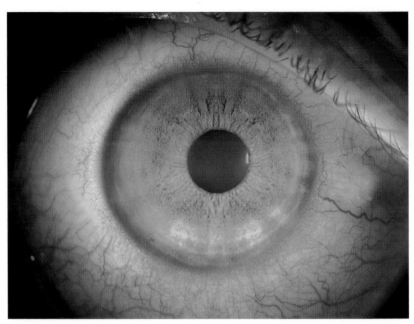

Figure 7.6   Marked bulbar and limbal conjunctival hyperaemia in an event of CLARE

Contact lens-induced acute red eye

CLARE is a sudden-onset, corneal infiltrative event observed during EW/CW of conventional hydrogel and silicone hydrogel lenses and always found associated with sleeping in lenses (Holden *et al.*, 1996; Sankaridurg *et al.*, 1996, 1999b; Nilsson, 1997). Typically the patient reports being woken from sleep with symptoms of irritation or pain, redness and watery eyes, or these symptoms are noticed soon after waking. The condition is normally unilateral. First reported by Zantos and Holden in 1978, CLARE was referred to as a 'red eye reaction' or 'non-ulcerative keratitis'. Mertz and Holden (1981) described a similar condition referred to as 'acute ocular inflammation'.

Clinically there is marked bulbar and limbal conjunctival hyperaemia with watery discharge (Figure 7.6). Mild conjunctival chemosis is sometimes seen. The defining feature of the condition is the presence of fine, diffuse, cellular infiltration of the peripheral to mid-peripheral cornea associated with clusters of faint, focal infiltrates (Figure 7.7). The infiltrates are limited to the anterior stroma. There is no lucid or clear interval between the diffuse infiltration and the limbus and infiltrates appear to be streaming in from the limbal vessels. The extent of involvement of the diffuse infiltration along the corneal circumference ranges from 10 to 360 degrees and most frequently 240 ± 113 degrees (median value) (Sankaridurg, 1999). The focal infiltrates are found interspersed among the diffuse infiltration or extend centrally into the clear cornea. Epithelial involvement, if present, is minimal and limited to punctate corneal staining. The posterior cornea is clear and anterior chamber involvement is rare. Vision is normally unaffected.

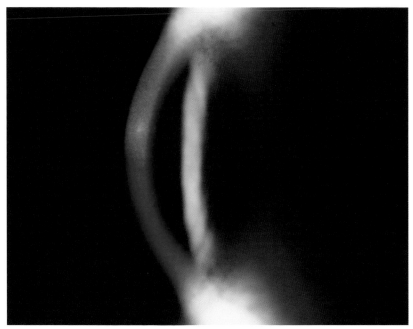

Figure 7.7   CLARE: diffuse infiltration extending in from the limbus in the superior quadrant (observed as granular, hazy area) associated with a focal infiltrate

Microbiological analysis of contact lenses retrieved at the time of CLARE revealed many lenses to be contaminated with significant levels of Gram-negative bacteria (Sankaridurg *et al.*, 1996). Occasionally Gram-positive bacteria were also seen (Sankaridurg *et al.*, 1999a) but, as described by Willcox *et al.* in Chapter 4, Gram-negative bacteria such as *Haemophilus influenzae*, *Serratia marcescens* and *Pseudomonas* spp. were most frequent.

Temporary discontinuation of lens wear until resolution of the corneal infiltrates is required. No medical therapy is required. The condition resolves to a clear cornea with no sequalae.

Incidence

CLARE has been reported with EW/CW of conventional hydrogel and silicone hydrogel lenses. Sudden onset, unilateral, non-infective acute red eye (ARE), with no epithelial involvement and an infiltrate pattern as seen in CLARE, has rarely if ever been reported in otherwise healthy non-wearers or daily lens wearers. Table 7.8 details the incidence of the condition from various studies.

Clinical features

Tables 7.9 and 7.10 describe the most frequently observed symptoms and signs for a group of 67 events of CLARE seen in the CCLRU/LVPEI clinical studies.

Table 7.8   Annualized incidence of CLARE

Lens type	Mode of wear	Description of event	Incidence (%)	Eyes/ people	Authors
Spectacles	–	CLARE	0	Eyes	CCLRU/LVPEI database
Soft	DW	CLARE	0	Eyes	CCLRU/LVPEI database
Soft	EW	Non-ulcerative keratitis	34.0 (2 years)	People	Zantos and Holden (1978)
Soft	EW	CLARE	12.3	People	Sankaridurg et al. (1999b)
Soft	EW	CLARE	1.0	Eyes	CCLRU database
Soft	EW	CLARE	7.0	Eyes	LVPEI database
Silicone hydrogel	CW	CLARE	0.8	Eyes	Nilsson (1997)
Silicone hydrogel	EW	CLARE	0.7	Eyes	Nilsson (1997)
Silicone hydrogel	CW	CLARE	12.8	Eyes	LVPEI database
Silicone hydrogel	CW	CLARE	2.5	Eyes	CCLRU database

Table 7.9   Symptoms of CLARE

Symptoms
- No symptoms before eye closure
- Patient woken from sleep by symptoms, or symptoms noticed soon after waking
- Irritation to moderate pain
- Redness, tearing, burning sensation and photophobia

Zantos and Holden (1978) reported that CLARE presents with pain (described as a scratchy sensation beneath the top lid), watering, red eye, light sensitivity and an occasionally sticky eye. The clinical signs included marked conjunctival and ciliary vessel engorgement and small patches of infiltrates scattered over the peripheral parts of the cornea. Minor atypical fluorescein staining was seen overlying some foci of infiltrates and debris was found trapped beneath the contact lens.

Risk factors and pathogenesis

CLARE is always associated with overnight wear of lenses (Zantos and Holden, 1978; Mertz and Holden, 1981; Holden et al., 1996; Sankaridurg et al., 1996, 1999a). Zantos and Holden (1978) and Mertz and Holden (1981) found debris trapped beneath the contact lens and also a tight lens during events of ARE. It was suggested that the condition may be an immunological reaction due to the accumulation of toxins on or beneath the lens. Cytological studies of debris specimens taken from subjects showing inflammation indicated the presence of mucus and a high concentration of inflammatory cells. However, recent studies (Sankaridurg, 1999) found no relationship between lens tightness (during the day) and the development of a CLARE response.

Table 7.10   Clinical signs of CLARE

Feature	Signs
Corneal infiltrate	
– Location	Peripheral to mid–peripheral
– Type	Fine, faint, cellular, diffuse infiltration (either sectorial or circumferential); fine clusters of focal infiltrates (low to moderate in number) interspersed amongst diffuse infiltration or beyond in the clear cornea
– Depth	Anterior stroma (subepithelial)
Overlying epithelium	No significant staining; if present, limited to punctate corneal staining
Corneal oedema	Uncommon
Anterior chamber reaction	Uncommon
Lid oedema	Uncommon
Bulbar/limbal redness	Moderate to severe; circumferential
Unilateral/bilateral	Commonly unilateral

Schematic representation

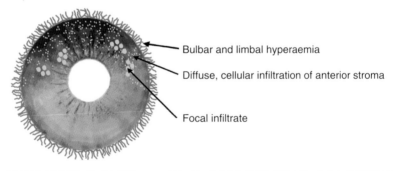

Bulbar and limbal hyperaemia

Diffuse, cellular infiltration of anterior stroma

Focal infiltrate

Baleriola-Lucas *et al.* (1991) reported that patients with CLARE had high levels of Gram-negative bacterial contamination of their lenses. Interestingly, in a study conducted at the CCLRU, 12 patients wore contact lenses overnight that were inadvertently contaminated with high levels of Gram-negative bacteria such as *P. aeruginosa* and *Serratia* spp. Five eyes of four subjects (21 per cent) developed a CLARE response and an additional seven eyes (29 per cent) developed infiltrates (Holden *et al.*, 1996). The authors suggested that endotoxin released from the bacteria on the lenses was the primary cause of the cellular infiltration seen during the CLARE response. More evidence supporting this link was found when contact lenses retrieved at the time of a CLARE event were found to be contaminated with significant levels of Gram-negative bacteria such as *H. influenzae* and Gram-positive bacteria such as *Streptococcus pneumoniae* (Sankaridurg *et al.*,

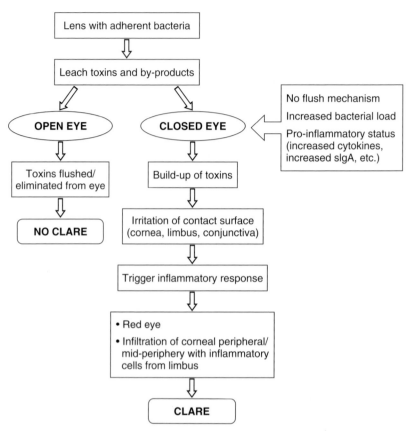

Figure 7.8   Possible sequence of events leading to a CLARE response (adapted from Sankaridurg, 1999)

1996, 1999a). Table 4.5 (Chapter 4) presents a list of bacteria isolated from the contact lenses during events of CLARE for studies conducted at the CCLRU/LVPEI.

Based on the evidence it appears that CLARE is an acute inflammatory reaction to toxins such as lipopolysaccharide, enzymes and other by-products leaching from bacteria present on the contact lens. The possible sequence of events leading to a CLARE are presented as a flow chart in Figure 7.8. A period of eye closure associated with bacterial contamination of the contact lens appears to be a crucial factor triggering the CLARE response. As described in Chapter 4, a number of changes occur in the external eye during eye closure and include the absence of flushing mechanisms of tears, decrease in the tear flow, and increase in pro-inflammatory cytokine levels such as interleukin-6 (IL-6), IL-8, granulocyte-macrophage colony-stimulating factor (GM-CSF), leukotriene B_4 (LTB$_4$) and platelet activation factor (PAF) (Thakur *et al.*, 1998) and an increase in secretory immunoglobulin A (sIgA) (Tan *et al.*, 1993). Also an increase in the bacterial load with overnight eye closure has been reported (Ramachandran *et al.*, 1995). All of these changes contribute to a pro-inflammatory state of the external eye during eye closure. A build-up of the bacterial toxins and by-products during the closed eye state, in combination with some of the above factors, triggers an inflammatory response resulting in the peripheral corneal infiltrative response that is CLARE (Figure 7.7). Evidence giving weight to this hypothesis was found when tears recovered from patients experiencing CLARE responses showed increased levels of cytokines and chemoattractants, particularly GM-CSF, IL-8, LTB$_4$ and PAF-like activity in comparison to control tears (Thakur and Willcox, 1998). In spite of significant levels of Gram-negative bacteria on the contact lens, no infection was seen in any of the events. In Chapter 4, Willcox *et al.* elucidate the factors that are responsible for these pathogens causing only an inflammatory episode rather than infection.

Severity as an eye disease

For 67 events of CLARE observed in the CCLRU/LVPEI clinical studies, the mean severity was 2.1 ± 0.7.

Management

CLARE necessitates discontinuation of lens wear and resolves simply on cessation of lens wear (Zantos and Holden, 1978; Sankaridurg *et al.*, 1999b) without the need for anti-inflammatory agents or antibiotics. Zantos and Holden (1978) reported that complete disappearance of infiltrates required one to two weeks. Sankaridurg *et al.* (1999b) reported that 17 per cent of events resolved by day four, 38 per cent by day seven, 67 per cent by day 14, 88 per cent by day 22 and the maximum time to resolution was day 45. The cornea was clear on resolution and there were no sequalae.

Recurrences of CLARE episodes are reported, with one study reporting that nearly 75 per cent of the patients are prone to having a recurrent attack (Sweeney *et al.*, 1993). They reported the probability of having a second episode of a CLARE to be as high as 0.73 and a third occurrence as high as 0.64 (Sweeney *et al.*, 1993). However, another study reported the probability of recurrence to be 0.13 (Sankaridurg, 1999). More importantly, reports suggest that recurrent events tend to occur in the immediate period following the first event. In a group of six subjects who had recurrent CLARE the time to recurrence was 2.0 ± 1.7 months following the first episode. Therefore, on resolution of a CLARE event and prior to recommencing EW, patients need to be counselled as to the possibility of recurrence. The sources of bacteria contaminating the contact lenses and leading to a CLARE response are believed to be other body sites, such as oropharynx or the nasolacrimal duct (Sankaridurg *et al.*, 1996, 1999a), or the domestic water supply (Willcox *et al.*, 1997). Instances of patients having cold-like symptoms preceding the CLARE event and the same organism seen on the contact lens being recovered from the throat support this hypothesis (Sankaridurg *et al.*, 1996). Contact lens wearers should therefore be made aware of the potential risk of developing events such as CLARE during and subsequent to periods of upper respiratory tract infection or acute illnesses such as influenza and advised to discontinue lens wear during such episodes.

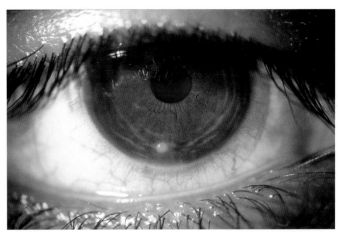

Figure 7.9   Circular, dense focal infiltrate on the eye at 6 o'clock meridian (mucus plug on the infiltrate)

Contact lens peripheral ulcer

CLPU, like CLARE, is mostly observed with EW, with some events in DW (Grant *et al.*, 1998). Events of CLPU have also been reported with CW of silicone hydrogels (Long *et al.*, 2000; Iruzubieta *et al.*, 2001). Depending on the stage at which they present, individuals with CLPU may present with or without symptoms. When symptoms are present, redness is the most frequently reported, followed by pain or soreness, irritation and watering (Grant *et al.*, 1998; Holden *et al.*, 1999; Sankaridurg, 1999). The condition is almost always unilateral and almost invariably consists of a single lesion.

As with the symptoms, the clinical presentation can vary depending on the stage at which the patient is seen. In its acute stage, CLPU is characterized by marked bulbar and limbal hyperaemia, often more severe in the quadrant corresponding to the area of corneal infiltration. A circular, well-circumscribed, dense, yellowish-white, focal corneal infiltrate ranging in diameter from 0.2 to 1.2 mm and located in the peripheral to mid-peripheral cornea is characteristic of the event (Figure 7.9). The infiltrate is always anterior stromal in depth and is associated with a complete loss of the overlying epithelium (defined by the presence of an epithelial defect overlying the infiltrate and rapid diffusion of fluorescein into the stroma; Figure 7.10). Fine, cellular, diffuse infiltration is seen extending in from the limbus and surrounding the focal infiltrate. The posterior cornea is clear. In severe cases the anterior chamber may show mild flare and cells. The condition resolves to an anterior stromal scar corresponding to the focal infiltrate. On occasions the patient may present with a focal infiltrate that is resolving. In such cases, the edges of the infiltrate show scarification or the epithelium overlying the infiltrate is intact or shows only punctate changes (Sankaridurg, 1999). The patient may also present for a routine aftercare visit with a well-circumscribed, focal, anterior, stromal scar representative of a resolved event (Grant *et al.*, 1998). Vision is normally unaffected.

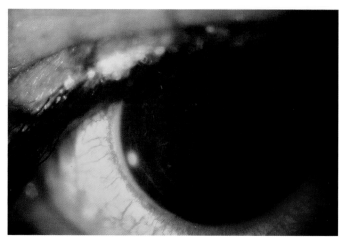

Figure 7.10   Event of CLPU: evaluation with fluorescein shows staining overlying the infiltrate and a glow surrounding the infiltrate indicative of stromal diffusion of the dye

Table 7.11   Annualized incidence of CLPU

Lens type	Mode of wear	Description of event	Incidence (%)	Eyes/people	Authors
Spectacles	–	CLPU	0	Eyes	CCLRU/LVPEI database
Soft	DW	CLPU	2.5	Eyes	LVPEI database
Soft	EW	CLPU	13.6	People	Sankaridurg *et al.* (1999b)
Soft	EW	CLPU	8.4	Eyes	LVPEI database
Soft	EW	CLPU	1.1	Eyes	CCLRU database
Silicone hydrogel	CW	CLPU	13.8	Eyes	LVPEI database
Silicone hydrogel	CW	CLPU	2.1	Eyes	CCLRU database

In its acute phase CLPU necessitates temporary discontinuation of lens wear until resolution of the corneal infiltrates. As with CLARE, CLPU simply resolves on cessation of lens wear without the need for any medical therapy. The anterior stromal scar is seen to persist for periods beyond six months from the onset of the event.

Incidence

Table 7.11 presents the incidence of CLPU. The condition is seen to occur during both DW and EW/CW with hydrogels including silicone hydrogels. A review of the literature suggests that some events described as microbial infections are likely to be events of CLPU (Schein and Poggio, 1990; Buehler *et al.*, 1992). Also the description of the clinical features of other entities such as 'sterile keratitis', 'peripheral corneal infiltrates' and 'infiltrates' is similar to those seen with CLPU.

Table 7.12   Symptoms with CLPU

Symptoms
- Redness
- Pain
- Watering
- Irritation
- Foreign body sensation
- Asymptomatic

'Peripheral corneal infiltrates' reported by Suchecki *et al.* (1996) were less than 1.5 mm in size, had anterior, stromal, cellular reaction in 75 per cent of events, were culture-negative in 50 per cent of events and 64 per cent of the events had corneal epithelial involvement. An anterior stromal cellular reaction was found in 75 per cent of the events. Ninety-four events of 'sterile keratitis' were reported by Bates *et al.* (1989) and 92 per cent of these events were peripheral in location. All events were associated with minimal symptoms, little discharge and small corneal lesions. Also nine events of 'paracentral infiltrates' which were culture-negative and had some features similar to events of CLPU were described by Mertz *et al.* (1990).

Clinical features

Tables 7.12 and 7.13 detail the clinical features of 43 events of CLPU seen in CCLRU/LVPEI clinical studies.

Grant *et al.* (1998) described CLPU to be a typically circular lesion and that fluorescein penetrated to the stroma if the ulcer was seen early in the episode, suggesting a full-thickness defect of the epithelium. Associated clinical signs included mild to moderate bulbar hyperaemia and epithelial and anterior stromal infiltrates surrounding the lesion. A large number of microcysts and endothelial bedewing were found associated with the event in some patients.

It is vital that CLPU be effectively distinguished from other events that occur in the peripheral cornea (Table 7.14). CLPU can mimic early MK and it is important to distinguish it from MK, which is potentially sight-threatening. Clinical features that are commonly associated with MK include increased severity of symptoms despite discontinuation of lens wear, lid oedema, purulent discharge, severe generalized bulbar and limbal redness, large, irregular focal infiltrate, satellite lesions, involvement of posterior cornea and endothelium and an anterior chamber response. These are not routinely seen with events of CLPU. Perhaps the most useful distinguishing features are that, with CLPU, the symptoms are milder and begin receding immediately on discontinuation of lens wear. CLPUs rapidly and simply resolve without treatment to leave a small, circumscribed scar, whereas MKs worsen if there is no medical intervention.

CLPU though, also being an inflammatory ulcer, is different from hypersensitivity-induced peripheral corneal diseases such as catarrhal ulcers or corneal phylctenulosis. Marginal corneal ulcers such as catarrhal ulcers are associated with

Table 7.13   Clinical signs of CLPU

Feature	Signs
Infiltrate	
– Location	Peripheral to mid-peripheral
– Type	Usually small, single, circular, dense, yellowish-white, focal infiltrate (up to 2 mm). Slight, fine diffuse infiltration surrounding focal infiltrate
– Depth	Anterior stroma (subepithelial)
Overlying epithelium	Full-thickness loss (when active)
Corneal oedema	Only if very severe, rarely clinically observed
Anterior chamber reaction	Only if severe
Lid oedema	Uncommon
Bulbar/limbal redness	Moderate; severe in the region corresponding to the focal infiltrate
Unilateral/bilateral	Unilateral
On resolution	Circular, anterior stromal scar which persists for more than six months beyond the event

Schematic representation

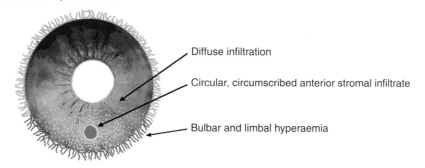

Diffuse infiltration

Circular, circumscribed anterior stromal infiltrate

Bulbar and limbal hyperaemia

Table 7.14   Differential diagnosis for CLPU

Conditions
- Early MK
- Catarrhal infiltrates or marginal keratitis
- Corneal phylectenulosis

Staphylococcus aureus on the lid margins and are commonly located at 2, 4, 8 and 10 o'clock meridians, and are usually oval with a tendency to spread in a concentric manner (Mondino, 1988). Also, the infiltrate is separated from the limbus by a distinct clear interval which, on occasions, is bridged by blood vessels (Figure 7.11).

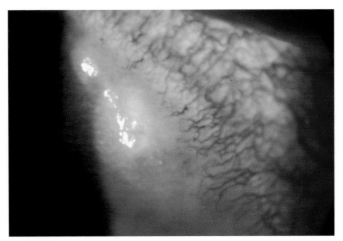

Figure 7.11   Marginal corneal ulcer characterized by an oval arcuate shaped infiltrate. Note blood vessels in the clear cornea approaching the infiltrate

CLPUs, on the other hand, occur at all meridians of the peripheral cornea (Grant *et al.*, 1998). Importantly, there is no clear interval with diffuse infiltrates seen streaming in from the limbus and enclosing the focal infiltrate. Blood vessels (or vascularization) are not seen with CLPU. CLPU is also different from corneal phylectenulosis in that there is an absence of raised nodular infiltrates and vascularization, which are features of events of phylectenulosis.

Stein *et al.* (1988) examined a series of 50 patients with culture-negative infiltrates and reported that minimal pain and anterior chamber reaction, absence of discharge and epithelial staining limited to superficial punctate keratitis were associated with this condition. A variety of causes such as preservatives in contact lens solutions and hypoxia were found. Interestingly, they also had events with arcuate infiltrates. None of the CLPUs were arcuate in shape and it therefore appears that, while events reported by Stein *et al.* encompass a broad spectrum of conditions with culture-negative infiltrates, CLPU is possibly just one of the entities.

Risk factors and pathogenesis

The aetiology of CLPU remains somewhat unclear; however, it is certain that it is not a corneal infection as both scrapings and biopsies show absolutely no evidence of micro-organisms (Holden *et al.*, 1999). Thus, unless it is caused by some extremely subtle organism, it would appear to be an 'inflammatory' ulcer, with the scarring being caused by post-inflammatory cicatrization. Biopsies of four CLPU events revealed a focal epithelial loss with thinning of the adjacent epithelium, an intact Bowman's layer, dense infiltration of the anterior stroma with polymorphonuclear leucocytes (PMNs) and an absence of micro-organisms (Holden *et al.*, 1999).

CLPUs can show contact lens contamination with significant numbers of Gram-positive bacteria prior to an event (Willcox *et al.*, 1995). However, the link is not consistent for micro-organisms isolated at the time of an event (Holden *et al.*, 1999). This may be partly due to the difficulty of harvesting lenses as many patients go through an episode without realizing it. There have also been reports of significant bacterial contamination of lenses by *Staphylococcus aureus* (Jalbert *et al.*, 2000) and *streptococcus pneumoniae* (Sankaridurg *et al.*, 1999a) at the time of the event. Recent observation of these ulcers with silicone hydrogel lenses indicates that they are not related to hypoxia and may be exacerbated by minor surface trauma.

The presence of full-thickness loss of the epithelium during active events of CLPU raises interesting contradictory hypotheses as to whether this epithelial injury precedes or follows the infiltrate. Epithelial trauma releases chemokines and other chemoattractants (Lausch *et al.*, 1996; Planck *et al.*, 1997), which could lead to leucocyte infiltration. However, it is also possible that epithelial loss is secondary to the focal infiltrate. The cellular enzymes and toxins and other products involved in the formation of the infiltrate could release factors which led to dissolution of the overlying epithelium. The latter scenario is unlikely given the finding that Bowman's layer remains intact between the infiltrate and the epithelial loss (Holden *et al.*, 1999). Regardless of the exact aetiology, the epithelial loss and the infiltrate occur almost simultaneously, as a sequential process has never been observed.

The reason for the peripheral location of these events on the cornea is not understood. The striking immunological differences between the central and peripheral cornea give credence to the theory that the condition is an antigen–antibody reaction. In the eye, Langerhans cells are present in the conjunctiva and at the limbus. There is a decrease in the density of Langerhans cells from the periphery to the centre of the cornea and the central cornea is normally devoid of Langerhans cells (Gillette *et al.*, 1982). Components of the complement pathway such as C1 are said to exist in the peripheral to central cornea in a ratio of 5:1 (Mondino, 1988). Also immunoglobulin, such as IgM, is found more in the peripheral than the central cornea. Antigens in the peripheral cornea are reported to be closer to conjunctival blood vessels and lymphatics than antigens in the central cornea, presumably enabling them to elicit an immune response more easily (Mondino, 1988).

For CLPU to occur, it is possible that the contact lens acts either as (1) a vector for the delivery of the antigen to the corneal surface (e.g. bacteria) or (2) a trap for antigenic material against the cornea (e.g. retrolental debris). Presumably the antigenic material, possibly in combination with epithelial trauma, then releases chemical signals such as pro-inflammatory cytokines. Due to the proximity to the limbus, the peripheral cornea is able to deliver the antigens more effectively than the central cornea, thereby eliciting an immune response which consists of inflammatory cells homing to the site of the antigen (Figure 7.12) and possibly preventing infection.

Severity as an eye disease

In 43 events of CLPUs observed in the CCLRU/LVPEI clinical studies, the mean severity of the condition was 2.3 ± 0.5.

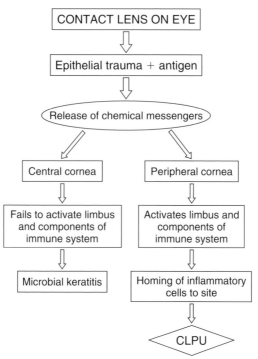

Figure 7.12   Flow chart depicting the possible sequence of events leading to a CLPU event (adapted from Sankaridurg, 1999)

Management

Events of CLPU are benign, self-limiting and resolving, leaving a small, round, sometimes 'bull's eye' (denser centre surrounded by a paler region) scar. Healed events are fairly commonly seen during extended lens wear (Sankaridurg, 1999). It is possible that in such circumstances the contact lens may have provided therapeutic insulation by acting as a bandage that masked patient symptoms and promoted healing. In addition to being benign and self-limiting, events resolve without the need for medical therapy. In a series of 19 active CLPUs, all events were found to resolve simply on discontinuation of lens wear. Twenty-one per cent resolved by day 7, 80 per cent by day 14 and all events by day 26. All events resolved to a subepithelial, circumscribed opacity which was present six months after the event (Sankaridurg, 1999). While Sweeney *et al.* (1993) did not find any recurrent events in their series of 12 events of CLPU, Sankaridurg (1999) reported the probability of having a second episode to be 0.33 and a third episode to be 0.14 in a study with an average wear time in EW of 13 ± 10 months. The time to recurrence following the first episode was 4.7 ± 4.2 months and ranged from 1.2 to 13 months. Therefore, as with CLARE, clinicians will need to warn patients of possible recurrences of the event if the patient recommences EW.

While evidence suggests that CLPU is a distinct non-infective entity, the similarity of initial appearance between a CLPU and early peripheral MK requires the

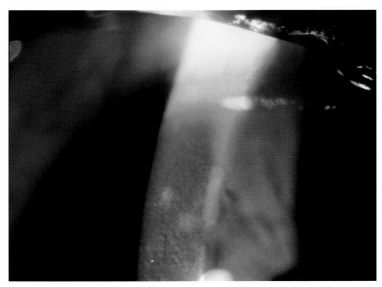

Figure 7.13   Event of IK: diffuse infiltration is seen in the superior quadrant and is associated with a focal infiltrate (from Sankaridurg, 1999)

clinician to take a conservative approach when managing CLPUs and (1) advise discontinuation of lens wear and prescribed prophylactic topical antibiotics; and (2) monitor the condition frequently, e.g. daily until resolution.

Infiltrative keratitis

IK is a general category for sudden-onset, symptomatic, infiltrative events observed during contact lens wear that are not categorized as MK, CLARE or CLPU. The condition reported in the following pages is distinct from the references in the literature to events of IK (Josephson and Caffery, 1979; Snyder, 1995). With IK the patient always reports symptoms with the most common being redness, pain, irritation and watering. Unlike events of CLARE, which are associated with sleep, patients with IK typically report the onset of symptoms to be later in the day and not associated with any sleep (Sankaridurg, 1999).

Mild to moderate bulbar and limbal conjunctival hyperaemia is seen and at times is accompanied by a watery discharge. The corneal signs are two-fold:

1. Some events have features suggestive of trauma (corneal erosion or epithelial defect) and on occasions a foreign body or foreign matter is seen on the cornea, trapped between the lens and eye. There is typically a corneal erosion with underlying infiltration corresponding to the location of the foreign body on the eye (Figure 7.13).

2. Some events present with faint, cellular, diffuse infiltration of the peripheral to mid-peripheral cornea (Figure 7.14). The infiltration is limited to the anterior stroma and is generally seen streaming in from the limbus. In a series of

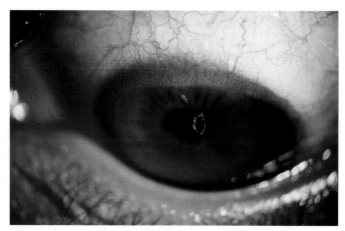

Figure 7.14   A corneal epithelial defect in the superior cornea which corresponded to a torn lens. Infiltrates (not depicted in the photo) were seen beneath the epithelial defect (from Sankaridurg, 1999)

21 events of IK observed with EW of disposable hydrogels, the extent of involvement of the corneal circumference with diffuse infiltration was 105 ± 84 degrees, ranging from 15 to 360 degrees (Sankaridurg, 1999). In addition to the diffuse infiltrates, focal infiltrates are also seen in many events and present either as (a) small clusters of cellular infiltrates which could be single or multiple, or (b) irregular, dense infiltrates. As with diffuse infiltrates, the focal infiltrates occur in the anterior stroma. In a majority of events, the epithelium overlying the infiltrates shows loss of continuity that ranges from mild punctate staining to frank epithelial defects. The posterior cornea and endothelium are not involved and the anterior chamber shows no activity. Vision is normally unaffected.

A percentage of the cases with clinical signs not associated with trauma have significant Gram-positive and Gram-negative bacteria isolated from the contact lenses during the event (Sankaridurg, 1999; see Chapter 4). In its acute phase the condition necessitates temporary discontinuation of lens wear and removal of the foreign body if present. IK resolves on cessation of lens wear with no medical therapy. In some events an opacity corresponding to the focal infiltrate or corneal erosion is seen as a sequel to the event (Sankaridurg, 1999).

Incidence

Table 7.15 lists the incidence of events of IK from CCLRU/LVPEI clinical studies. As can be seen from the table, the incidence of IK appears to be greater with silicone hydrogel lens wear in comparison to conventional lenses and it is thought that this could partly be due to the material properties of silicone hydrogel lenses, which produce greater mechanical interaction, resulting in trauma, irritation and inflammation of the cornea.

Table 7.15 Annualized incidence of IK

Lens type	Mode of wear	Description of event	Incidence (%)	Eyes/ people	Authors
Spectacles	–	IK	0	Eyes	CCLRU/LVPEI database
Soft	DW	IK	1.3	Eyes	LVPEI database
Soft	EW	IK	9.7	People	Sankaridurg et al. (1999b)
Disposable soft	EW	IK	4.0	Eyes	LVPEI database
Disposable soft	EW	IK	2.1	Eyes	CCLRU database
Silicone hydrogel	CW	IK	17.8	Eyes	LVPEI database
Silicone hydrogel	CW	IK	5.6	Eyes	CCLRU database

Table 7.16 Symptomatology for IK

Symptoms
- Redness
- Mild to moderate irritation or pain
- Watering
- Foreign body sensation

Clinical features

Tables 7.16 and 7.17 detail the clinical features of 57 events of IK observed in CCLRU/LVPEI clinical studies.

Risk factors and pathogenesis

There is possibly more than one mechanism leading to the development of IK. In some events the stimulus for development of corneal infiltrates is readily apparent, with trauma to the cornea evidently inducing the infiltration. It is possible that in these events either the foreign body or the epithelial compromise led to the infiltrative response. Corneal epithelial cells in disease states such as alkali burns are known normally to produce several cytokines such as IL-1, IL-6, IL-8 (Elner et al., 1991; Wilson et al., 1992; Sotozono et al., 1997) and lipid inflammatory mediators LTB_4 and 12-hydroxy-5,8,14-eicosatrienoic acid (12-HETE) (Husted et al., 1997; Thakur and Willcox, 1998; Chapter 4). When released these inflammatory cytokines can lead to infiltration by PMNs.

In other cases the clinical signs resemble those seen in CLARE, suggesting that a bacteria-driven response may be the cause. In a series of 21 events of IK, five patients with IK had a CLARE response either prior to or after the event (Sankaridurg, 1999) and some of these had Gram-negative bacteria on their lenses. Grimmer (1992) conducted a retrospective study of patients wearing hydrogel lenses of various water contents and found that medium- and high-water-content lenses were associated with a greater incidence of IK. Grimmer (1992) postulated that medium- and high-water-content materials may allow bacteria and viruses to adhere more readily to the protein that builds up on these surfaces.

Table 7.17   Clinical signs of IK

Feature	Signs
Corneal infiltrate	
– Location	Peripheral to mid-peripheral cornea
– Type	(1) Corneal erosion or defect with underlying diffuse infiltration – foreign body may be present
	(2) Faint, cellular diffuse infiltration with possibly small focal infiltrate(s)
– Depth	Anterior stroma (subepithelial)
Overlying epithelium	Involvement ranges from slight to severe
Corneal oedema	None
Anterior chamber reaction	None
Lid oedema	None
Bulbar/limbal redness	Slight to moderate, localized
Unilateral/bilateral	Unilateral
On resolution	May leave behind an opacity

Schematic representation

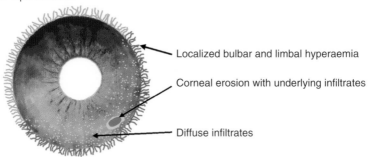

Localized bulbar and limbal hyperaemia

Corneal erosion with underlying infiltrates

Diffuse infiltrates

Severity as an eye disease

In 67 events observed in the CCLRU/LVPEI clinical studies, the severity of the condition was rated as 1.2 ± 0.7.

Management

IK resolves simply on discontinuation of lens wear without the need for treatment. In a series of 19 events of IK, 45 per cent of the events resolved by day 7 and all events had resolved by day 20 (Sankaridurg *et al.*, 1999b). The resolution time for IK is less than for CLARE and CLPU, suggesting that the reaction is less severe. Some events resolve with an opacity corresponding to the infiltrate or the corneal erosion.

Figures for the probability of developing a recurrent event (0.07) suggest that the prognosis for continuing in lens wear without developing another event is good (Sankaridurg, 1999). However, it is possible that some of these patients may develop more symptomatic events such as CLARE and therefore patients need to be counselled regarding the possibility of recurrence, the importance of good hygiene practices with lens wear and the need for discontinuation of lens wear during any periods of acute illness.

Contact lens-induced papillary conjunctivitis

CLPC, an inflammatory condition of the upper tarsal conjunctiva commonly referred to in the literature as giant papillary conjunctivitis (GPC), is a major cause for discontinuation from lens wear. The condition is characterized by mucus discharge, redness of the upper tarsus and presence of polygonal to irregular papillae which are either distributed evenly across the entire tarsus or localized to a few areas on the tarsus, usually corresponding to the site of the contact lens edge. The term GPC implies very large papillae that are not often seen with contact lens wear, unless the condition is severe or advanced. GPC is associated with wear of ocular prostheses, protruding nylon sutures, scleral buckles, elevated corneal deposits and filtering blebs (Srinivasan *et al.*, 1979; Sugar and Meyer, 1981; Dunn *et al.*, 1990; Heidemann *et al.*, 1993). CLPC was first reported by Spring in 1974, who described the condition to be an allergic reaction affecting the upper lid of soft contact lens wearers. Since then CLPC has been reported with the use of hard or PMMA lenses (Allansmith *et al.*, 1978), RGP (Douglas *et al.*, 1988; Schnider *et al.*, 1988; Alemany and Redal, 1991) and most commonly with soft lenses (Allansmith *et al.*, 1978; Mackie and Wright, 1978; Soni and Hathcoat, 1988; Hart *et al.*, 1989; Alemany and Redal, 1991; Roth, 1991; Sankaridurg *et al.*, 1999b, 2000). Also, events of CLPC have been reported with silicone hydrogel lenses (Nilsson, 1997; Skotnitsky *et al.*, 2000; Fonn *et al.*, 2002).

CLPC is characterized by acute ocular discomfort and lens intolerance which, when severe, lead to patients dropping out of lens wear. The features that contribute and result in ocular discomfort and intolerance include itching, mucus or ropy discharge, excessive movement of lens on eye, increased deposition of lens surface and blurred vision due to lens mislocation and mucus coatings on lens. On discontinuation of lens wear, most symptoms of CLPC disappear rapidly over days; however, the ocular signs take longer to subside and, importantly, some papillae may still remain. Recurrences of CLPC are likely on resumption of lens wear. To minimize recurrences, patients have often been managed by reducing their wear time in lenses and successful outcomes have also been reported in patients who changed to frequent replacement or daily disposable lenses (Strulowitz and Brudno, 1989; Bucci *et al.*, 1993).

Incidence

The incidence of CLPC is seen to vary widely, with estimates ranging from as little as 1.5 per cent (Lamer, 1983) to as much as 47.5 per cent (Alemany and Redal, 1991). The incidence is seen to vary with the type of lens used, the lens material,

Table 7.18   Annualized incidence of CLPC

Lens type	Mode of wear	Description of event	Incidence (%)	Eyes/ people	Authors
Conventional soft	EW	GPC (year 1)	13.0	People	Boswall et al. (1993)
Conventional soft	EW	GPC (year 2)	18.0	People	Boswall et al. (1993)
Conventional soft	EW	GPC (year 3)	18.0	People	Boswall et al. (1993)
Disposable soft	EW	GPC (year 1)	1.6	People	Boswall et al. (1993)
Disposable soft	EW	GPC (year 2)	2.3	People	Boswall et al. (1993)
Disposable soft	EW	GPC (year 3)	4.8	People	Boswall et al. (1993)
Disposable soft	DW	CLPC	0	Eyes	Levy et al. (1997)
Disposable soft	EW	CLPC	2.0	Eyes	Levy et al. (1997)
Disposable soft	EW	GPC (year 1)	16.0	Eyes	Maguen et al. (1991)
Disposable soft	EW	GPC (year 3)	4.0	Eyes	Maguen et al. (1991)
Soft	EW	CLPC	6.4	People	Sankaridurg et al. (1999b)
Disposable soft	EW	CLPC	4.1	Eyes	LVPEI database
Disposable soft	EW	CLPC	1.1	Eyes	CCLRU database
Silicone hydrogel	CW	CLPC	5.9	Eyes	LVPEI database
Silicone hydrogel	CW	CLPC	6.8	Eyes	CCLRU database

wearing schedule and lens care regimen but, overall, CLPC occurs more often with soft contact lens wear than with wear of RGP lenses (Alemany and Redal, 1991) and more often with EW than with DW (Levy et al., 1997). Table 7.18 summarizes the incidence of CLPC with different lens types and wear modalities.

Clinical features

Tables 7.19 and 7.20 detail the clinical feature of events of CLPC. CLPC can be either unilateral or bilateral. The ocular sign that defines CLPC is the presence of one or more papillae on the upper tarsal conjunctiva. Papillae are usually associated with increased tarsal redness and it is possible that the patient may be asymptomatic in the early stages. If the condition progresses, signs can worsen and the patient becomes symptomatic. Itching with lens wear is the defining symptom and often worsens as the duration in lens wear progresses. As mentioned before, other symptoms include a stringy or ropy mucus discharge, excessive movement of the lens, frequent mislocation of the lens on the eye and blurred vision. If no action is taken symptoms worsen with time, leading to lens intolerance.

In order to facilitate examination and diagnosis, Allansmith and colleagues divided the surface of the central tarsus into three equally sized zones (Allansmith et al., 1977). The junctional conjunctiva, which contains no tarsal plate, was disregarded. Papillae can occur as a small cluster of localized papillae in one or two zones of the central tarsal conjunctiva (Figure 7.15) or randomly distributed across the entire tarsus (Figure 7.16). Skotnitsky et al. (2002) have reported that a greater number of CLPC cases with silicone hydrogel lenses were localized in nature. Papillae can range in size from being small discrete elevations of less than 0.5 mm to large papillae of >2 mm in size.

Table 7.19 Symptoms of CLPC (in the order of most frequent to less frequent[a])

Symptoms
● Itchiness or irritation
● Mucus discharge (stringy or ropy)
● Excessive movement of lens on eye
● Blurred vision (due to lens mislocation or discharge or coatings on lens)
● Foreign body sensation
● Redness

[a] From Sankaridurg (1999).

Table 7.20 Clinical features of CLPC

Feature	Signs
Papillae	
– Location	Upper tarsal conjunctiva
– Type	Polygonal, hyperaemic, elevations ranging in size from 0.5 to >2 mm
– Distribution	Localized to region corresponding to the lens edge on the tarsus or evenly distributed across the tarsus
Lid oedema	Not common
Bulbar/limbal redness	Not common; may be present in severe cases
Other features	Stringy or ropy discharge
Unilateral/bilateral	Can be bilateral

Schematic representation

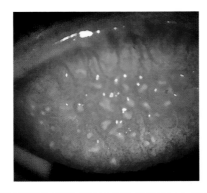

Allansmith *et al.* (1977) categorized the condition into four distinct stages: (1) preclinical, characterized by minimal patient symptoms and no ocular signs; (2) early clinical, characterized by mild symptoms and mild hyperaemia and early papillae; (3) moderate, characterized by moderate to severe symptoms and elevated

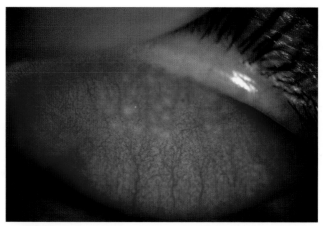

Figure 7.15   Localized papillae seen close to the lid margin in an event of CLPC. Note the hyperaemia surrounding the papillae

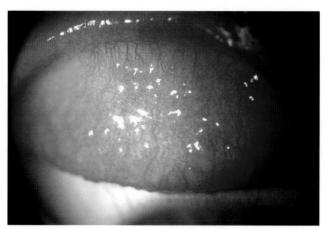

Figure 7.16   Papillae scattered across the entire tarsus in an event of CLPC

papillae and moderate to severe coatings on the lens; and (4) severe, characterized by total lens intolerance and large papillae.

CLPC needs to be differentially diagnosed from vernal conjunctivitis. Vernal conjunctivitis is common in young children and adults and is most frequently seen in spring. In vernal conjunctivitis, the papillae are distributed evenly across the entire tarsus and are cobblestone in appearance (sometimes up to 8 mm in diameter). Importantly, limbal involvement, such as Horner–Trantas dots or elevated gelatinous appearance of the limbus, is common. Corneal involvement in the form of punctate keratitis is also common and shield ulcers are sometimes seen.

Risk factors and pathogenesis

Histologically GPC is characterized by the presence of mast cells and eosinophils in the substantia propria and basophils in the epithelium and substantia propria

(Allansmith *et al.*, 1978). While the pathological features have been well characterized, the aetiology remains unclear. Theories have been put forward suggesting that GPC is either a delayed hypersensitivity reaction (Allansmith *et al.*, 1978) or an IgE-mediated immediate hypersensitivity reaction (Donshik and Ballow, 1983; Barishak *et al.*, 1984).

Whatever the mechanism, it is widely held that deposits, such as protein on the lenses, are the major risk factor for the development of GPC (Fowler *et al.*, 1979; Douglas *et al.*, 1988; Allansmith, 1990). Other suggested risk factors include lower patient age (Hart *et al.*, 1989), increased periods of lens wear (Allansmith, 1990), infrequent replacement of lenses (Allansmith, 1990) and the wearing of larger lenses (Allansmith, 1990). In this context, frequent replacement and disposable lenses have been advocated as reducing GPC (Grant *et al.*, 1987; Driebe, 1989; Gruber, 1989; Sagan, 1989; Bleshoy *et al.*, 1994). However, there have been several reports of CLPC with EW of disposable hydrogels (see Table 7.18; Rao *et al.*, 1996). This suggests that either: (1) mechanisms other than deposits on the lens surface could be responsible for the pathogenesis of the condition; or (2) deposits with even short-term exposure can induce CLPC. Factors which have hitherto not been looked at closely but which may explain the pathogenesis of CLPC include mechanical trauma from the lens surface or lens edges. This hypothesis is strengthened by the observation that GPC is seen where there is mechanical irritation of the tarsus with exposed sutures, elevated blebs and calcific plaques (Srinivasan *et al.*, 1979; Sugar and Meyer, 1981; Heidemann *et al.*, 1993).

Management

The conventional approach to management of CLPC commonly involves:

1. cleaning or replacement of lenses to minimize risk from lens surface deposition;
2. reducing wearing time in lenses to reduce exposure;
3. changing lens material or type; and
4. adjunctive drug therapy.

However, this management is based on the presumption that lens surface deposition is the major risk factor for development of the condition. If trauma from the lens surface or the lens edge rather than the surface deposition is a risk factor, then continuing in the same lens type may not alleviate the condition. In such a situation discontinuation of lens wear until the condition subsides and then reintroducing the patient to a different lens type is probably the best option.

Superior epithelial arcuate lesions

SEALs are whitish, arc-like lesions found located on the superior cornea in the area normally covered by the upper lid and are within 1–3 mm of the superior limbus (Figure 7.17). SEALs are sometimes referred to in the literature as superior arcuate keratopathy (Young and Mirejovsky, 1993) or an epithelial split (Malinovsky *et al.*, 1989).

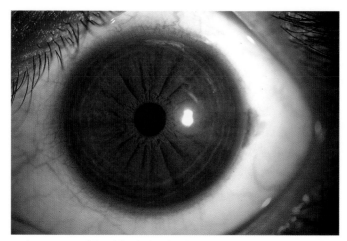

Figure 7.17   Arcuate, greyish–white lesion in the superior cornea close to limbus (approximately 11.30 to 12.30 o'clock meridian) characteristic of SEAL

SEALs are commonly asymptomatic and unilateral but can also be bilateral. In some cases patients may report discomfort associated with lens wear. On direct examination using white light on a slit-lamp biomicroscope, the edges of a SEAL are often raised and irregular. There is usually a clear region between the SEAL and the limbus and the lesion can vary in length from 1 mm to up to 5 mm and is found located between 10 and 2 o'clock meridians on the cornea.

SEALs are most easily observed using sodium fluorescein and a Wratten no. 12 filter. The lesion stains intensely with fluorescein and the clinical picture varies from arcuate-shaped staining to an epithelial 'split' (full epithelial depth) or a band. Also some events may be associated with redness of the limbus and diffuse, subepithelial infiltration immediately beneath or surrounding the lesion. Arcuate-shaped epithelial or subepithelial opacities without overlying staining have also been observed (Horowitz *et al.*, 1985) and may represent a later stage of the condition where the epithelial damage has healed but subepithelial disruption from the infiltrates is still evident. There are no reports of permanent scarring resulting from SEALs.

Incidence

Because they are often asymptomatic, SEALs may often be undiagnosed; thus the true incidence remains difficult to determine. Also, very few reports exist in the literature of events of SEALs. Reported incidences vary from 0 to 8 per cent of eyes (Table 7.21). Hine *et al.* (1987) reported an incidence of 5 per cent in eyes of 200 presbyopic and young myopic patients with soft contact lenses on both DW and CW schedules. Sankaridurg *et al.* (1999b) reported an incidence of 0.9 per cent in 330 young neophytes wearing disposable hydrogel lenses on a CW schedule.

A number of SEALs have been reported with wear of silicone hydrogel lenses (Nilsson, 1997; Dumbleton *et al.*, 2000; Long *et al.*, 2000; Iruzubieta *et al.*,

Table 7.21   Incidence of SEALs

Lens type	Mode of wear	Description of event	Incidence (%)	Eyes/people	Authors
Spectacles	–	SEAL	0	Eyes	CCLRU/LVPEI database
Conventional soft	DW	SEAL	5.0	Eyes	Hine et al. (1987)
Daily disposable	DW	SEAL	0	Eyes	LVPEI database
Disposable soft	EW	SEAL	1.3	People	Sankaridurg et al. (1999b)
Disposable soft	EW	SEAL	0	Eyes	CCLRU database
Disposable soft	EW	SEAL	0.4	Eyes	LVPEI database
Soft	DW + EW	Epithelial splitting	6.0	Eyes	Watanabe (1999)
Silicone hydrogel	CW	SEAL	18.7	Eyes	LVPEI database
Silicone hydrogel	CW	SEAL	3.6	Eyes	CCLRU database

Table 7.22   Symptoms of SEALs

Symptoms
- Commonly asymptomatic
- If symptomatic, can present with edge awareness or irritation and/or foreign body sensation

2001; Jalbert et al., 2001), suggesting that these events may be a frequent occurrence with silicone hydrogel lenses in comparison to conventional soft lenses. In a group of 504 patients randomized to either 30-night or seven-night CW with silicone lenses, the incidence in the 30-night group was 0.4 per cent. No events were seen in the seven-night group. Dumbleton et al. (2000) reported the incidence to be 4.5 per cent. The increased incidence of SEALs with silicone hydrogels appears to be related to material properties and mechanical interaction with the corneal surface and is explained in detail in the following sections.

Clinical features

The clinical features of events of SEALs as seen in CCLRU/LVPEI clinical studies are given in Tables 7.22 and 7.23.

Risk factors and pathogenesis

SEALs are essentially a complication of soft contact lens wear and have not been associated with rigid lenses. Various risk factors have been suggested and can be separated into two main categories: (1) lens wearer or patient characteristics; and (2) lens characteristics. Table 7.24 lists these risk factors.

From these observations, two possible aetiologies have been suggested. The first is mechanical trauma resulting from inadequate lens flexure in the region overlying the superior lid (Young and Mirejovsky, 1993). Young and Mirejovsky suggest that,

Table 7.23   Clinical signs of SEALs

Feature	Signs
Epithelial lesion	
– Location	Superior cornea; peripheral
– Type	Arc-shaped, greyish-white epithelial lesion with heaped edges. Diffuse infiltrates underlying lesion possible
– Depth	Epithelium and anterior stroma
Overlying epithelium	Significant staining, immediate diffusion into surrounding tissues
Corneal oedema	None
Anterior chamber reaction	None
Lid oedema	None
Bulbar/limbal redness	None
Unilateral/bilateral	Unilateral
On resolution	Clear cornea

Schematic representation

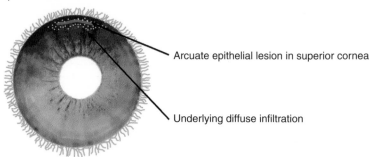

Arcuate epithelial lesion in superior cornea

Underlying diffuse infiltration

Table 7.24   Suggested risk factors for SEALs

Risk factors:
- Tight eyelids (Josephson 1978a; Horowitz *et al.*, 1985)
- Oriental race (Josephson 1978a, 1978b)
- Low positioned upper lid (Josephson 1978b)
- Steep corneas (Kline and Deluca, 1977)
- Large corneal sagittal height (Young and Mirejorsky, 1993)
- Newly dispensed lens (Hine *et al.*, 1987)
- Lathe-cut hydrogels (Josephson 1978b; Malinovsky *et al.*, 1989)
- Stiffer lenses with a higher modulus (Young and Mirejorsky, 1993)
- Thick lenses (Horowitz *et al.*, 1985; Young and Mirejorsky, 1993)
- An equal centre to edge thickness ratio (Hine *et al.*, 1987)
- Monocurve lens design (Young and Mirejorsky, 1993)

in cases where the elastic modulus of the lens material is high or alternatively where the lens periphery is thick, the lens is unable to flex and align with the flatter periphery of the cornea and stands away from the eye, vaulting the limbus. However, due to lid pressure the lens is forced to flex but assumes a compromised position with an area of misalignment in the superior cornea and presses against the epithelium and causes mechanical irritation. The authors also hypothesized that the pressure results in tear fluid thinning in this area, causing greater frictional forces on the cornea. In another hypothesis, localized hypoxia exacerbated by the position of the pressure and thickness of the lens edge leading to development of SEALs was suggested (Josephson, 1978a, 1978b). However, the occurrence of SEALs with silicone hydrogel lenses suggests that mechanical irritation rather than oxygen availability is more likely to play a role in the aetiology of these events.

Management

When SEALs are detected the patient should discontinue lens wear until staining and any infiltration resolve. Patients can be refitted with lenses but require more frequent monitoring visits due to the high probability of recurrence and the asymptomatic nature of the event. If SEALs recur, a different lens material/design should be tried. There does not seem to be a unique pattern for recurrence of SEALs. In Hine's study (Hine *et al.*, 1987), 50 per cent of the subjects suffered from a second episode when redispensed with the same lens type but there was no recurrence when subsequently refitted with a different lens and/or care system. Thirteen per cent of subjects had recurrent episodes with the same and different lens type or care system. Because of this apparent predisposition for developing SEALs with some subjects, these individuals need to be closely monitored for second occurrences of epithelial lesions when refitted.

In the event of repeated recurrences (three or more events), discontinuation of soft lens wear and refitting with rigid lenses is an alternative as SEALs have not been reported with rigid lens wear.

As mechanical interactions producing damage to the superior cornea are a risk factor, it was suggested that punctate staining in this region could be a precursor to SEALs. In a CCLRU study, 70 per cent of reported SEAL cases were preceded by punctate staining in the superior area; however, 40 per cent of cases of punctate staining in the superior cornea did not progress to a full SEAL (CCLRU database). Cases demonstrating superior staining, suggestive of an arcuate pattern, should therefore be considered at risk of developing SEALs and be monitored more closely.

It has been suggested that SEALs tend to happen in a short period following insertion of a new lens (Horowitz *et al.*, 1985; Hine *et al.*, 1987), so practitioners should pay particular attention to the superior cornea when monitoring newly fitted or newly dispensed lenses.

Corneal erosions

Corneal erosions or epithelial abrasions can be observed in association with lens wear as a consequence of mechanical injury or physiological damage. Corneal

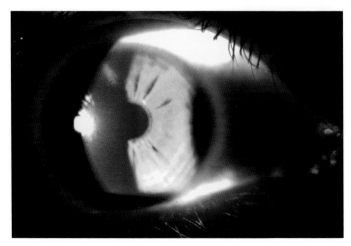

Figure 7.18 Area of corneal erosion in the superior cornea close to the limbus

damage from a contact lens is usually limited and anterior to Bowman's membrane. Injury can also result from foreign objects trapped between the corneal surface and the contact lens.

Incidence

Because the clinical picture and causes of corneal erosions are wide-ranging and often poorly defined in clinical trials, to our knowledge there are no good data available on the incidence of corneal erosions associated with contact lens wear. Some prevalence figures are reported below.

Clinical features

The clinical features of corneal erosions are widespread, depending on the extent (size and depth) of the injury. Superficial erosions of the first one to three epithelial layers are often asymptomatic, as the sparse innervation of the surface epithelium may allow cells to be dislodged without causing distress (Bergmanson, 1992). Deep abrasions (Figure 7.18) are symptomatic and will cause moderate to severe pain, watering and blepharospasm (Bergmanson, 1992).

Risk factors and pathogenesis

Although mechanical erosions are more prevalent with rigid lens wear, they are still found in conjunction with soft lens use and seem to be more prevalent with EW. In a recent large study ($n = 23\,068$), the prevalence of corneal erosions was 0.1 per cent in EW disposable lens users and 0 per cent in DW disposable lens users (Hamano *et al.*, 1994). Ultra-thin soft high-water-content lenses have been linked with the production of epithelial erosions (Holden *et al.*, 1986). Diabetic subjects are probably more at risk of developing corneal erosions as abnormalities in their basement membrane and increased epithelial fragility have been shown (O'Leary and Millodot, 1981).

The pathogenesis of corneal erosions is multifactorial: lens defects, poor lens finish, poor fit, overwear, poor insertion or removal techniques and foreign bodies (Bergmanson, 1992). One suggested aetiology closely resembled the hypothesis for SEALs with lens dehydration, thinning or loss of post-lens tear film, and mechanical damage or desiccation of the underlying epithelium as possible mechanisms (Holden *et al.*, 1986). It is therefore possible that factors associated with the production of SEAL reactions may also be more likely to induce corneal erosions in contact lens wearers. The reader should refer to the previous section on SEALs for a comprehensive review of these risk factors.

Management

The main concern with management of corneal erosions is with prevention of contamination, as the weakened epithelium may be more susceptible to secondary infections. The wound should be examined for any trace of foreign matter, especially in known foreign body-related injuries. Contact lens wear should be discontinued for large superficial lesions (>0.5 mm) or any deep abrasions. A superficial abrasion usually heals in 24 hours and deeper lesions can take up to several days. The length of time of discontinuation should be sufficient to allow complete healing of the epithelium to avoid the risk of corneal epithelial erosions occurring subsequently. Contact lens wear may be continued with small (<0.5 mm) superficial abrasions under close monitoring. Scarring is unlikely as usually Bowman's membrane is not involved and also there is no infiltration which causes disorganization of stromal lamellae.

Prophylactic antibiotics can be considered in severe cases but practitioners should remember that preservatives included in antibiotic preparations can delay the natural healing process. In severe cases, with anterior chamber involvement (cells and flare), the use of cycloplegics is indicated to reduce pain and to prevent mitosis and posterior synechiae. Patching of corneal abrasions in contact lens wearers is contraindicated (Clemons *et al.*, 1987). The patch provides a suitable environment for bacteria present around the wound and significantly increases the risk of development of MK (Clemons *et al.*, 1987). Corneal infiltration is a rare complication of corneal erosions (Ionides *et al.*, 1997); steroid therapy remains contraindicated in most cases of epithelial abrasions, as it may also lead to the development of MK (Chalupa *et al.*, 1987). Patients should be advised to use systemic analgesics as needed.

NON–SIGNIFICANT ADVERSE EVENTS (ASYMPTOMATIC)

Asymptomatic infiltrative keratitis (AIK)

AIK is a mild corneal infiltrative event observed with both DW and EW of hydrogel lenses, including silicone hydrogel lenses and also during non-lens wear.

Table 7.25   Annualized incidence of AIK

Lens type	Mode of wear	Description of the event	Incidence (%)	Eyes/ people	Authors
Spectacles	–	AIK	0	Eyes	CCLRU database
Spectacles	–	AIK	0.8	Eyes	LVPEI database
Soft	DW	AIK	1.3	Eyes	CCLRU database
Soft	DW	AIK	2.5	Eyes	LVPEI database
Soft	EW	AIK	1.9	Eyes	CCLRU database
Soft	EW	AIK	4.19	Eyes	LVPEI database
Silicone hydrogel	CW	AIK	10.7	Eyes	LVPEI database
Silicone hydrogel	CW	AIK	3.1	Eyes	CCLRU database

As the terminology indicates, the event is asymptomatic and is observed at routine aftercare visits. While commonly unilateral, bilateral events can also occur.

Clinically the conjunctiva is usually normal; however, some events can present with mild bulbar and limbal hyperaemia. There is no watering. Corneal signs include the presence of either: (1) faint, cellular, diffuse infiltration of mainly the peripheral cornea with or without small, focal infiltrates; or (2) small, focal infiltrates. As with events of IK, the overlying epithelium often shows loss of continuity in the region overlying the infiltrates and is commonly punctate in nature. When diffuse infiltration is present, it appears to be streaming in from the limbal blood vessels and the median involvement of the corneal circumference is 65 ± 30 degrees (median $\pm$ semi-interquartile). The focal infiltrates are small and range in size from 0.1 to 0.3 mm. The infiltration is limited to the anterior stroma and there is no activity in the anterior chamber.

Vision is not affected and the condition is seen to resolve rapidly without any sequelae.

Incidence

Table 7.25 presents the incidence from the CCLRU/LVPEI clinical studies. The condition presents during spectacle wear, DW and EW of disposable hydrogels and CW with silicone hydrogel lenses. Figure 7.19 shows a photograph of an event of AIK.

In clinical studies conducted with prototype silicone hydrogels at the CCLRU and the LVPEI, AIK has been noted. Also, while many other studies reported the presence of infiltrates with silicone hydrogels, it is not known if these infiltrates were symptomatic or asymptomatic in nature (Nilsson, 1997; Brennan et al., 2002).

Clinical features

There are no patient symptoms. The clinical signs of the condition are similar to those seen with events of IK (Table 7.26).

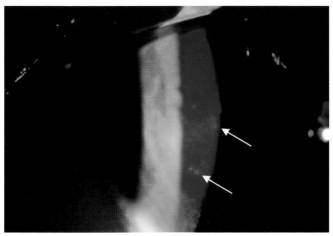

Figure 7.19   Photograph shows multiple focal infiltrates in an event of AIK (cornea)

Table 7.26   Clinical signs of AIK

Feature	Signs
Corneal infiltrate – Location – Type – Depth	 Peripheral to mid-peripheral Mild to moderate fine diffuse infiltration with possibly small focal infiltrate or small, focal infiltrates Anterior stroma (subepithelial)
Overlying epithelium	Often punctate staining
Corneal oedema	None
Anterior chamber reaction	None
Lid oedema	None
Bulbar/limbal redness	Slight to moderate, localized
Unilateral/bilateral	Commonly unilateral
On resolution	Clear cornea

Schematic representation

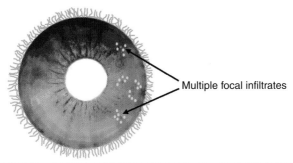

Multiple focal infiltrates

Risk factors and pathogenesis

In a series of 19 events of AIK, 37 per cent had either significant Gram-positive or Gram-negative contamination of contact lenses at the time of the event (Sankaridurg *et al.*, 1999a). The organisms isolated were the same as those recovered from contact lenses of patients with CLARE (see Chapter 4), suggesting that AIK could possibly be a variant or a precursor to CLARE. It is possible that, when patients continue to sleep in lenses that are contaminated with these bacteria, the subclinical response could develop into a more symptomatic, acute response such as CLARE. However, this theory does not explain the episodes of infiltrates seen in non-lens wearers. It is likely that in spectacle wear the infiltrative response could be a normal ocular defence response to environmental antigens such as dust, toxic fumes or bacteria.

While epithelial involvement is a feature in all AIKs, staining is relatively mild and punctate in nature. It is possible that this staining is not a precursor to the development of the infiltrative response.

Severity as an eye disease

In a series of 40 events of AIK observed in the CCLRU/LVPEI clinical studies, the mean severity rating was only 0.7 ± 0.4.

Management

The condition is seen to resolve rapidly on discontinuation of lens wear, with complete resolution achieved by day 7 in 71 per cent of the events and 100 per cent resolved by day 11 (Sankaridurg *et al.*, 1999a). No medical intervention is required. Disruption to lens wear is not routinely indicated; however, events associated with redness, diffuse infiltration or multiple focal infiltrates need to be treated cautiously and the clinician may do well to discontinue these subjects from lens wear and monitor them until resolution. In events where a CLARE-like lens contamination aetiology is suspected, precautionary measures, as with CLARE, should be taken.

Asymptomatic infiltrates (AI)

AIs appear to be faint clusters of a few inflammatory cells in both lens and non-lens wearers. Bilateral events are common.

As with AIK, the condition is observed at routine aftercare visits. The conjunctiva is normal and the corneal signs include the presence of small, focal infiltrates less than 0.2 mm in size (Figure 7.20). Usually single, these infiltrates are commonly seen in the periphery but could be located anywhere on the cornea. The infiltrates are limited to the anterior stroma. The epithelium overlying the infiltrates is intact and the condition resolves rapidly with no sequelae.

Incidence

Table 7.27 presents the incidence of the condition. The condition occurs in both lens and non-lens wearers and there is little variation in the incidence with various

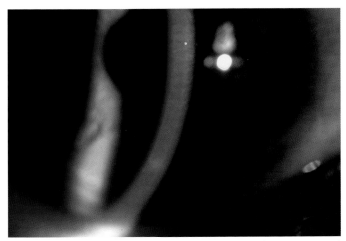

Figure 7.20 A single focal infiltrate located in the slit section (below the pupil) in an event of AI

Table 7.27 Annualized incidence of AI

Lens type	Mode of wear	Description of the event	Incidence (%)	Eyes/ people	Authors
Spectacles	–	AI	–	Eyes	CCLRU database
Spectacles	–	AI	6.7	Eyes	LVPEI database
Disposable soft	DW	AI	6.8	Eyes	CCLRU database
Disposable soft	DW	AI	8.5	Eyes	LVPEI database
Disposable soft	EW	AI	4.6	Eyes	CCLRU database
Disposable soft	EW	AI	5.9	Eyes	LVPEI database
Silicone hydrogel	CW	AI	6.9	Eyes	LVPEI database
Silicone hydrogel	CW	AI	10.2	Eyes	CCLRU database

modes of lens wear. Also, events of AI have been noted in clinical studies conducted with silicone hydrogels at CCLRU and LVPEI.

Clinical features

The condition is asymptomatic. The clinical signs are presented in Table 7.28.

Risk factors and pathogenesis

As with AIK, no definite risk factors have been identified to date and the pathogenesis of the condition remains unclear. Hickson and Papas (1997) reported that they observed several normal non-lens wearers with small, faint, subepithelial infiltrates. They called this entity subepithelial microinfiltrates and estimated their size to be approximately 40 μm. They suggested that these observations were within the normal physiological range of the corneal response. AIs appear

Table 7.28   Clinical signs of AI

Feature	Signs
Infiltrate – Location – Type – Depth	Commonly peripheral; can be present anywhere on the cornea Small, focal infiltrates (normally 0.2 mm in size) and/or mild diffuse infiltration Anterior stroma (subepithelial)
Overlying epithelium	Intact
Corneal oedema	None
Anterior chamber reaction	None
Lid oedema	None
Bulbar/limbal redness	None
Unilateral/bilateral	Can be bilateral
On resolution	Clear cornea

Schematic representation

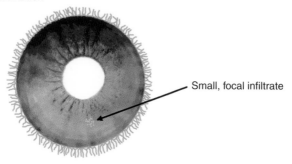

Small, focal infiltrate

to be larger than those reported by Hickson and Papas. Many of the infiltrates are commonly 0.1–0.2 mm in size. There is no association with microbial contamination of the contact lens (Sankaridurg, 1999) and they may be a normal subclinical response to environmental antigens.

Severity as an eye disease

In 153 events of AIs observed in the CCLRU/LVPEI the severity of the condition was rated to be 0.3 ± 0.2.

Management

The condition does not require discontinuation from lens wear; however, if multiple infiltrates are observed, the clinician may want to discontinue lens wear and monitor until resolution. AIs resolve rapidly, with all events resolving by day 11

(Sankaridurg, 1999). Similar rates of occurrence of AIs between lens wearers and non-lens wearers suggest that the condition is not a result of lens wear and that one would continue to see these events with silicone hydrogel lens wear.

SUMMARY

For contact lenses truly to challenge spectacles they need to provide excellent vision, be extremely comfortable and cause no adverse events. Silicone hydrogel lenses that virtually eliminate hypoxia have enabled us to test the feasibility of a truly convenient lens – the major unfulfilled challenge. It is hoped that, because epithelial metabolism is virtually normal, the cells will function normally, synthesizing the key elements that make the cornea resistant to infection.

The contrary argument is that tear stasis under a soft lens may prolong the contact of virulent organisms with the cornea and induce infection, despite a metabolically healthy epithelium. Only time, and large closely monitored studies, will tell. It is very important, however, that we minimize the risk of adverse events. This can best be achieved with excellent surface wettability, good 'stress-free' design and careful fitting. These factors are more critical with silicone hydrogel lenses intended for CW, in order to minimize epithelial trauma. As bacterial adherence is a risk factor for many adverse events, the type and nature of the lens surface and the deposits the lens surface attracts will also be important.

Proper patient hygiene and careful instructions on lens handling are also critical to avoid contamination and adverse events. The most important 'rules' for patients are as follows:

- If a lens is removed from the eye for any time it should be properly cleaned and disinfected.
- If an eye becomes red or sore, the lens should be removed and advice sought immediately.

The current generation of silicone hydrogel lenses will not eliminate adverse responses; thus patient selection, careful lens fitting, appropriate diagnosis and proper patient management of adverse events will be key to maximizing the success with this modality.

REFERENCES

Adams, C. P., Cohen, E. J., Laibson, P. R. *et al.* (1983) Corneal ulcers in patients with cosmetic extended wear contact lenses. *Am. J. Ophthalmol.*, **96**, 705–709

Alemany, A. L. and Redal, P. (1991) Giant papillary conjunctivitis in soft and rigid lens wear. *Contactologica*, **13**, 14–17

Alfonso, E., Mandelbaum, S., Fox, M. J. and Forster, R. K. (1986) Ulcerative keratitis associated with contact lens wear. *Am. J. Ophthalmol.*, **101**, 429–433

Allansmith, M. R. (1990) Giant papillary conjunctivitis. *J. Am. Optom. Assoc.*, **61**, 42–46

Allansmith, M. R., Whitney, C. R., McClellan, B. H. and Newman, L. P. (1973) Immunoglobulins in the human eye. *Arch. Ophthalmol.*, **89**, 36–45

Allansmith, M. R., Korb, D. R., Greiner, J. V. *et al.* (1977) Giant papillary conjunctivitis in contact lens wearers. *Am. J. Ophthalmol.*, **83**, 697–708

Allansmith, M. R., Korb, D. R. and Greiner, J. V. (1978) Giant papillary conjunctivitis induced by hard or soft contact lens wear: quantitative histology. *Ophthalmology*, **85**, 766–778

Baleriola-Lucas, C., Grant, T., Newton-Howes, J. *et al.* (1991) Enumeration and identification of bacteria on hydrogel lenses from asymptomatic patients and those experiencing adverse responses with EW. *Invest. Ophthalmol. Vis. Sci.*, **32**(s), 739

Barishak, Y., Zavaro, A., Samra, Z. and Sompolinsky, D. (1984) An immunological study of papillary conjunctivitis due to contact lenses. *Curr. Eye. Res.*, **3**, 1161–1168

Bates, A. K., Morris, R. J., Stapleton, F. *et al.* (1989) Sterile corneal infiltrates in contact lens wearers. *Eye*, **3**, 803–810

Bennett, H. G., Hay, J., Kirkness, C. M. *et al.* (1998) Antimicrobial management of presumed microbial keratitis: guidelines for treatment of central and peripheral ulcers. *Br. J. Ophthalmol.*, **82**, 137–145

Bergmanson, J. P. G. (1992) Contact lens-induced epithelial pathology. In *Clinical Contact Lens Practice* (eds E. S. Bennett and B. A. Weissman). J. B. Lippincott, Philadelphia, Ch. 60

Bleshoy, H., Guillon, M. and Shah, D. (1994) Influence of contact lens material surface characteristics on replacement frequency. *Int. Cont. Lens Clin.*, **21**, 82–94

Boswall, G. J., Ehlers, W. H., Luistro, A. *et al.* (1993) A comparison of conventional and disposable EW contact lenses. *J. Cont. Lens Assoc. Ophthalmol.*, **19**, 158–165

Brennan, N. A., Coles, M-L., Comstock, T. L. *et al.* (2002) A 1-year prospective clinical trial of balafilcon a (PureVision) silicon hydrogel contact lens used on a 30-day continuous wear schedule. *Ophthalmology*, **109**, 1172–1177

Brown, S. I., Bloomfield, S., Pearce, D. B. and Tragakis, M. (1974) Infections with the therapeutic soft lens. *Arch. Ophthalmol.*, **91**, 275–277

Bucci, F., Jr, Lopatynzky, M., Jenkins, P. *et al.* (1993) Comparison of the performance of the Acuvue disposable contact lens and CSI lens in patients with giant papillary conjunctivitis. *Am. J. Ophthalmol.*, **115**, 454–459

Buehler, P. O., Schein, O. D., Stamler, J. F. *et al.* (1992) The increased risk of ulcerative keratitis among disposable soft contact lens users. *Arch. Ophthalmol.*, **110**, 1555–1558

Cavanagh, H. D., Ladage, P. M., Li, S. L. *et al.* (2002) Effects of daily and overnight wear of a novel hyper oxygen-transmissible soft contact lens on bacterial binding and corneal epithelium: a 13 month clinical trial. *Ophthalmology*, **109**(11), 1957–1959

Chalupa, E., Swarbrick, H. A., Holden, B. A. and Sjostrand, J. (1987) Severe corneal infections associated with contact lens wear. *Ophthalmology*, **94**(1), 17–22

Chatterjee, A., Kwartz, J., Ridgway, A. E. A. and Storey, J. K. (1995) Disposable soft contact lens ulcers: a study of 43 cases seen at Manchester Royal Eye Hospital. *Cornea*, **14**(2), 138–141

Cheng, K. H., Leung, S. L., Hoekman, H. W. *et al.* (1999) Incidence of contact-lens-associated microbial keratitis and its related morbidity. *Lancet*, **354**, 181–185

Cheung, J. and Slomovic, A. R. (1995) Microbial etiology and predisposing factors among patients hospitalized for corneal ulceration. *Can. J. Ophthalmol.*, **30**, 251–255

Cheung, S. N., Cho, P. and Edwards, M. H. (2002) Contact lens practice in Hong Kong in the new millennium. *Clin. Exp. Optom.*, **85**, 358–364

Clemons, C. S., Cohen, E. J., Arentsen, J. J. *et al.* (1987) *Pseudomonas* ulcers following patching of corneal abrasions associated with contact lens wear. *J. Cont. Lens Assoc. Ophthalmol.*, **13**, 161–164

Cohen, E. J., Laibson, P. R., Arentsen, J. J. and Clemons, C. S. (1987) Corneal ulcers associated with cosmetic EW of contact lenses. *Ophthalmology*, **94**, 109–113

Cohen, E. J., Fulton, J. C., Hoffman, C. J. *et al.* (1996) Trends in contact lens associated corneal ulcers. *Cornea*, **15**, 566–570

Cooper, R. L. and Constable, I. J. (1977) Infective keratitis in soft contact lens wearers. *Br. J. Ophthalmol.*, **61**, 250–254

Cowell, B. A., Willcox, M. D. P., Hobden, J. A. *et al.* (1998) An ocular strain of *Pseudomonas aeruginosa* is inflammatory but not virulent in the scarified mouse model. *Exp. Eye Res.*, **67**, 347–356

Cruz, O. A., Sabir, S. M., Capo, H. and Alfonso, E. C. (1993) Microbial keratitis in childhood. *Ophthalmology*, **100**, 192–196

Dart, J. K. G. (1988) Predisposing factors in microbial keratitis: the significance of contact lens wear. *Br. J. Ophthalmol.*, **72**, 926–930

Dart, J. K. J., Stapleton, F. and Minassian, D. (1991) Contact lenses and other risk factors in microbial keratitis. *Lancet*, **338**, 650–653

Dixon, J. M., Young, C. A., Baldone, C. A. *et al.* (1966) Complications associated with the wearing of contact lenses. *J.A.M.A.*, **195**, 901–903

Donnenfeld, E. D., Cohen, E. J., Arentsen, J. J. *et al.* (1986) Changing trends in contact lens associated corneal ulcers: an overview of 116 cases. *J. Cont. Lens Assoc. Ophthalmol.*, **12**(3), 145–149

Donshik, P. C. and Ballow, M. (1983) Tear immunoglobulins in giant papillary conjunctivitis induced by contact lenses. *Am. J. Ophthalmol.*, **96**, 460–466

Douglas, J. P., Lowder, C. Y., Lazorik, R. and Meisler, D. M. (1988) Giant papillary conjunctivitis associated with RGP contact lenses. *J. Cont. Lens Assoc. Ophthalmol.*, **14**, 143–147

Driebe, W. T. (1989) Disposable soft contact lenses. *Surv. Ophthalmol.*, **34**, 44–46

Dumbleton, K., Fonn, D., Jones, L. *et al.* (2000) Severity and management of contact lens related complications with continuous wear of high *Dk* silicone hydrogel lenses. *Optom. Vis. Sci.*, **77**, 216

Dunn, J. P., Mondino, B. J., Weissman, B. A. *et al.* (1989) Corneal ulcers associated with disposable hydrogel contact lenses. *Am. J. Ophthalmol.*, **108**, 113–117

Dunn, J. P., Jr, Weissman, B. A., Mondino, B. J. and Arnold, A. C. (1990) Giant papillary conjunctivitis associated with elevated corneal deposits. *Cornea*, **9**, 357–358

Eichenbaum, J. W., Felstein, M. and Podos, S. M. (1982) Extended wear aphakic soft contact lenses and corneal ulcers. *Br. J. Ophthalmol.*, **66**, 663–666

Elner, V. M., Streiter, R. M. and Pavilack, M. A. (1991) Human corneal interleukin-8: IL-1 and TNF-induced gene expression and secretion. *Am. J. Pathol.*, **139**, 977–988

FDA Federal Register (1995) Vol. 60, no. 40, pp. 11284–11287

Ficker, L., Hunter, P., Seal, D. *et al.* (1989) *Acanthamoeba* keratitis occuring with disposable contact lens wear. *Am. J. Ophthalmol.*, **108**(4), 453

Fleiszig, S. M., Lee, E. J., Wu, C. *et al.* (1998) Cytotoxic strains of *Pseudomonas aeruginosa* can damage the intact corneal surface in vitro. *J. Cont. Lens Assoc. Ophthalmol.*, **24**, 41–47

Fonn, D., MacDonald, K. E., Richter, D. and Pritchard, N. (2002) The ocular response to extended wear of a high *Dk* silicone hydrogel contact lens. *Clin. Exp. Optom.*, **85**, 176–182

Fowler, S. A., Greiner, J. V. and Allansmith, M. R. (1979) Soft contact lenses from patients with giant papillary conjunctivitis. *Am. J. Ophthalmol.*, **88**, 1056–1061

Gebauer, A., McGhee, C. N. and Crawford, G. J. (1996) Severe microbial keratitis in temperate and tropical Western Australia. *Eye*, **10**, 575–580

Gillette, T. C., Chandler, J. W. and Greiner, J. V. (1982) Langerhans cells of the ocular surface. *Ophthalmology*, **89**, 700–711

Gorlin, A. I., Gabriel, M. M., Wilson, L. A. and Ahearn, D. G. (1995) Binding of *Acanthamoeba* to hydrogel contact lenses. *Curr. Eye Res.*, **15**, 151–155

Grant, T., Kotow, M. and Holden, B. A. (1987) Hydrogel EW: current performance and future options. *Contax*, 5–8

Grant, T., Chong, M. S., Vajdic, C. *et al.* (1998) Contact lens induced peripheral ulcers during hydrogel contact lens wear. *J. Cont. Lens Assoc. Ophthalmol.*, **24**, 145–151

Graves, A., Henry, M., O'Brien, T. P., *et al.* (2001) *In vitro* susceptibilities of bacterial ocular isolates to fluoroquinolones. *Cornea*, **20**, 301–305

Grimmer, P. R. (1992) Soft contact lens water content and five common post-fitting complications: are there relationships? *Clin. Exp. Optom.*, **75**, 182–187

Gruber, E. (1989) The best reasons to include disposable contact lenses in your practice. *Spectrum*, 31–36

Hamano, H., Hori, M., Hamano, T. *et al.* (1983) Effects of contact lens wear on mitosis of corneal epithelium and lactate content in aqueous humor of rabbit. *Jpn J. Ophthalmol.*, **27**, 451–458

Hamano, H., Watanabe, K., Hamano, T. *et al.* (1994) A study of the complications induced by conventional and disposable contact lenses. *J. Cont. Lens Assoc. Ophthalmol.*, **20**, 103–108

Hart, D. E., Schkolnick, J. A., Bernstein, S. *et al.* (1989) Contact lens induced giant papillary conjunctivitis: a retrospective study. *J. Am. Optom. Assoc.*, **60**, 195–204

Heidemann, D. G., Dunn, S. P. and Siegal, M. J. (1993) Unusual causes of giant papillary conjunctivitis. *Cornea*, **12**(1), 78–80

Hickson, S., Papas, E. (1997) Prevalence of idiopathic corneal anomalies in non-contact lens wearing population. *Optom. Vis. Sci.*, **74**, 1–5.

Hine, N., Back, A. and Holden, B. (1987) Aetiology of arcuate epithelial lesions induced by hydrogels. *Trans. BCLA Conference*, pp. 48–50

Holden, B. A., Sweeney, D. F., Vannas, A. *et al.* (1985) Effects of long-term extended contact lens wear on the human cornea. *Invest. Ophthalmol. Vis. Sci.*, **26**, 1489–1501

Holden, B. A., Sweeney, D. F. and Seger, R. G. (1986) Epithelial erosions caused by thin high water content lenses. *Clin. Exp. Optom.*, **69**, 103–107

Holden, B. A., La Hood, D., Grant, T. *et al.* (1996) Gram-negative bacteria can induce contact lens induced acute red eye (CLARE) responses. *J. Cont. Lens Assoc. Ophthalmol.*, **22**, 47–52

Holden, B. A., Reddy, M. K., Sankaridurg, P. R. *et al.* (1999) Contact lens-induced peripheral ulcers with EW of disposable hydrogel lenses: histopathologic observations on the nature and type of corneal infiltrate. *Cornea*, **18**, 538–543

Horowitz, G. S., Lin, J. and Chew, H. C. (1985) An unusual corneal complication of soft contact lens. *Am. J. Ophthalmol.*, **100**, 794–797

Husted, R. C., Conners, M. S., Connors, R. A. *et al.* (1997) Quantitative analysis of 12-hydroxy-5,8,14-eicosatrienoic acid (12-HETrE) in rabbit aqueous humor and corneal extracts and in human tears. *Invest. Ophthalmol. Vis. Sci.*, **38**, s285

IACLE (2003) International Association of Contact Lens Educators Database

Ionides, A. C., Tuft, S. J., Fergusin, V. M. *et al.* (1997) Corneal infiltration after recurrent corneal epithelial erosion. *Br. J. Ophthalmol.*, **81**(7), 537–540

Iruzubieta, M. J. J. R, Ripoll, N. J., Chiva, O. E. *et al.* (2001) Practical experience with a high *Dk* lotrafilcon A fluorosilicone hydrogel extended wear contact lens in Spain. *CLAO J.*, **27**, 41–46

Jalbert, I., Willcox, M. D. and Sweeney, D. F. (2000) Isolation of *Staphylococcus aureus* from a contact lens at the time of a contact lens-induced peripheral ulcer: case report. *Cornea*, **19**, 116–120

Jalbert, I., Sweeney, D. F. and Holden, B. A. (2001) Epithelial split associated with wear of a silicone hydrogel contact lens. *CLAO J.*, **27**, 231–233

Jones, L., Dumbleton, K., Woods, C. and Joseph, J. (2002) Practitioner perspectives towards recommendation of daily disposable and continuous wear lenses. *Optom. Vis. Sci.*, **79**, 6

Josephson, J. E. (1978a) Comments on: Pitting stain with soft Hydrocurve lenses (L. Kline and T. Deluca). *J. Am. Optom. Assoc.*, **49**, 445

Josephson, J. E. (1978b) A corneal irritation uniquely produced by hydrogel lathed lenses and its resolution. *J. Am. Optom. Assoc.*, **49**, 869–870

Josephson, J. E. and Caffery, B. E. (1979) Infiltrative keratitis in hydrogel lens wearers. *Int. Cont. Lens Clin.*, September–October, 47–69

Kent, H. D., Sanders, R. J., Arentsen, J. J. *et al.* (1989) *Pseudomonas* corneal ulcer associated with disposable soft contact lenses. *J. Cont. Lens Assoc. Ophthalmol.*, **15**, 264–265

Kenyon, E., Polse, K. A. and Seger, R. G. (1986) Influence of wearing schedule on EW complications. *Ophthalmology*, **93**, 231–236

Killingsworth, D. W. and Stern, G. A. (1989) *Pseudomonas* keratitis associated with the use of disposable soft contact lenses. *Arch. Ophthalmol.*, **107**, 795

Kline, L. N. and Deluca, T. I. (1977) Pitting stain with soft contact lenses: Hydrocurve® thin series. *J. Am. Optom. Assoc.*, **48**, 372–376

Lam, D. S. C., Houang, E., Fan, D. S. P. *et al.* (2002) Hong Kong Microbial Keratitis Study Group: incidence and risk factors for microbial keratitis in Hong Kong; comparison with Europe and North America. *Eye*, **16**, 608–618

Lamer, L. (1983) EW contact lenses for myopes: a follow-up study of 400 cases. *Ophthalmology*, **90**, 156–161

Lausch, R. N., Chen, S. H., Tumpey, T. M. *et al.* (1996) Early cytokine synthesis in the excised mouse cornea. *J. Interf. Cytok. Res.*, **16**, 35–40

Lemp, M. A., Blackman, H. J., Wilson, L. A. *et al.* (1984) Gram negative corneal ulcers in elderly aphakic eyes with extended wear lenses. *Ophthalmology*, **91**(1), 60–63

Levy, B., McNamara, N., Corzine, J. and Abbott, R. L. (1997) Prospective trial of daily and EW disposable contact lenses. *Cornea*, **16**, 274–276

Liesegang, T. J. and Forster, R. K. (1980) Spectrum of microbial keratitis in South Florida. *Am. J. Ophthalmol.*, **90**, 38–47

Lim, L., Loughnan, M. S. and Sullivan, L. J. (2002) Microbial keratitis associated with extended wear of silicone hydrogel lenses. *Br. J. Ophthalmol.*, **86**, 355–357

Long, B., Robirds, S. and Grant, T. (2000) Six months of in practice experience with a high *Dk* lotrafilcon A soft contact lens. *Cont. Lens Ant. Eye*, **23**, 112–118

Mackie, I. A. and Wright, P. (1978) Giant papillary conjunctivitis (secondary vernal) in association with contact lens wear. *Trans. Ophthalmol. Soc. UK*, **98**, 3–9

Macrae, S., Herman, C., Stulting, R. D. *et al.* (1991) Corneal ulcer and adverse reactions rates in pre-market contact lens studies. *Am. J. Ophthalmol.*, **111**, 457–465

Madigan, M. (1990) Cat and monkey cornea as models for extended hydrogel contact lens wear in humans. PhD thesis, University of New South Wales

Madigan, M. C. and Holden, B. A. (1988) Factors involved in loss of epithelial adhesion (EA) with long-term continuous hydrogel lens wear. *Invest. Ophthalmol. Vis. Sci.*, **29**(s), 253

Madigan, M. C. and Holden, B. A. (1992) Reduced epithelial adhesion after extended contact lens wear correlated with reduced hemidesmosome density in cat cornea. *Invest. Ophthalmol. Vis. Sci.*, **33**, 314–323

Madigan, M. C., Holden, B. A. and Kwok, L. S. (1987) EW of contact lenses can compromise corneal epithelial adhesion. *Curr. Eye Res.*, **6**, 1257–1260

Maguen, E., Tsai, J. C., Martinez, M. *et al.* (1991) A retrospective study of disposable EW lenses in 100 patients. *Ophthalmology*, **98**, 1685–1689

Maguen, E., Rosner, I., Caroline, P. *et al.* (1992) A retrospective study of disposable EW lenses in 100 patients: year 2. *J. Cont. Lens Assoc. Ophthalmol.*, **18**, 229–231

Maguen, E., Rosner, I., Caroline, P. *et al.* (1994) A retrospective study of disposable EW lenses in 100 patients: year 3. *J. Cont. Lens Assoc. Ophthalmol.*, **20**, 179–182

Malinovsky, V., Pole, J. J., Pence, N. A. and Howad, D. (1989) Epithelial splits on the superior cornea in hydrogel contact lens patients. *Int. Cont. Lens Clin.*, **16**, 252–255

Matthews, T. D., Frazer, D. G., Minassian, D. C. *et al.* (1992) Risks of keratitis and patterns of use with disposable contact lenses. *Arch. Ophthalmol.*, **110**, 1559–1562

McClellan, K. A., Bernard, P. J. and Billson, F. A. (1989) Microbial investigations in keratitis at the Sydney Eye Hospital. *Aust. NZ J. Ophthalmol.*, **17**, 413–416

Mertz, G. W. and Holden, B. A. (1981) Clinical implications of EW research. *Can. J. Optom.*, **43**, 203–205

Mertz, P. H. V., Bouchard, C. S., Mathers, W. D. *et al.* (1990) Corneal infiltrates associated with disposable EW soft contact lenses: a report of nine cases. *J. Cont. Lens Assoc. Ophthalmol.*, **16**, 269–272

Miller, M. J. and Ahearn, D. G. (1987) Adherence of *Pseudomonas aeruginosa* to hydrophilic contact lenses and other substrata. *J. Clin. Microbiol.*, **25**, 1392–1397

Mondino, B. J. (1988) Inflammatory diseases of the peripheral cornea. *Ophthalmology*, **95**, 463–472

Mondino, B. J., Weissman, B. A., Farb, M. D. *et al.* (1986) Corneal ulcer associated with daily wear and extended wear contact lenses. *Arch. Ophthalmol.*, **98**, 1767–1770

Morgan, P. and Efron, N. (2000) Trends in UK contact lens prescribing 2000. *Optician*, **219**(5749), 22–23

Morgan, P. and Efron, N. (2001) Trends in UK contact lens prescribing 2001. *Optician*, **221**(5803), 38–39

Morgan, P., Efron, N., Woods, C. *et al.* (2002) Survey results from six countries provide a snapshot of contact lens prescribing around the world. *Cont. Lens Spectrum*, July

Nilsson, S. E. (1997) Seven-day extended wear and 30-day continuous wear of high oxygen transmissibility soft silicone hydrogel contact lenses: a randomized 1-year study of 504 patients. *CLAO J.*, **23**, 185–191

Nilsson, S. E. G. and Montan, P. G. (1994) The hospitalised cases of contact lens induced Keratitis in Sweden and their relation to lens type and wear schedule: results of a three year retrospective study. *J. Cont. Lens Assoc. Ophthalmol.*, **20**, 97–101

O'Leary, D. J. and Millodot, M. (1981) Abnormal epithelial fragility in diabetes and in contact lens wear. *Acta Ophthalmol.*, **59**, 827

Ormerod, L. D. (1987) Causation and management of microbial keratitis in subtropical Africa. *Ophthalmology*, **94**, 1662–1668

Ormerod, L. D. and Smith, R. E. (1986) Contact lens associated microbial keratitis. *Arch. Ophthalmol.*, **104**, 79–83

Patrinely, J. R., Wilhelmus, K. R., Rubin, J. M. *et al.* (1985) Bacterial keratitis associated with extended wear soft contact lenses. *CLAO J.*, **11**(3), 234–236

Perlman, E. M. and Binns, L. (1997) Intense photophobia caused by *Arthrographis kalrae* in a contact lens-wearing patient. *Am. J. Ophthalmol.*, **123**(4), 547–549

Planck, S. R., Rich, L. F., Ansel, J. C. *et al.* (1997) Trauma and alkali burns induce distinct patterns of cytokine gene expression in the rat cornea. *Ocular Immun. Inflamm.*, **5**, 95–100

Poggio, E. C. and Abelson, M. (1993) Complications and symptoms in disposable EW lenses compared with conventional soft DW and soft EW lenses. *J. Cont. Lens Assoc. Ophthalmol.*, **19**, 31–39

Poggio, E. C., Glynn, R. J., Schein O. D. *et al.* (1989) The incidence of ulcerative keratitis among users of DW and EW soft contact lenses. *N. Engl. J. Med.*, **321**, 779–783

Ramachandran, L., Sharma, S., Sankaridurg, P. R. *et al.* (1995) Examination of the conjunctival microbiota after 8 hours of eye closure. *J. Cont. Lens Assoc. Ophthalmol.*, **21**, 195–199

Rao, G. N., Naduvilath, T. J., Sankaridurg, P. R. *et al.* (1996) Contact lens related papillary conjunctivitis in a prospective randomised clinical trial using disposable hydrogels. *Invest. Ophthalmol. Vis. Sci.*, **37**s, 1129

Roth, H. W. (1991) Studies on the etiology and treatment of giant papillary conjunctivitis in contact lens wearers. *Contactologia*, **13E**, 55–60

Ruben, M. (1976) Acute eye disease secondary to contact lens wear. *Lancet*, January, 138–140

Sagan, W. (1989) The hidden potential of the disposable lens. *Spectrum*, **4**, 39–41

Sankaridurg, P. R. (1999) Corneal infiltrative conditions with EW of disposable hydrogels. PhD thesis, University of New South Wales, Sydney, Australia

Sankaridurg, P. R., Willcox, M. D. P, Sharma, S. *et al.* (1996) *Haemophilus influenzae* adherent to contact lenses associated with production of acute ocular inflammation. *J. Clin. Microbiol.*, **34**, 2426–2431

Sankaridurg, P. R., Sharma, S., Willcox, M. *et al.* (1999a) Colonization of hydrogel lenses with *Streptococcus pneumoniae*: risk of development of corneal infiltrates. *Cornea*, **18**, 289–295

Sankaridurg, P. R., Sweeney, D. F., Sharma, S. *et al.* (1999b) Adverse events with extended wear of disposable hydrogels: results for the first thirteen months of lens wear. *Ophthalmology*, **106**, 1671–1680

Sankaridurg, P. R., Sweeney, D. F. and Gora, G. (2000) Adverse events with daily disposable contact lens and spectacle wear from a propective clinical trial. *Invest. Ophthalmol. Vis. Sci.*, Suppl., S74

Schaefer, F., Bruttin O., Zografos, L. and Guex-Crosier, Y. (2001) Bacterial keratitis: a prospective clinical and microbiological study. *Br. J. Ophthalmol.*, **85**, 842–847

Schein, O. D. and Poggio, E. C. (1990) Ulcerative keratitis in contact lens wearers. *Cornea*, **1**(s), 55–58

Schein, O. D., Glynn, R. J., Poggio, E. C. *et al.* (1989) The relative risk of ulcerative keratitis among users of DW and EW soft contact lenses: a case-control study. *N. Engl. J. Med.*, **321**, 773–778

Schnider, C. M., Zabiewicz, K. and Holden, B. A. (1988) Unusual complications association with RGP EW. *Int. Cont. Lens Clin.*, **15**, 124–129

Seal, D. V., Kirkness, C. M., Bennett, H. G. B. *et al.* (1999) Population based cohort study of microbial keratitis in Scotland: incidence and features. *Cont. Lens Ant. Eye*, **22**, 49–57

Sharma, S., Ramachandran, L. and Rao, G. N. (1995) Adherence of cysts and trophozoites of *Acanthamoeba* to unworn rigid gas permeable and soft contact lenses. *J. Cont. Lens Assoc. Ophthalmol.*, **21**, 247–251

Sharma, S., Gopalakrishnan, S., Aasuri, M. *et al.* (2003) Trends in contact lens-associated microbial keratitis in southern India. *Ophthalmology*, **110**, 138–143

Skotnitsky, C., Kalliris, A., Sankaridurg, P. R. *et al.* (2000) Contact lens induced papillary conjunctivitis (CLPC) is either local or general. *ICLC*, **27**, 193–195

Skotnitsky, C., Sankaridurg, P. R., Sweeney, D. F. *et al.* (2002) General and local contact lens induced papillary conjunctivitis. *Clin. Exp. Optom.*, **85**, 193–197

Snyder, C. (1995) Infiltrative keratitis with contact lens wear a review. *J. Am. Optom. Assoc.*, **66**, 160–177

Solomon, O. D., Loff, H., Perla, B. *et al.* (1994) Testing hypothesis for risk factors for contact lens-associated infectious keratitis in an animal model. *CLAO J.*, **20**(2), 109–113

Soni, P. S. and Hathcoat, G. (1988) Complications reported with hydrogel EW contact lenses. *Am. J. Optom. Physiol. Opt.*, **65**, 545–551

Sotozono, C., He, J., Matsumoto, Y. *et al.* (1997) Cytokine expression in the alkali-burned cornea. *Curr. Eye Res.*, **16**, 670–676

Spilker, B. (1991) Terminology. In *Guide to Clinical Trials*. Raven Press, New York, p. 567

Spoor, T. C., Hartel, W. C., Wynee, P. *et al.* (1984) Complications of continuous-wear contact lenses in a nonreferral population. *Arch. Ophthalmol.*, **102**, 1312–1313

Spring, T. F. (1974) Reaction to hydrophilic lenses. *Med. J. Aust.*, **1**, 449–450

Srinivasan, B. D., Jakobiec, F. A. and De Voe, A. G. (1979) Giant papillary conjunctivitis with ocular prosthesis. *Arch. Ophthalmol.*, **97**, 892–895

Stapleton, F., Dart, J. K. G. and Minassian, D. (1993) Risk factors with contact lens related suppurative keratitis. *J. Cont. Lens Assoc. Ophthalmol.*, **19**, 204–210

Stein, R. M., Clinch, T. E., Cohen, E. J. *et al.* (1988) Infected vs sterile corneal infiltrates in contact lens wearers. *Am. J. Ophthalmol.*, **105**, 632–636

Stern, G. A., Weitzenkorn, D. and Valenti, J. (1982) Adherence of *Pseudomonas aeruginosa* to the mouse cornea. *Arch. Ophthalmol.*, **100**, 1956–1958

Stern, G. A., Lubniewski, A. and Allen, C. (1985) The interaction between *Pseudomonas aeruginosa* and the corneal epithelium: an electron microscopic study. *Arch. Ophthalmol.*, **103**, 1221–1225

Strulowitz, L. and Brudno, J. (1989) The management and treatment of giant papillary conjunctivitis with disposables. *Spectrum*, **4**, 45–46

Suchecki, J. K., Ehlers, W. H. and Donshik, P. C. (1996) Peripheral corneal infiltrates associated with contact lens wear. *J. Cont. Lens Assoc. Ophthalmol.*, **22**, 41–46

Sugar, A. and Meyer, R. F. (1981) Giant papillary conjunctivitis after keratoplasty. *Am. J. Ophthalmol.*, **91**, 239–242

Sweeney, D. F., Grant, T., Chong, M. S. *et al.* (1993) Recurrence of acute inflammatory conditions with hydrogel EW. *Invest. Ophthalmol. Vis. Sci.*, **34**(s), 1008

Tan, K. O., Sack, R. A., Holden, B. A. and Swarbrick, H. A. (1993) Temporal sequence of changes in tear film composition during sleep. *Curr. Eye Res.*, **12**, 1001–1007

Thakur, A. and Willcox, M. D. P. (1998) Cytokine and lipid inflammatory mediator profile of human tears during contact lens associated inflammatory diseases. *Exp. Eye Res.*, **67**, 9–19

Thakur, A., Willcox, M. D. P. and Stapleton, F. (1998) The proinflammatory cytokines and arachidonic acid metabolites in human overnight tears: homeostatic mechanisms. *J. Clin. Immunol.*, **18**, 61–70

Upadhyay, M. P., Rai, N. C., Brandt, G. and Shreshta, R. B. (1982) Corneal ulcers in Nepal. *Graefes Arch. Clin. Exp. Ophthalmol.*, **219**, 55–59

Watanabe, K. (1999) The classification of epithelial complications resulting from contact lens use. In *Current Opinions in the Kupto Cornea Club* (eds S. Kinoshita and Y. Ohashi), Volume III, The Hague, The Netherlands, Kugler Publications

Weissman, B. A., Mondino, B. J., Pettit, T. H. *et al.* (1984) Corneal ulcers associated with extended wear soft contact lenses. *Am. J. Ophthalmol.*, **97**, 476–481

Wilhelmus, K. R. (1987) Review of clinical experience with microbial keratitis associated with contact lenses. *J. Cont. Lens Assoc. Ophthalmol.*, **13**, 211–214

Wilhelmus, K. R. (1996) Bacterial keratitis. In *Ocular Infection and Immunity* (eds J. S. Pepose, G. N. Holland and K. R. Wilhelmus). Mosby, St Louis, MO, pp. 970–1032

Wilhelmus, K. R., Robinson, M. M., Font, R. A. *et al.* (1988) Fungal keratitis in contact lens wearers. *Am. J. Ophthalmol.*, **106**, 708–714

Willcox, M. D. P., Sweeney, D. F., Sharma, S. *et al.* (1995) Culture negative peripheral ulcers are associated with bacterial contamination of contact lenses. *Invest. Ophthalmol. Vis. Sci.*, **36**(s), 152

Willcox, M. D. P., Power, K. N., Stapleton, F. *et al.* (1997) Potential sources of bacteria that are isolated from contact lenses during wear. *Optom. Vis. Sci.*, **74**, 1030–1038

Wilson, S. E., He, Y. G. and Lloyd, S. A. (1992) EGF, EGF receptor, basic FGF, TGF beta-1 and IL-1alpha mRNA in human corneal epithelial cells and stromal fibroblasts. *Invest. Ophthalmol. Vis. Sci.*, **33**, 1756–1765

Young, G. and Mirejovsky, D. (1993) A hypothesis for the aetiology of soft contact lens-induced superior arcuate keratopathy. *Int. Cont. Lens. Clin.*, **20**, 177–180

Zantos, S. G. and Holden, B. A. (1978) Ocular changes associated with continuous wear of contact lenses. *Aust. J. Optom.*, **61**, 418–426

Chapter **8**

Where do silicone hydrogels fit into everyday practice?

Noel A. Brennan, M–L. Chantal Coles and Anna K. Dahl

INTRODUCTION

We have known for many years that contact lenses can offer patients a feeling of 'freedom' with vision correction. Numerous market surveys (market research reports by GFK Sweden AB, 1996, 1998, 2002) have shown that what patients really want from their vision correction is to forget all about it and to be able to correct their vision with convenience, safety, comfort and for extended periods.

In response to these desires the contact lens industry has spent much time developing new lens materials capable of sustaining both extended wear (EW – up to seven nights) and continuous wear (CW – up to 30 nights). Lenses made from these materials should have the comfort of a hydrogel, the oxygen transmissibility of a silicone lens, and the surface properties at least equivalent to a polymethyl methacrylate (PMMA) lens. Meeting these targets has been the aim of the contact lens industry for many years.

CW is not new but the unique silicone hydrogel materials have heralded an era of success for this modality. When practitioners were first introduced to silicone hydrogels, many were sceptical as they did not know what to expect from these products. Several years of clinical experience have now established that silicone hydrogels do satisfy patients' needs and practitioners can offer their patients the freedom that they expect when they opt for contact lens wear.

In this chapter we aim to bridge the gap between science and the patient by presenting a guide to prepare practitioners for the use of silicone hydrogels in contact lens practice and by including the clinical experience from the contact lens clinics of the Contacta group in Sweden.

THE HISTORY OF EW AND CW WITH HYDROGEL LENSES

The first generation of CW soft contact lenses (SCLs) that came to market in the 1970s were made from lathe-cut, high-water-content materials. These lenses were worn for two to four weeks and were then taken out, cleaned, disinfected and reinserted. Lenses were replaced with a new lens after six months to one year of wear.

These lenses became very popular all over the world because they enabled patients to wear lenses overnight and continuously. However, soon after these lenses were introduced, an increase in the number of contact lens complications, including giant papillary conjunctivitis (GPC) (Spring, 1974; Allansmith *et al.*, 1977) and microbial keratitis (MK) (Adams *et al.*, 1983; Hassman and Sugar, 1983; Musch *et al.*, 1983; Mondino *et al.*, 1986; Smith and Macrae, 1989), became evident. Holden and colleagues' study of patients from a large contact lens practice in Göteborg, Sweden, established that long-term EW with these SCLs resulted in chronic physiological changes to all layers of the cornea (Holden *et al.*, 1985, 1986). There were also complications associated with contact lens deposits, tight fits and allergic reactions to contact lens solutions. The main shortcomings of the lenses were inadequate oxygen supply, surface spoilation and inferior mechanical properties. Attempts were made to circumvent some of these problems by changing lenses more often, and by using smaller-diameter lenses and flatter fits to improve tear exchange.

The second generation of EW was launched with the development of the disposable soft lens, which was worn on an EW basis for up to 14 days, then replaced. This ensured that the eye was routinely presented with clean lenses (Kame, 1988; Driebe, 1989). Disposable lenses, particularly those used for seven days or less, did reduce the incidence of non-infectious conditions such as contact lens-induced acute red eye (CLARE) and papillary conjunctivitis (Boswall *et al.*, 1993; Hamano *et al.*, 1994; Kotow *et al.*, 1987; Marshall *et al.*, 1992; Poggio and Abelson, 1993), but these adverse events were not eliminated (Dunn *et al.*, 1989; Ficker *et al.*, 1989; Maguen *et al.*, 1991, 1992, 1994; Suchecki *et al.*, 1996; Sankaridurg *et al.*, 1999) and the relative risk of MK with disposable lenses remained similar to conventional lens types (Nilsson and Montan, 1994a, 1994b; Schein *et al.*, 1994). Non-compliance may be a key factor in this equation.

While the experience with neither EW nor CW was successful in the minds of practitioners, the demand for these contact lenses did not diminish. The Swedish Contact Lens Association and contact lens companies conducted a survey to look at patient attitudes to conventional lens wear and, more particularly, the reasons for lens wear dropout market research reports by GFK Sweden AB (1996, 1998, 2002). The most frequent reasons given for discontinuation from lens wear were that lenses were uncomfortable, harmful to the eyes, difficult to handle and prone to cause dry eyes. However, despite these issues, patients were still keen to embrace CW if it could be made more safe, comfortable and decreased the need for handling of their lenses (market research reports by GFK Sweden AB, 1996, 1998, 2002). Curiously, one publication by Buckley *et al.* (1997) reported practitioner satisfaction with EW despite an infection rate similar to that of the landmark papers by Schein and coworkers (Poggio *et al.*, 1989; Schein *et al.*, 1989).

The widespread concern over the safety of sleeping in lenses, and the mounting research that indicated the higher risk of infection with this modality, caused the USA Food and Drug Administration (FDA) to reduce the maximum number of nights of wear from 30 to seven. By the 1990s clinical opinion was still polarized on the risk–benefit equation of EW. During this decade EW with SCLs was rarely prescribed in Sweden and other countries, although some contact lens practitioners continued to prescribe EW in the USA (Barr, 1998a).

WHAT ARE THE NEEDS OF A CONTACT LENS PATIENT?

As optometrists working with contact lens fitting we sometimes forget to ask patients what they really want from their contact lenses. It is easy just to fit the lens types that we are used to. However, by giving patients what they really want we ensure that we increase their satisfaction and, therefore, the chance of the patient staying in lens wear.

Most patients don't really know the difference between all the types of materials and modalities available, or about the issues of safety, risk factors, comfort or discomfort associated with each lens type. It is the eyecare professional's job to keep patients informed and to recommend a lens that is best suited to a patient's particular needs and health status. One survey has shown that 81 per cent of contact lens wearers in Europe would probably or definitely buy a CW lens, as long as it was recommended by their practitioner (van Cranenburgh, 1999).

IS CW RIGHT FOR YOUR PRACTICE?

All practitioners contemplating CW should ask themselves the following two questions:

1. Is it clinically and ethically legitimate to offer silicone hydrogel materials for CW in practice?
2. Is the provision of silicone hydrogels for CW a worthy application of the clinical skills of contact lens practitioners?

This first question relates to issues of safety of CW balanced against the advantages to be gained from the wearing pattern, the popular demand for this modality and the assessment of the risk–benefit ratio. The second question relates to the scope of the practice, practitioner competence and profitability of CW. We shall bear these questions in mind as we explore the application of silicone hydrogels in practice.

Practitioners seek to provide the highest possible quality of service to their patients. Some may feel that prescribing CW presents a significant risk to their patient population and, therefore, choose against this mode of practice. However, with consumer awareness in general at an all-time high, the failure to make available the CW option to patients might be seen as an unreasonable restriction on quality of service and create the perception of the practitioner being 'out of touch'. Competitive forces, including other corrective options such as refractive surgery or fellow practitioners prepared to fit CW, should not be underestimated.

There is documented overlap between patient interest in refractive surgery and contact lens wearers (Migneco and Pepose, 1996). The Contacta group in Sweden found that patients who are initially interested in laser surgery as a permanent means of correcting their vision are no longer interested if they experience CW with silicone hydrogels. This concurs with data from the Cornea and Contact Lens Research Unit (CCLRU) showing that 66 per cent of their patients have considered laser surgery and only 32 per cent are still interested after wearing silicone hydrogels (Skotnitsky *et al.*, 1999). In addition to convenience, patients also demand that their choice of vision correction is safe. In comparison to laser surgery, vision loss with contact lens wear is relatively rare. The loss of two or more lines of best corrected visual acuity (BCVA) with low-*Dk* soft EW is estimated at 0.8 per 10 000 wearers, whereas the rate of loss of two or more lines of BCVA with laser surgery is many hundred-fold greater (Holden *et al.*, 2003). The approximation of loss of BCVA with contact lens wear was based on the mean of annual estimates, whereas the loss of BCVA with laser surgery was derived from the mean of several studies that conducted a single course of treatment per eye. The difference in vision loss between contact lens wear and laser surgery is because MK is the only sight-threatening complication associated with contact lens wear, whereas there are many more sight-threatening adverse events that can occur with laser surgery.

Refereed publications detailing the exact demand for CW are few and far between. Data presented by CIBA Vision suggest that from 53 to 71 per cent of patients, depending on country, would like to be able to sleep or nap in their lenses (Barr, 1998a). Unpublished data from Bausch & Lomb put the figure at 62 per cent for current contact lens patients in the USA and 73 per cent in France. Most critics agree that there is a strong demand and that the interest in refractive surgery arises largely from the same population that desires CW of contact lenses but thus far has not been afforded access to it.

A number of papers have considered the financial success that contact lenses can bring to practice (Ziegler, 1997; Barr, 1998b; Marrioneaux and Gwin, 1998). Successful promotion of contact lens practice can increase the number of referrals per patient and provide additional revenue through accessory sales of sunglasses, prescription glasses and solutions. The availability of lenses which meet our expectations for CW should add additional support to the arguments for the financial viability of contact lens practice.

The introduction of silicone hydrogels is likely to increase the success and therefore the demand for CW, which should be a bonus for the eyecare practice. Professional services will necessarily be more complex and, therefore, it is reasonable to charge accordingly for these services. With heavy discounting on many disposable lenses and competition from mail-order and Internet contact lens suppliers, the opportunity to provide a unique service in the form of professional care is likely to be welcomed by contact lens practitioners. There is a clear value addition to this product compared to previous products which should also translate into higher practice turnover.

Aside from the question of providing practice viability and business growth, CW can impact on the professional fulfilment that a practitioner enjoys in a number of ways. The complexities involved with conducting a practice using silicone hydrogels for CW or even daily wear (DW), over the simplistic requirements of caring for disposable lens patients in DW, can add to job satisfaction. CW patients also tend to be enthusiastic and appreciative of the services provided, which provides personal reward for the practitioner.

Certain preparations should be made before launching into full-scale CW practice. While the steps are relatively easy to take, care should be exercised to ensure that appropriate systems are in place. The practitioner entering into CW practice should be aware that the commitment is serious and requires a substantial undertaking of time and energy to ensure adequate provision of patient care. A thorough review of the practice and its systems is recommended. The following is a guide to aid the practitioner in this review. For some of these points practitioners may need simply to confirm the adequacy of their existing systems.

UPDATING PRACTITIONER KNOWLEDGE

Realistic assessment of practitioner competency to handle CW is an important step in setting up practice. Many practitioners may already be equipped to handle most aspects of CW, given the availability of excellent contact lens continuing education worldwide. Simple revision may be all that is required.

An easy self-assessment test can be conducted to establish proficiency with CW. A well-prepared fitter should be able to identify and enumerate striae, folds and microcysts and to evaluate the regularity of the endothelial matrix. If there is any deficiency in this area, practitioners should seek additional training before fitting CW lenses. Practical training workshops and continuing education sessions taught by professionals in the field should then be attended to secure knowledge in this area.

Additional understanding of the differential diagnosis of complications, general pathology, microbiology, immunology and pharmacology can be a powerful asset in the prevention, handling and treatment of adverse events. Some of this information is contained in this book. Continuing education courses can also be of benefit in this regard.

EDUCATION OF OFFICE STAFF

Well-informed support staff form an essential component of the contact lens practice and are one of the keys to safe CW. Education should include instructions on methods for responding to enquiries about CW with detailed, factual information. Staff should encourage potential wearers to arrange an appointment to provide a detailed assessment of their suitability for this lens type.

Appropriate handling of enquiries from patients fitted with CW lenses is also important. Instruction to staff on appointment scheduling should include the appropriate time of day, length of consultation, frequency of visits and urgency of the care requirement. The benefits and risks of silicone hydrogels and CW should be fully explained to staff so that they can provide well-informed advice to patients.

We recommend that staff be highly familiar with the Information Sheet and Informed Consent form, a version of which is included in the Appendix to this chapter. Familiarity with the three-point plan presented in that documentation for dealing with problems should be of assistance in advising patients. This plan involves an assessment of symptoms so as to advise on the need to:

1. remove lenses temporarily;
2. remove lenses until the next appointment, which should be arranged for the earliest convenient time; or
3. seek immediate contact with the contact lens practitioner.

In addition to being positive and enthusiastic, staff should be well informed about all contact lens types that are available so that they can provide the best information to the patients. Staff should also be competent in providing advice about handling of lenses, wearing and replacement schedules, contact lens cleaning and maintenance and the need for good compliance with instructions. Regular meetings between practitioners and support staff will ensure that all staff are kept up to date with current lens practice and patient attitudes.

UPGRADING OF IN-OFFICE SYSTEMS

Smooth-running systems should be devised for organizing patients. These systems should include patient recall, follow-up contact by phone or letter of those who fail to keep appointments, maintenance of trial lens stocks and other supplies, and upkeep of documentation as described elsewhere in this chapter.

The practitioner should also review appointment scheduling and the overall capacity of handling the work in terms of efficiency and volume. The availability of silicone hydrogel lenses may create an increase in the number of patients interested in contact lens wear in general, which will require the scheduling of more appointments. Each individual CW patient requires a more intensive aftercare programme, which increases the average chair time and staff time per patient. 'On-call' time for after-hours emergency contact adds to the burden. A review of fees for service should be undertaken to reflect this increased burden of time and responsibility.

PURCHASE OF ADDITIONAL EQUIPMENT

The well-equipped consulting room should be adequate for handling most aspects of CW. Obviously a visual acuity tester, keratometer, biomicroscope and phoropter or trial lens set are essential. The practitioner should also obtain a grading scale system, such as those published by the CCLRU or Efron. The grading system should be kept at hand in the consulting room to aid in the recording of appearance of the various ocular physiological indicators.

Optional items are a video or photographic slit-lamp, corneal topographer and pachometer. These help in the assessment of lens fit, corneal response and corneal swelling but are not essential items of equipment for fitting CW.

Fitting silicone hydrogel lenses requires acquisition of one or more trial lens sets available from the manufacturing companies. Provision of these trial sets will likely vary from country to country and there may be different-size trial sets available. Further information should be sought from your local company representatives. Trial lens sets may need to be purchased, but such an expense for practitioners who wish to integrate silicone hydrogel lens fitting into their contact lens practice is likely to be reasonable. The alternative is to order single trial lenses from the manufacturer, an exercise which can be tedious and time consuming for both the practitioner and the patient.

EMERGENCY CARE

The patient should have access to the practitioner or a representative of the practitioner at all times in case of emergency such as infection or acute red eye (ARE). Indeed, we consider 24-hour access as mandatory for undertaking CW practice. Options for access include a pager or mobile phone. We do not recommend answering machines, as a delay of any time may be of significance in the development of an adverse reaction. To aid in access and maintain recreation time for the practitioner, it is advisable to rotate the on-call practitioner within a practice or set up co-operative arrangements with neighbouring practices. As a guide for planning manpower to accommodate round-the-clock access, out-of-hours contact is likely to be made by less than 5 per cent of patients over a 12-month period and these are most often of limited consequence.

Mechanisms for dealing with emergency situations should be well established prior to beginning a CW practice. If the practitioner has access to therapeutic drugs, the system will initially revolve around ensuring 24-hour per day access as described above. A destination hospital facility should be identified and communication with the attending physicians should be established. Where the practitioner does not have access to therapeutic drugs, clear instruction and provision of suitable documentation should be provided to facilitate attendance at an emergency outpatient clinic specializing in eyecare. In more remote areas, establishment of a working relationship with a local ophthalmologist who is fully conversant with this new modality of lens wear is the recommended route for practitioners. The establishment of this relationship in other circumstances is also prudent, since lack of familiarity with the advantages of silicone hydrogels by attending physicians at an emergency centre may lead to undermining of patient confidence in a practitioner's prescription and instructions.

DOCUMENTATION

Special attention should be directed to record keeping. More information on this topic is presented in detail below under the heading 'Liability'.

It is in the interest of the practitioner to establish clear practice guidelines for all patients eligible to be fitted with silicone hydrogel lenses, and to prepare specific guidelines and aftercare procedures for ongoing CW in individual patients.

Considerations for establishing such guidelines are presented below in the sections entitled 'Patient selection issues' and 'Aftercare'.

In addition to ensuring the quality of clinical record keeping, preparation of additional documentation is necessary and responsible in a CW contact lens practice. We suggest the production of a documentation set which contains six essential elements. An example of a documentation set is provided in the Appendix to this chapter. Further discussion on documentation is presented below in the sections entitled 'Patient information and instruction' and 'Liability'.

PATIENT EXPECTATIONS WITH CW

The presentation of the CW concept to patients is likely to be met with a dichotomy of responses. Those who have not been prejudiced against the notion usually respond positively to the prospect of the convenience which CW affords. Indeed, so attractive is the concept that caution should be exercised by the practitioner to guard against the patient considering CW as a cure-all.

There is another group of patients who have been duly warned by practitioners, friends or in press articles about the dangers of sleeping with contact lenses. This second group is likely to maintain a deep-rooted scepticism and require considerable reassurance from the practitioner who wishes to pursue CW.

It is very important to present CW to the patient in context with other corrective devices and procedures such as spectacles, DW contact lenses including one-day disposables, and refractive surgery. Each of the various refractive options has its advantages and disadvantages, and failure to make this information transparent to the CW candidate is both unreasonable and potentially dangerous from a legal perspective. It is also important that the patient understands silicone hydrogels are equally acceptable for use on a DW or flexible EW schedule as well as for up to 30 nights' CW.

The most rewarding aspect of fitting CW contact lenses for the practitioner is genuinely to assist those people who have functional issues with other forms of refractive correction. A frequent response to the question of the importance of wearing contact lenses is to overcome a sense of vulnerability felt, in particular, by many high myopes. Comments regularly heard include the desire to be able to read the bedside clock at night or to be able to respond in the middle of the night to an emergency situation without needing to search for a refractive aid. Patients also talk about a reluctance to bother with insertion and removal with DW, problems handling flimsy lenses and dropping or losing their lenses.

In practice, the majority of contact lens wearers are known to be female. This is possibly because males seem reluctant to engage in the procedures necessary to care for contact lenses. The availability of a more convenient modality may encourage a greater proportion of males to wear contact lenses. Initial experience with silicone hydrogels indicates that there is at least an equal proportion of male to female wearers, with some practices reporting a higher percentage of male wearers.

PATIENT SELECTION ISSUES

Selecting suitable patients is one of the more difficult components of achieving successful CW. In this situation it is probably more important to fit the right patient to the lens rather than the right lens to the patient. Successful selection of candidates relies on attention to ocular status and general health issues, lifestyle and demographic considerations, as well as motivational and personality factors. A well-structured case history will supply the answers to most questions. The flexible wear approach to silicone hydrogels makes them particularly useful across a wide range of needs as they offer improved corneal health to daily wearers, those looking for flexible EW options and to those who prefer CW.

HISTORY AND ADDITIONAL INFLUENCES PERTINENT TO THE INDIVIDUAL

Patients should be encouraged to provide details regarding their past ocular and general health. Those who are diabetic, who have diseases which may compromise immunity, who have conditions requiring intake of steroids or other systemic medication, or those who suffer from severe seasonal allergies, previous reactions to solutions or to hydrogel contact lens wear should be advised against CW and offered alternative modalities or forms of correction.

Previous success or failure with EW is an uncertain indicator of success with the modality. The CCLRU have reported that the adverse responses will recur in 15 per cent of patients who have experienced ARE and 35 per cent of patients who have experienced contact lens-related peripheral ulceration (CLPU).

Motivational factors to CW can assist in the selection of the suitable patient. These should also be identified during the case history. It is recognized that motivation is one of the means to achieving successful lens wear. Of the factors most readily linked to motivation, the magnitude of refractive error is the most apparent (Efron et al., 1988). Patients with higher refractive errors find spectacles provide important functional and cosmetic limitations. But other key issues in motivation are improvement of self-image and vocational, lifestyle or recreational factors.

Convenience is an important motivational aspect as well as a controversial one. The hassle of inserting, removing and maintaining lenses on a daily basis can be a deterrent of considerable proportion to consistent DW of contact lenses. However, the desire for convenience per se in contact lens wear is not a sufficient condition for fitting CW as the desire for convenience may be linked to a propensity for non-compliant behaviour. Compliance with instructions is essential to minimize the risks associated with CW. Non-compliant behaviour has been clearly linked with complications, at least in DW patients (Collin and Carney, 1986). However, compliance is a difficult aspect to predict and the practitioner should be alert to the balance between a genuine desire to improve one's quality of life versus such undesirable attributes as untidiness or negligence.

Practitioners should also be aware that wearing lenses beyond the recommended replacement frequency can decrease patient satisfaction with lens wear. A survey of US and Canadian SCL wearers ($n = 1014$) reports a high level of non-compliance with frequency of replacement (Jones, 2002). Fifty-four per cent of patients on a two-week replacement schedule and 45 per cent of patients on a four-week replacement schedule were non-compliant, and eight per cent of all patients reported that their practitioners supported their non-compliance by recommending replacement frequencies not advised by the manufacturers. Jones and colleagues found that the non-compliance of these patients was associated with reduced comfort and quality of vision and increased symptoms of dryness.

Certain demographic factors have been associated with an increased risk of complications with EW. Dart et al. (1991) reported that males have a higher relative risk of infectious keratitis than females, and persons in non-professional occupations are more likely to suffer from corneal infections than professionals. Smokers have a higher incidence of infectious keratitis and infiltrative keratitis than non-smokers (Schein et al., 1989; Cutter et al., 1996). There has also been the surprising finding of a greater incidence of adverse events in younger people (Brennan and Mullen, 2001; du Toit et al., 2002). Preliminary evidence from the cases of MK with silicone hydrogels suggest that young males (under 30 years of age) are at a greater risk of infection, and swimming without goggles while wearing contact lenses is a potential risk factor (Holden et al., 2003). While these demographic factors do not immediately eliminate candidates from CW, these factors should be weighed into the equation when selecting patients.

Another important factor which may affect the practitioner's decision to fit a given patient is access to emergency care. Patients who live in remote areas or who have careers or hobbies that may regularly place them out of contact of specialist services are not good candidates for CW. Patient education is essential in these cases.

REFRACTIVE ERROR

Clearly the patient must fall within the spherical parameter range available from the contact lens manufacturer. Initially lenses will be available only in spherical form and the normal clinical criteria for fitting astigmats with spherical lenses should apply. Presbyopic patients require special consideration in much the same way as patients being fitted with traditional hydrogel materials. Generally, silicone hydrogel lenses are not suitable for patients with more than 1.00 D of cyl.

Previously, fitting high myopes and hypermetropes with EW lenses was strongly advised against because the lens thickness profiles required to provide the appropriate power impacted upon the oxygen transmissibility of lenses. Higher-water-content lenses were required as the power of the lens rose to maintain optimal average oxygen transmissibility (Brennan et al., 1991). This effect becomes less important with silicone hydrogels because of the inherent high permeability of the materials.

OCULAR STATUS

The physiological status and integrity of the cornea is a most important consideration in selecting a patient for CW. A cautious biomicroscopic evaluation will

Table 8.1 Pre-fit checklist on ocular health

Characteristic	Requirement
Comfort	Grade 3 (comfortable) or better
Subjective vision rating	Grade 3 (good) or better
Visual acuity	Within 1 line of best spectacle acuity
Hypoxic effects	No microcysts or vacuoles[a]
	No striae or signs of visible oedema
Limbal vascularization	<0.5 mm vessel penetration
Corneal staining	None[b]
Endothelial polymegethism	≤Grade 1
Changes in corneal curvature	No irregular corneal distortion or warpage[b]
Infiltrates	None[b]
Bulbar and palpebral conjunctiva redness	≤Grade 1
Palpebral conjunctival papillae	≤Grade 1
Conjunctival staining	≤Grade 1

[a]Existing wearers may show some degree of microcysts, vacuoles or corneal distortion or warpage and clinical judgement should be used to assess suitability for fitting.
[b]EW lenses should not be fitted until staining or infiltrates are resolved.

confirm or eliminate any doubts that may have been raised during the case history and must weigh heavily in the final selection. It is imperative that only patients with normal ocular health be fitted with CW lenses. Signs of inflammation are a risk factor for further problems with CW.

Table 8.1 presents a list of pre-fit ocular health conditions which should be verified before prescribing CW. The absence of corneal staining as a prerequisite for fitting CW lenses may be an issue of some debate. Since one-fifth of non-symptomatic patients will at any given time exhibit corneal staining (Norn, 1972), it may be argued that a minimum amount of corneal staining may not be a contraindication for CW fitting. However, incidental staining resolves quickly, so if suspected the patient should be rebooked to verify that the region of staining is clear. Where staining is not incidental, for example in the case of mild dry eye which produces punctate band staining, we recommend treatment of the condition prior to fitting CW. The presence of small peripheral infiltrates should be treated in a similar fashion to staining. The practitioner is advised to wait for the infiltrate to clear prior to initiating CW. Any blepharitis or meibomian gland dysfunction should be treated prior to fitting CW.

Palpebral conjunctival status should be considered as well as vascularization, infiltrates, abrasions, ocular physiology and pathology. The quality of the tear layer is likely to have important ramifications for success in any form of contact lens wear. Indeed, dryness is recognized as the major symptom experienced by SCL wearers (Brennan and Efron, 1989). Patients with treatable signs should be identified and the problem adequately corrected prior to fitting, otherwise these patients should also be advised to refrain from attempting extended contact lens wear and a daily disposable lens might represent a preferred alternative.

SELECTING THE RIGHT LENS

With the introduction of silicone hydrogel lenses there is no reason to provide a patient interested in CW of SCLs with any other type of lens for spherical correction. Rigid gas-permeable (RGP) lenses still remain an option for astigmatic patients, particularly now that these lenses have FDA approval for CW.

With regard to surface properties, the desired quality of the lens is that it should maintain its surface wetting between blinks and remain relatively free of build-up. The advantages of disposable lenses, with regard to reduced inflammatory conditions, have been proven and incorporation of the disposability concept into silicone hydrogel lenses was inevitable. As described in detail in Chapter 1 on silicone hydrogel materials, surface modification such as plasma treatment is required to enable the lenses to wet and resist deposition. The silicone component of the dual-phase material would otherwise lead to poor wetting, discomfort and surface build-up. There is insufficient published information to determine differences between the lenses from different manufacturers, but the disposal of lenses after 30 days reduces the impact of lens build-up, thereby minimizing discomfort and untoward effects on the eyelids such as papillary conjunctivitis. The quality and reproducibility of the surface coatings are excellent but the practitioner should be alert for possible variations in quality that may impact on wetting and deposition. There may be some patient–lens combinations which are simply unsatisfactory.

Silicone hydrogel lenses are more easily handled than traditional hydrogels of the same thickness because of the stiffness of the silicone component. This interesting facet will be pleasing to both practitioners and patients as it will greatly facilitate the handling of the lens. In our experience the lenses also tend to be more damage-resistant than traditional hydrogels.

One of the most prominent aspects of lens selection from a practitioner standpoint is optimizing lens fit. This is of sufficient concern to warrant a separate section, as presented below.

FITTING AND DELIVERY OF SILICONE HYDROGEL LENS

As with all SCLs, the end result in silicone hydrogel contact lens fitting must be comfort and good visual acuity as well as little disturbance to the tear layer, cornea, conjunctiva and eyelids. To meet these criteria, careful lens selection is essential.

FITTING PROCEDURE

Trial lens fitting should always be performed prior to allowing a patient to undertake CW. The practitioner selects a preliminary trial lens after the following procedures:

- best correction of refractive error;
- keratometry readings; and

■ careful biomicroscopic assessment of all the anterior eye tissues in steady state.

Currently two companies provide silicone hydrogel lenses; one has two base curve options available (8.4 or 8.6 mm). Dumbleton *et al.* (2002) recommend that eyes with steeper corneal curvature (>45.50 D) may be more comfortable with the 8.4 mm base curve for lotrafilcon A.

Before insertion, practitioners should check trial lenses for correct inversion and to ensure that they are wet, clean, clear and undamaged. Once in place the selected lens is assessed for optimal centration, corneal coverage and movement by biomicroscopy. The lens should centre well with complete corneal coverage. Edge lift or fluting of the edge is unacceptable; therefore, try the other steeper base curve or the other lens type. If the lens is uncomfortable it should not be dispensed as the problem tends to remain, unlike RGP lens wear in which adaptation is likely to occur.

Adequate lens mobility with CW is considered to be important for success.

The aim of maximizing lens movement is to allow as much tear exchange as possible behind the lens (refer to Chapter 3). This is not for the purpose of increasing oxygenation, which is marginally affected at best by increasing movement. Increasing tear exchange is considered to be important because it may help reduce corneal inflammatory and infectious conditions. During closed-eye wear the post-lens tear film is depleted and the lens becomes immobile (Bruce and Mainstone, 1996). Stagnation of tears allows extended bacterial presence at the epithelial interface. One of the key predisposing factors in infection appears to be time of contact, even in the presence of an intact cornea (Fleiszig *et al.*, 1998). Infiltrative keratitis may also be induced by the failure to clear away debris from underneath a lens during closed-eye wear (Mertz and Holden, 1981; Zantos, 1984).

Clinical findings seem consistent with these theories as regards adequate lens movement. In Scandinavia, where disposable lenses were pioneered, SCLs are fitted loosely as a standard. This clinical practice may have benefits which include low numbers of ARE (Nilsson, 1983), reduced numbers of infections (Nilsson and Persson, 1986; Donshik, 1994; Nilsson and Montan, 1994a, 1994b) and reduced numbers of microcysts (Holden *et al.*, 1987).

Minimal lens movement is unlikely to cause significant problems with DW, and many US manufacturers seek to minimize soft lens movement so as to maximize comfort. However, it is generally considered good practice to fit CW lenses as mobile as is functional. Ideally movement should be of the order of 0.3 mm or greater. If the lens does not show adequate movement it should not be supplied.

In our experience silicone hydrogel lenses tend to show good movement. This is likely the result of mechanical and surface properties as well as design. The addition of lens lubricants to the care regimen may also assist in mobilizing lenses. During fitting, excessive reflex tearing can be responsible for the lens becoming apparently immobile on the eye. If this is noticed during trial fit of these lenses the lens should be removed and rinsed and the eye allowed to recover from the initial irritation. If adequate movement cannot be demonstrated, it is essential that a period of trial DW be undertaken with review after the lens has been in the eye for some time to allow assurance of adequate movement.

Although not essential, the concept of a short adaptation to the lens in DW is prudent if the patient has not worn contact lenses previously. This enables the patient to become proficient at handling the lenses and allows the practitioner to make a precautionary evaluation of the impact of silicone hydrogel materials on the eyes. We recommend a period of one week of DW with reassessment prior to beginning CW. At the one-week visit lens movement and corneal integrity should be checked to ensure satisfactory performance before commencing CW.

DISPENSING

There are differing opinions as to the preferred frequency for lens removal with CW. At this stage the practitioner may choose a flexible wear schedule for up to a maximum of 30 nights CW as conditions seem appropriate for a given patient. Both of the manufacturers of silicone hydrogel lenses currently available recommend 30-day replacement of lenses although some practitioners prefer a seven-day removal schedule. It is inadvisable for patients to extend the wearing time beyond 30 days because of an increased likelihood of deposit-related problems and decreased patient satisfaction due to decreased comfort.

A spare pair of lenses should be made available to patients to guard against the temptation to wear an unsuitable lens. While acknowledging this advantage, we suggest that the supply of lenses should be geared around the next scheduled aftercare visit as a means of securing patient compliance. Availability of silicone hydrogel lenses through third-party outlets may render this option unworkable in the future. Ideally supply of lenses should be restricted by government regulation as a safety measure. Another alternative to aid in regular review of patients is to restrict the contact lens prescription to a period of six months.

The patient instruction sheet provided in the Appendix gives details of care and maintenance of the contact lenses and is discussed below in the section entitled 'Patient information and instruction'. This aspect of wear should be emphasized and the practitioner should provide instruction both verbally and by demonstration, as well as providing the written instructions. A care kit containing solutions for rubbing, rinsing and storage, a contact lens case and lubricating eye drops should be provided.

A standard multi-action solution is adequate for the rubbing, rinsing and storage components. Surfactant cleaners with abrasive components are not currently recommended for use with the coating on silicone hydrogel lenses. Hydrogen peroxide systems are also acceptable. Enzyme cleaning appears to be an acceptable procedure. The following components of the care and maintenance should be emphasized: rubbing and rinsing, renewal of solution with each removal of the contact lens from the eye, case care and regular case replacement. Since lenses will be removed at longer intervals rather than on a daily basis, extra care should be taken to ensure that patients do not use solutions beyond the expiry date. Where lenses are to be used for 30-night periods and then disposed of, solutions should still be dispensed as an encouragement to patients to remove and clean the lenses where circumstances necessitate this action. Solutions and cases still require regular replacement and monitoring by the practitioner.

When prescribing silicone hydrogels on a DW basis, practitioners should be cautious of the potential for toxic-type corneal staining resulting from the use of some multipurpose solutions, in particular those containing polyaminopropyl biguanide (PHMB) (Jones *et al.*, 2002).

Patients should be advised to look at their eyes every night before sleep and in the morning on awakening. The patient should confirm that their eyes 'look good, feel good and see well'. If there is discomfort prior to sleep the lens should not be worn overnight. If patients are physically unwell, they should refrain from overnight wear.

Patients are also advised to use lubricating drops liberally, especially before bedtime and upon eye opening. This action will minimize debris behind the lens and reduce the duration of binding upon eye opening. The improved mobility should result in better tear exchange. Patient use of these drops tends to fluctuate in frequency over time. The only caveat in using comfort drops is maintenance of sterility of the dropper tip of the container. Contamination of the container will potentially result in the introduction of pathogenic organisms into the eye. Unit dose saline is one effective method of avoiding such contamination.

AFTERCARE

The early period of CW should be accompanied by frequent contact with the patient. Following lens delivery and instructions on care and warning signs, 24-hour and one-week assessments should be made. This practice also aids in establishing good patient morale and confidence, allows the practitioner to keep track of the patient's early progress, and reassures the patient that the ongoing care is a partnership between practitioner and patient. Our experiences in the early phases of clinical trials have demonstrated that this feature was important with this new lens wear modality.

A standard aftercare regimen is outlined in Table 8.2. The aftercare programme is scheduled in cognizance of the clinical experience that adverse effects occur most frequently within the first six months. For all visits it is advisable that the patient be seen early in the morning soon after awakening with contact lenses in situ. We prefer the appointment to be within the first hour after awakening, preferably within half an hour. This allows the practitioner to assess the eye and lens in a state which is regarded as the most illustrative of the stress that the lens places on the eye. Striae, and thus overnight swelling, lens binding and subsequent movement and the amount and clearance of debris can all be reasonably assessed.

Reinforcement of all safety procedures is essential at all aftercare visits. Human nature dictates that the impact of instruction and informational material is rapidly forgotten. Re-education about potential risks and the steps to take to avoid problems is essential at each aftercare visit. This consists of refreshing the patient's memory of the potential hazards of failing to follow instructions, e.g. by showing

Table 8.2   Recommended schedule of appointments

1. Initial visit	Examine lens fit, check for debris under the lens and wettability of the surface Recommend a week of DW for new lens wearers or those new to EW
2. First night of EW	Appointment should be made in the morning Assess the patient's history and vision Slit-lamp examination with and without lenses Rewetting eye drops can be recommended to patients who experience discomfort on waking or to those such as smokers who are at more risk of poor lens wettability
3. One week	Ensure patients are satisfied and confident with their lenses and wear schedule Examine the cornea for any signs of poor fit or mechanical interaction of the lens with the cornea (especially causing superior epithelial arcuate lesions). It is important to ensure that the lens is not too loose Pay particular attention to vision as some patients may experience a small change in refraction and some patients who have a history of EW with low-Dk soft lenses may have a slight shift in their refractive error
4. One and three months	Appointments should be made at the end of the wear schedule before changing to a new lens Look for signs of hypoxia (microcysts) and vascularization
5. Six months	This is the first opportunity to assess whether the patient is best suited to the wear schedule The level of comfort, convenience and confidence that patients have with their lenses and wear schedule should be assessed in detail The cornea, limbal area, conjunctiva and upper lid tarsus plate should be fully examined The conjunctiva and the limbus area should be white and clear

them a poster of serious complications. The care and maintenance procedures and daily routine should be reviewed at each aftercare visit.

Aftercare examinations should consist of vision assessment and, if indicated, a full refraction. The small change in refractive error (myopic creep) that is associated with EW of low-Dk hydrogels does not occur with CW of silicone hydrogels, and several authors have found that some silicone hydrogel wearers with previous lens experience can have a reduction in myopia after a short period of continuous wear (Dumbleton *et al.*, 1999; Jalbert *et al.*, 1999; McNally and McKenney, 2002). A history and ocular examination with and without the lenses in place are also essential. The most important aspect of this is the slit-lamp examination. It is also important to remember the value of ophthalmoscopy for non-contact lens-related issues, which can sometimes be overlooked in contact lens aftercare. Additional testing should be performed as indicated by signs and symptoms.

Detailed slit-lamp examination is the pillar around which successful CW practice is built. The reader is referred to the CCLRU Standards for Success in

Table 8.3   The successful EW patient

Characteristic	Requirement
Wear time	Ability to wear the contact lenses for six or more nights consecutively
Comfort	Grade 3 (comfortable) or better
Subjective vision rating	Grade 3 (good) or better
Visual acuity	Within 1 line of best spectacle acuity
Hypoxic effects	⩽10 microcysts or vacuoles
	No striae 1 hour after eye opening
	No endothelial folds
Vascularization	⩽0.5 mm vessel penetration
Endothelial polymegethism	⩽1 grade increase (CCLRU grading scale)
Changes in corneal curvature or refractive error	No irregular corneal distortion or warpage
	⩽± 0.50 D in flat K and/or ± 0.75 D in steep K
	⩽± 0.50 D sphere and/or ± 0.75 D cyl in spectacle refraction
Corneal staining	⩽Grade 2 type of staining (macropunctate)
	⩽Grade 1 depth of staining (superficial epithelial involvement)
	⩽Grade 1 extent of staining (1–15% surface involvement)
Lens adherence	No signs 1 hour after eye opening
Eyelid changes	⩽1 Grade increase in papillae or redness of superior palpebral conjunctiva
Bulbar redness	⩽1 Grade increase
Patient appearance	No unacceptable change

Contact Lenses as a basis for assessing the success of individual patients (Terry *et al.*, 1993). Although these standards were developed prior to the introduction of silicone hydrogels, the principles essentially remain applicable. These, combined with the use of a grading scale, provide a practical and structured method for assessing patients. As an aid to understanding the principles outlined in the paper of Terry and colleagues we have reproduced the essential findings in Table 8.3. Comments provided below should be considered in conjunction with the CCLRU Standards paper.

The Terry Standards paper does not include reference to infiltrative conditions, on the basis that such occurrences were considered to be immediate signs of individual failure in EW. Review of the categorization of inflammatory conditions seen with contact lens wear has led to the development of a separate CCLRU document (CCLRU and L. V. Prasad Eye Institute (LVPEI) Guide to Corneal Infiltrative Conditions seen in Contact Lens Practice; see Chapter 7) and this excellent guide is recommended for assessing infiltrative conditions in clinical practice.

Superior arcuate staining, CLPU and lesser infiltrative conditions can be asymptomatic and, as such, will not result in patients seeking care. The slit-lamp examination should be sufficiently attentive so as to identify the possibility of such conditions and allow appropriate action to be taken.

Corneal oedema can be assessed through examination of the CW patient soon after awakening following overnight wear. Assessment of chronic hypoxia is probably best achieved through consideration of the corneal epithelial microcystic response and endothelial irregularity. The number of microcysts is clearly linked to the oxygen transmissibility of the lens being worn, although the time course of the development adds a second dimension for consideration. With traditional hydrogel lens wear there is a delay of several weeks before the appearance of microcysts. Typically, on cessation of CW, the initial period of epithelial recovery is marked by a proliferation of microcysts over several weeks. Where patients are swapped from traditional hydrogel lens EW into silicone hydrogel lens CW, this short-term 'recovery' effect is similarly noticed. Thus, while microcysts are a useful indicator of chronic hypoxia, the time course effects should be factored into the clinical equation.

Endothelial irregularity was found to be a significant correlate of chronic oxygen deprivation in presenting hydrogel contact lens daily wearers and is, therefore, a useful way of assessing the impact of hypoxia (Brennan and Coles, 1998). We consider this to be a useful predictor of the likelihood of corneal exhaustion syndrome; however, this breakdown in physiology, which seems to be more of a DW phenomenon, should be contrasted to the adverse outcomes with either EW or CW, which are more often inflammatory in nature. In grading endothelial health, assessment should be based upon a number of parameters. These include examination of the regularity of cells using an appropriate grading scale. It is also valid to assess pleomorphism (irregularity of cell shape), the number of rosettes, lack of smoothness of the endothelium which is indicated by waves or regions of darkness in the specular reflection (especially visible when the angle between the illumination and observation system is increased), blebbing and variations in the brightness between and within individual cells.

The lens should also be examined both on and off the eye for irregularities and deposition. Deposits should be assessed and the care and maintenance system and replacement programme tailored accordingly. Other defects demand immediate lens replacement and investigation into the causes of lens damage.

PATIENT INFORMATION AND INSTRUCTION

We advocate the use of a six-element documentation kit, consisting of:

1. an information brochure;
2. the practitioner–patient agreement;
3. the instruction sheet;
4. a question and answer sheet;
5. the Informed Consent; and
6. emergency documentation.

Guidelines for documentation are presented in the Appendix to this chapter. Each element is relatively short and to the point, maximizing the opportunity of the patient to comprehend and use the information. The practitioner can amend the format of the documentation but we recommend ensuring that these separate elements are incorporated. The information presented in the Appendix is a guide only and separate advice should be sought concerning the content and wording from the professional association or qualified legal practitioners to suit the specific needs of the legislation in a given country.

The aim of the information and documentation kit is to provide details of what the patient can expect from the practitioner, clear instructions to follow to avoid complications, information on the support network available and a description of the repercussions of non-compliance and as an aid in avoiding legal action, as detailed below. The patient should read the instruction sheet in the presence of the practitioner and be encouraged to ask questions. The questions and answers to these questions should also be recorded. An important point of emphasis in the instructions is to advise the patient of steps to follow in the event of any symptom. A patient who does not appear to understand the instructions, or who indicates an unwillingness to follow the advice, should not be prescribed CW lenses.

The Informed Consent form should be signed and witnessed and the additional pages initialled. The formality of this procedure adds emphasis to the need of the patient to view CW as a therapeutic modality rather than a simple cosmetic device.

ANTICIPATING ADVERSE EFFECTS

Despite these best efforts severe problems still arise. In particular, the occurrence of severe inflammatory conditions such as CLARE and CLPU are difficult to pre-empt.

Careful patient selection and prudent aftercare are key elements to avoiding CW complications. The section above on patient selection details the important aspects of ocular examination to minimize risk. At aftercare the patient should be evaluated against the criteria listed for success in CW in Table 8.2 and those who do not meet these criteria should be discontinued, at least temporarily. Care should be taken, as mentioned above, to identify those conditions which are asymptomatic but which can be observed with the slit-lamp.

However, avoidance of problems is likely best achieved not via slit-lamp skill but by communication with the patient. This involves the proactive instruction to patients on how to avoid risks (Figure 8.1). These include the points which have been mentioned elsewhere in this chapter but which deserve reinforcement – that patients should not sleep with a lens which is causing discomfort, particularly if it has already been taken out and rinsed, and they should not sleep in their lenses if they are unwell. Where the lens is uncomfortable, or if some adverse reaction seems to be occurring, it is essential that the patient contact the practitioner and that the practitioner be available 24 hours per day. This response can allow early intervention in adverse events with accompanying restriction of the extent of the sequelae. As ocular pathogens in domestic and recreational water may place lens wearers at risk, patients should be recommended to wear goggles when swimming in lenses. Examples of the different types of educational materials that can be given to patients are shown in Figure 8.2.

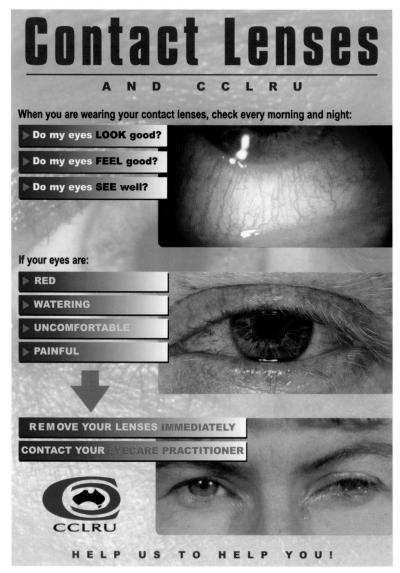

Figure 8.1   A sample of an in-office poster to remind patients to assess the status of their eyes morning and night, to be aware of potential problems related to contact lens wear and to remove their lenses and get in touch with their contact lens practitioners immediately in the event of a problem arising (courtesy of CCLRU)

LIABILITY

The decision to prescribe lenses is ultimately in the hands of the practitioner. The experts who have contributed to this book have provided their opinions to the best of their knowledge and can provide further advice should the need arise. CW carries risks which have been clearly explained in this book. Despite care and

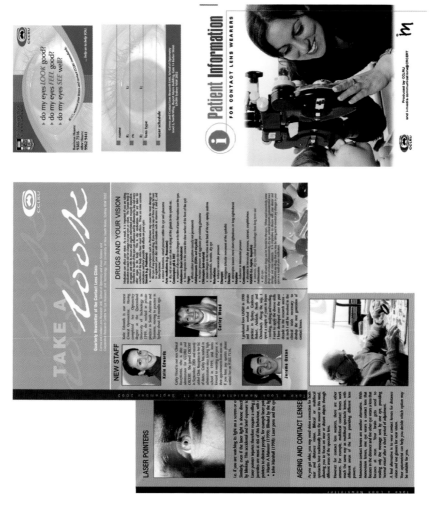

Figure 8.2   The different types of educational material that can be given to patients include: newsletters, one-page brochures outlining the dos and don'ts of lens wear, and credit-card-sized reminders to contact practitioners in emergencies and to wear goggles while swimming with contact lenses (courtesy of CCLRU)

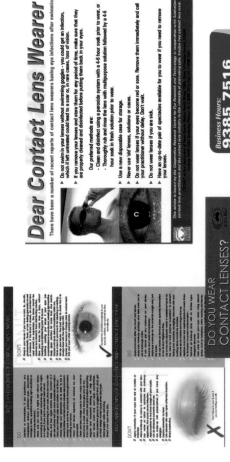

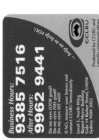

Figure 8.2 *Continued*

vigilance on behalf of the practitioner, complications will still arise. The practitioner is advised to minimize the extent of legal liability by ensuring that an accepted standard of clinical care is provided and by following a range of standard procedures. Several of these points have already been outlined in this document and they are summarized here to provide a checklist for the clinician:

- provision of a practitioner–patient agreement, Informed Consent form and instruction sheet;
- accurate and complete record keeping;
- establishment of a clear aftercare programme;
- careful and thorough examination of the patient at all aftercare visits;
- clear and documented advice to the patient on all aspects of ocular health and contact lens care; and
- procedures to deal with complications, in particular having a practitioner on call 24 hours per day.

Use of a practitioner–patient agreement and Informed Consent form such as that provided in the Appendix form an integral part of minimizing legal exposure. It should be noted that the Informed Consent form does not mitigate against liability for negligence or unprofessional conduct. However, it does provide a basis for an understanding on which the patient and practitioner can work together to provide maximum possible care for the patient and will hopefully deter nuisance, frivolous and irresponsible lawsuits.

Record keeping deserves specific comment. Records must be impeccably maintained to reflect the quality of care provided by the attending practitioner. As in all practitioner–patient relationships, the patient record is the only proof of the interaction that takes place in a consulting room and, in the event of legal action, can become a practitioner's greatest defence. Records must be complete, thorough and accurate to be of value. All the essential steps required in the fitting and aftercare of CW patients should be documented, visits must be clearly dated and incidental enquiries to clinical and support staff outside the consulting room should also be recorded. Attempts to contact patients who fail to attend for follow-up visits must be recorded. Cases where patients fail to attend aftercare visits or are non-compliant and cases where problems or adverse events have occurred should be given particularly detailed attention.

Ultimately disputes regarding the quality of care provided by a practitioner are judged against the standard of care that would be provided by one's colleagues. There is sufficient support amongst experts to suggest that fitting silicone hydrogels in CW is a reasonable professional practice. Professional misconduct is more likely to be judged not so much for fitting CW but for fitting it to the wrong individual or where it is perceived that appropriate care has not been provided.

THE SWEDISH EXPERIENCE WITH SILICONE HYDROGELS

In 1998 a prospective randomized study of 504 patients from 25 optometric practices in Sweden was conducted to assess the performance and complication

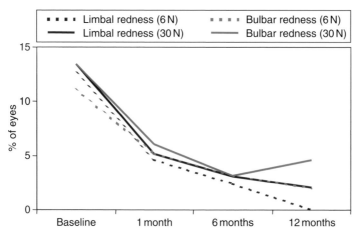

Figure 8.3   Percentage of eyes with a significant ($p < 0.001$) decrease in redness (grade 1–4) after commencing seven- or 30-day wear with silicone hydrogel lenses (adapted from Nilsson S. E. G. (2001) Seven-day extended wear and 30-day continuous wear of high-oxygen-transmissibility soft silicone hydrogel lenses: a randomized one-year study of 504 patients. *CLAO J.*, **27**, 125–136)

rates of silicone hydrogel lenses for CW in the market place (Nilsson, 2001). Initially practitioners were sceptical about the new lenses and were unconvinced that patients would be able to wear their lenses for 30 days without removal. The majority of practitioners did not usually fit EW and all patients were experienced SCL wearers.

Patients wore silicone hydrogel lenses either for 30 days CW ($n = 353$) or for seven days EW ($n = 151$) and were examined eight times: at the initial visit, after one night, one week, one month, three months and every three months thereafter for up to one year. There were no differences in the rate of subjective symptoms or complaints, or complications between patients in each of the wear schedules, and there were no cases of MK. Eighty per cent of all patients did not report any symptoms or complaints at the follow-up exams and when they were reported included predominantly dryness and discomfort. Anterior segment changes related to hypoxia were minimal and both limbal and bulbar hyperaemia decreased significantly soon after patients began wearing silicone hydrogel lenses (Figure 8.3). The most common clinically significant positive slit-lamp findings related to lens wear for the 30- and seven-day wearers were: corneal staining, corneal infiltrates, slight epithelial oedema and tarsal conjunctival abnormalities (Figure 8.4).

Patients from both wear schedules judged their comfort, visual quality, freedom from dryness and lens handling as excellent and the rate of discontinuation from lens wear was low. Of those who discontinued for lens-related reasons, 7.6 per cent were from the 30-day group and 13.2 per cent were from the seven-day group.

Nilsson's study highlighted to practitioners that 30-day CW with silicone hydrogel lenses can be recommended to patients as a first choice for vision

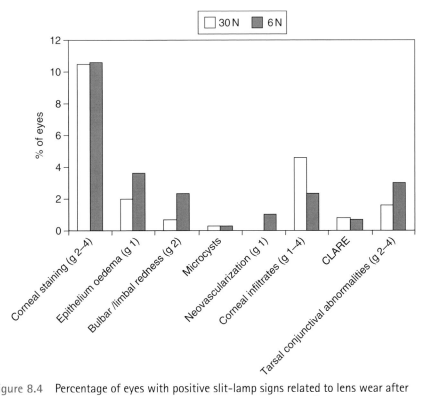

Figure 8.4 Percentage of eyes with positive slit-lamp signs related to lens wear after 12 months of seven- or 30-day wear with silicone hydrogel lenses (adapted from Nilsson S. E. G. (2001) Seven-day extended wear and 30-day continuous wear of high oxygen transmissibility soft silicone hydrogel lenses: a randomized 1-year study of 504 patients. *CLAO J.*, 27,125–136)

correction. In Sweden, optometrists have had nearly five years of experience with fitting silicone hydrogels and nearly 95 per cent of Swedish patients wearing silicone hydrogels now do so on a CW schedule. From this experience we have found that fitting 10–20 patients should give practitioners the experience necessary to understand fully how patients respond to silicone hydrogel lens wear.

For the patients who have not worn contact lenses before, we usually start with one to two weeks DW. This period is important for the patient to learn how to handle the lenses; however, too long a period of DW can sometimes result in a lack of motivation. No more than two weeks should be needed before moving to CW. For contact lens patients transferring to silicone hydrogels, we start on CW from the first day, and then the patient goes through our follow-up schedule. We do not find it necessary to start with DW at all. There do not appear to be any differences between RGP lens patients and soft lens patients, except that the number of soft lens patients is much higher. Regardless of wear history, all our patients follow the same schedule when they are transferred to silicone hydrogels.

Initially it is necessary to assess a patient's response to silicone hydrogels after three months of wear; after that, a recall every six months is all that is needed. Our recommendations for the first fit are:

1. Put the trial lens on. You may have to increase the power a little, for both myopic and hyperopic eyes. For example for −4.0 D increase the power to −4.25 D, and for +4.0 D increase the power to +4.25 D.
2. Look at the fit of the lens. Movement should be similar to that seen with conventional SCLs. Lenses that fit too flat may result in edge lift (fluting) and a lens with a steeper curve or a lens of different type should be tried.
3. Lenses that are too steep may result in problems with debris caused by minimal tear exchange under the lens. There should be no debris under the lens when the patient leaves after the first visit. Tear exchange should be sufficient to remove debris from both the front and back surfaces of the lens.
4. There should be good wettability on the surface when the patient leaves your practice. An examination of the lipid layer in the tear film is important to assess likely deposit problems. Patients with a 'thick' tear film may get problems with poor wettability and dry eye syndrome. We find that some patients have problems with lipid sticking to the lens surface, which can lead to poor wettability.

CONCLUSION

CW of silicone hydrogel lenses presents exciting new professional and business opportunities for eyecare practitioners. We now have a chance to provide patients with the 'freedom' they want with their vision correction. However, the decision to fit and manage CW patients requires considerable planning, expertise and dedication. Practitioners need to work with all designs on the market to find the best product and fit for each patient.

Well-informed optometrists and educated staff are important to the success of silicone hydrogel lenses. The follow-up schedule is also important to ensure continued safety and comfort for the patient. An office recall system for those who fail to attend the follow-up visit is also needed. We have provided here a guide and some useful written materials for the clinical practice of CW. The rest is up to you, the practitioner.

APPENDIX: DOCUMENTATION KIT FOR CW PRACTICE

We recommend preparation of a six-element documentation kit for CW practice as detailed below. The following information provides guidelines and samples for the various components of the documentation kit.

INFORMATION BROCHURE

The information brochure should be informative and accurate and can be used by the practitioner to generate awareness of the new-generation CW materials.

It should stress that detailed information about the possibility of CW for partic-ular patients requires a comprehensive examination. This brochure can be given to CW candidates by support staff, who can direct further questioning to the practitioner. Since the brochure can be promotional for the practice, a variety of formats are possible.

PRACTITIONER–PATIENT CW AGREEMENT (SAMPLE)

This agreement is between _____ (the patient) and _____ (the eyecare practi-tioner) and applies to the provision of contact lenses by the practitioner to be worn by the patient on an extended basis (sleeping in contact lenses for one or more consecutive nights).

You have indicated a desire to wear contact lenses on a CW basis. This means that you are choosing to sleep with your contact lenses on your eyes for one or more consecutive nights. The lenses that you will be using are made of a silicone hydrogel combination. This means that they have silicone, plastic and water com-ponents. They have been approved for CW of up to 30 days by the appropriate authorities in the USA, Europe and this country. Clinical trials comparing the new silicone-based contact lenses to the currently available non-silicone-based lenses have shown that this new lens material helps to maintain good eye health and reduces the redness which occurs as a result of overnight wear.

If you have any medical or eye-related conditions, are currently being treated for a medical or ocular condition or know of any reason which may invalidate your con-senting to this agreement, it is your duty to advise your practitioner.

Your practitioner has conducted a thorough eye examination to determine initial measurements of your eyesight, the health of your eyes, your contact lens prescription and spectacle prescription. He or she has asked you questions regard-ing your eyecare history. From this, he or she has determined your suitability to wear your contact lenses on a continuous basis. If you have any questions you should ensure that you have obtained satisfactory answers to these questions before entering into this agreement.

Follow-up visits

You should attend all follow-up visits scheduled by the practitioner. At these visits your eyesight and the health of your eyes will again be assessed. If the practitioner notices any signs or symptoms which require further monitoring, they will be treated until the condition clears. If any adverse event occurs, you will be referred for treatment to an eye specialist.

Instruction sheet

You have been provided with an instruction sheet which you should read care-fully. It is essential that you follow the instructions laid out in that document to minimize the risks of complications from CW.

Complications

It is impossible to predict all possible complications that may occur with any kind of contact lens wear. However, some risks are inherent to extended overnight contact lens wear including:

- swelling of the sensitive clear part of the front of the eye known as the cornea;
- small blood vessels growing into the cornea;
- small bumps on the inside of the eyelids;
- accumulation of debris or mucus on or behind the lens which may temporarily affect vision or comfort;
- internal inflammation of the eye;
- abrasions of the front surface of the eye;
- infections with potentially harmful micro-organisms; and
- inflammation of the cornea.

Most of these conditions are reversible. However, permanent vision loss can occur if one of the more serious side effects such as corneal infection occurs. You can reduce such risks by following the steps laid out on the instruction sheet.

If it is determined that use of these lenses presents new risks to your eyes or the possibility of undesirable side effects, you will be advised of this information so that you may determine whether or not you wish to continue wearing the lenses on an extended basis.

Alternatives to CW

The benefit of wearing contact lenses on an extended basis is the correction of your vision at all times that the lenses are on your eyes. Other procedures you may consider for such a purpose are eyeglasses, hard, soft or RGP contact lenses currently on the market or refractive surgery.

Discontinuation

This agreement is restricted to your decision to attempt CW of silicone-based SCLs. Of course, you are free to discontinue wear at any time for any reason. These decisions will not affect your future care from the practitioner in any way. If you wish to discontinue CW, you are responsible for notifying your eyecare practitioner upon discontinuation.

If you are unsure of any part of this agreement, your eyecare practitioner will be glad to answer any questions that you may have. If you have any additional questions later, please feel free to contact him or her on the following numbers.

[24-hour contact number, mobile telephone or pager number to be provided here]

Any complaints regarding this agreement or the conduct of the practitioner providing your eyecare can be addressed *in writing* to the relevant registration body of this state/province:

[provide details of authority]

You will be given a copy of this form to keep.

QUESTION AND ANSWER SHEET

A separate blank sheet should be appended to the documentation kit, which provides the opportunity to record any questions that the patient may have and the answers provided.

INSTRUCTION SHEET (SAMPLE)

Wearing and cleaning schedule

You can wear these lenses without interruption for [x] days, then remove them and clean and disinfect them according to the care and maintenance instructions below. You will be given a written copy of your lens care instructions. You should replace the lenses with a new pair after [y] days.

Care and maintenance of the lenses

Always wash hands thoroughly with a soap recommended by the eyecare practitioner before handling the lenses or touching your eyes.

Lenses should be cleaned after removal from the eye by placing the lens in the palm of the hand with a small amount of product [z]. Rub both surfaces of each lens for 20 seconds before rinsing with product [a]. The lens should then be stored in the lens case provided with freshly replaced product [b]. It is essential to replace all solutions prior to their expiration date.

The lens case

The lens case should be cleaned every month and rinsed and air-dried following removal of lenses. The lens case should be replaced every three months.

Follow-up visits

Aftercare visits will be scheduled at 24 hours, seven days, one, three and six months after initial dispensing of your contact lenses. Further examinations may be arranged by the practitioner. You are expected to attend for all of these visits in order to ensure appropriate follow-up and minimize risks to your eyesight.

What to do in the event of a problem

In the event that you experience problems with lens wear, you should rate the problem on the following three-step scale and act as indicated in the instructions which follow.

Three-point guide to problem management

1. *Pain, severe discomfort or aversion to bright lights.* Notify your eyecare practitioner without delay on the contact number indicated. Failure to do so immediately may result in permanent or partial loss of vision.

2. *Discomfort, eye redness, blurred vision or ocular discharge.* Remove your contact lenses and make an appointment for an examination at your earliest convenience. Do not recommence contact lens wear until you are advised that it is safe to do so by your practitioner. If the problem does not diminish within an hour after removal of the contact lens, you should notify your eyecare practitioner immediately.

3. *Minor irritation or minor blurring of vision.* Remove the contact lens, clean it in the prescribed manner and reinsert it. If the symptoms persists, you should arrange for an appointment as soon as possible and cease lens wear until then. If the irritation or blur is eliminated by removal and cleaning, then you should make a note of the event so that you can report it to your practitioner at your next scheduled visit.

Warning

Failure to adhere to the above instructions can lead to serious complications including vision loss.

Dos and Don'ts

Do check your eyes every morning and night.
Do use comfort drops.
Do call your practitioner if you have any questions.
Do call your practitioner if you experience discomfort which is not eliminated by lens removal and rinsing.
Do not delay in calling your practitioner if you experience pain, severe discomfort or aversion to bright lights.
Do not sleep in your lenses if your eye is uncomfortable.
Do not continue to wear the lens if discomfort is not alleviated by removal and rinsing.
Do not sleep in your lenses if you are unwell.
Do not use a damaged lens.
Do not swim in your contact lenses without using goggles.

INFORMED CONSENT (SAMPLE)

Patients must be at least 18 years of age and have full legal capacity to sign this document.

This agreement is between _____ (the patient) and _____ (the eyecare practitioner) and applies to the provision of contact lenses by the practitioner to be worn by the patient on an extended basis (sleeping in contact lenses for one or more consecutive nights).

Basic procedures of lens care, alternative vision correction and cleaning and disinfection methods and the advantages and disadvantages of CW have been explained to me by my eyecare practitioner. I have read the 'Information sheet' and the 'Instruction sheet', appended hereto, prior to signing this informed consent and understand the importance of following these instructions. By signing this informed consent, I agree that I understand the possible complications and benefits that may occur as a result of wearing my lenses on a CW basis. Although it is impossible for my eyecare practitioner to inform me of every possible complication, he or she has answered all my questions to my satisfaction and has assured me that he or she will advise me of new risks if they develop and will answer any further enquiries I may have about this product or my rights as a patient/customer/consumer. *Should any complications or emergencies occur*, I agree to contact my contact lens practitioner at the following contact numbers:

[24-hour contact number, mobile telephone or pager number to be provided here]

You are making a decision whether or not to wear contact lenses on an extended basis. Your signature indicates that you have agreed to wear the lenses in such a way as is prescribed, that you have read and understood the information provided above and that you are willing to follow the advice of your eyecare practitioner and that included in this instruction sheet.

Patient name:
Patient signature:
Date: //
Practitioner name:
Practitioner signature:
Date: //
Witness name:
Witness signature:
Date: //

EMERGENCY INFORMATION

We recommend providing the patient with a credit-card-size emergency information card. The following information should be provided:

- three-point problem instruction;
- practitioner contact numbers;
- emergency clinic phone number and address;
- details of lenses being worn;
- details of removal and replacement schedules;
- details of care and maintenance system.

REFERENCES

Adams, C., Cohen, E., Laibson, P. *et al.* (1983) Corneal ulcers in patients with cosmetic extended-wear contact lenses. *Am. J. Ophthalmol.*, **96**, 705–709

Allansmith, M. R., Korb, D. R. and Greiner, J. V. W. (1977) Giant papillary conjunctivitis in contact lens wearers. *Am. J. Ophthalmol.*, **83**, 697–708

Barr, J. (1998a). The 1997 annual report on contact lenses. *Cont. Lens Spectrum*, **13**, 23–33

Barr, J. (1998b). Renewed optimism about contact lens profitability. *Cont. Lens Spectrum*, **13**, 29–32

Boswall, G. J., Ehlers, W. H., Luistro, A. *et al.* (1993) A comparison of conventional and disposable EW contact lenses. *CLAO J.*, **19**, 158–165

Brennan, N. and Coles, M. L. (1998) Clinical endothelial regularity index as an indicator of chronic hypoxia. *Optom. Vis. Sci.*, **75**, S164

Brennan, N. A. and Efron, N. (1989) Symptomatology of HEMA contact lens wear. *Optom. Vis. Sci.*, **66**, 834–838

Brennan, N. A. and Mullen, B. (2001) Increased susceptibility of younger people to adverse reactions with silicone-hydrogel contact lens continuous wear. *Optom. Vis. Sci.*, **78**, S229

Brennan, N., Efron, N., Weissman, B. and Harris, M. (1991) Clinical application of the oxygen transmissibility of powered contact lenses. *CLAO J.*, **17**, 169–172

Bruce, A. and Mainstone, J. (1996) Lens adherence and postlens tearfilm changes in closed-eye wear of hydrogel lenses. *Optom. Vis. Sci.*, **73**, 28–34

Buckley, C. A., Buckley, C. J. and Griffiths, J. (1997) Extended wear disposable soft contact lenses as an alternative to photorefractive keratectomy: report of 4 years experience. *Aust. NZ J. Ophthalmol.*, **25**, 111–116

Collin, M. and Carney, L. (1986) Patient compliance and its influence on contact lens wearing problems. *Am. J. Optom. Physiol. Opt.*, **63**, 952–956

Cutter, G., Chalmers, R. and Roseman, M. (1996) The clinical presentation, prevalence, and risk factors of focal corneal infiltrates in soft contact lens wearers. *CLAO J.*, **22**, 30–36

Dart, J., Stapleton, F. and Minassian, D. (1991) Contact lenses and other risk factors in microbial keratitis. *Lancet*, **338**, 650–653

Donshik, P. (1994) Lower incidence of contact lens related ulcers in Sweden: is patient education a key? *CLAO J.*, **20**, 210–211

Driebe, W. J. (1989) Disposable soft contact lenses. *Surv. Ophthalmol.*, **34**, 44–46

Dumbleton, K. A., Chalmers, R. L., Richter, D. B. *et al.* (1999) Changes in myopic refractive error in nine months' extended wear of hydrogel lenses with high and low oxygen permeability. *Optom. Vis. Sci.*, **76**, 845–849

Dumbleton, K., Chalmers, R., McNally, J. *et al.* (2002) Effect of lens base curve on subjective comfort and assessment of fit with silicone hydrogel continuous wear contact lenses. *Optom. Vis. Sci.*, **79**, 633–637

Dunn, J. J., Mondino, B., Weissman, B. *et al.* (1989) Corneal ulcers associated with disposable hydrogel contact lenses. *Am. J. Ophthalmol.*, **108**, 113–117

du Toit, R., John, T., Sweeney, D. F. *et al.* (2002) Association of age, gender and ethnicity with the incidence of adverse responses with extended wear of silicone hydrogel lenses. *Optom. Vis. Sci.*, **79**, S9

Efron, N., Brennan, N. and Sek, B. (1988) Wearing patterns with HEMA contact lenses. *Int. Cont. Lens Clin.*, **15**, 344–350

Ficker, L., Hunter, P., Seal, D. and Wright, P. (1989) *Acanthamoeba* keratitis occurring with disposable contact lens wear. *Am. J. Ophthalmol.*, **108**, 453

Fleiszig, S. M., Lee, E. J., Wu, C. *et al.* (1998) Cytotoxic strains of *Pseudomonas aeruginosa* can damage the intact corneal surface *in vitro*. *CLAO J.*, **24**, 41–47

Hamano, H., Watanabe, K., Hamano, T. *et al.* (1994) A study of the complications induced by conventional and disposable contact lenses. *CLAO J.*, **20**, 103–108

Hassman, G. and Sugar, J. (1983) *Pseudomonas* corneal ulcer with extended-wear soft contact lenses for myopia. *Arch. Ophthalmol.*, **101**, 1549–1550

Holden, B. A., Sweeney, D. F., Vannas, A. *et al.* (1985) Effects of long-term extended contact lens wear on the human cornea. *Invest. Ophthalmol. Vis. Sci.*, **26**, 1489–1501

Holden, B. A., Sweeney, D. F., Swarbick, H. A. *et al.* (1986) The vascular response to long-term extended contact lens wear. *Clin. Exp. Optom.*, **69**, 112–119

Holden, B., Swarbrick, H., Sweeney, D. *et al.* (1987) Strategies for minimising the effects of extended contact lens wear: a statistical analysis. *Am. J. Optom. Physiol. Optics*, **64**, 781–189

Holden, B., Sweeney, D., Sankaridurg, P. *et al.* (2003) Microbial keratitis and vision loss with contact lenses. *Eye Cont. Lens*, **29**, S131–134

Jalbert, I., Holden, B., Keay, L. *et al.* (1999) Refractive and corneal power changes associated with overnight lens wear: differences between low Dk/t hydrogel and high Dk/t silicone hydrogel lenses. *Optom. Vis. Sci.*, **76**, S234

Jones, L. (2002) Comfort and compliance with frequent replacement soft contact lenses. *Optom. Vis. Sci.*, **79**, S259

Jones, L., MacDougall, N. and Sorbara, G. (2002) Asymptomatic corneal staining associated with the use of balafilcon silicone-hydrogel contact lenses disinfected with a polyamino-propyl biguanide-preserved care regimen. *Optom. Vis. Sci.*, **79**, 753–761

Kame, R. (1988) Disposability: an alternative to problems with hydrogel contact lenses. *Int. Cont. Lens Clin.*, **12**, 371–376

Kotow, M., Holden, B. and Grant, T. (1987) The value of regular replacement of low water content contact lenses for extended wear. *J. Am. Optom. Assoc.*, **58**, 461–464

Maguen, E., Tsai, J.C., Martinez, M. *et al.* (1991) A retrospective study of disposable extended-wear lenses in 100 patients. *Ophthalmology*, **98**, 1685–1689

Maguen, E., Rosner, I., Caroline, P. *et al.* (1992) A retrospective study of disposable extended wear lenses in 100 patients: year 2. *CLAO J.*, **18**, 229–231

Maguen, E., Rosner, I., Caroline, P. *et al.* (1994). A retrospective study of disposable extended wear in 100 patients: year 3. *CLAO J.*, **20**, 179–182

Marrioneaux, S. and Gwin, N. (1998) The golden opportunity in contact lenses. *Cont. Lens Spectrum*, **13**, 27–32

Marshall, E., Begley, C. and Nguyen, C. (1992) Frequency of complications among wearers of disposable and conventional soft contact lenses. *Int. Cont. Lens Clin.*, **19**, 55–59

McNally, J. and McKenney, C. (2002) A clinical look at a silicone hydrogel extended wear lens. *Cont. Lens Spectrum*, 38–41

Mertz, G. and Holden, B. (1981) Clinical implications of extended wear research. *Can. J. Optom.*, **43**, 203–205

Migneco, M. and Pepose, J. (1996) Attitudes of successful contact lens wearers towards refractive surgery. *J. Refract. Surg.*, **12**, 128–133

Mondino, B., Weissman, B., Farb, M. and Pettit, T. (1986) Corneal ulcers associated with daily wear and extended wear contact lenses. *Am. J. Ophthalmol.*, **102**, 58–65

Musch, D., Sugar, A. and Meyer, R. (1983) Demographic and predisposing factors in corneal ulceration. *Arch. Ophthalmol.*, **101**, 1545

Nilsson, K. (1983). Preventing extended wear problems, the Swedish way. *Cont. Lens Forum.*, **8**, 21–29

Nilsson, S. (2001) Seven-day extended wear and 30-day continuous wear of high oxygen transmissibility soft silicone hydrogel contact lenses: a randomized 1-year study of 504 patients. *CLAO J.*, **27**, 125–136

Nilsson, S. and Montan, P. (1994a) The hospitalized cases of contact lens induced keratitis in Sweden and their relation to lens type and wear schedule: results of a three-year retrospective study. *CLAO J.*, **20**, 97–101

Nilsson, S. and Montan, P. (1994b) The annualized incidence of contact lens induced keratitis in Sweden and its relation to lens type and wear schedule: results of a three-month prospective study. *CLAO J.*, **20**, 225–230

Nilsson, S. and Persson, G. (1986) Low complication rate in extended wear of contact lenses. *Acta Ophthalmol.*, **64**, 88–92

Norn, M. S. (1972) Vital staining of cornea and conjunctiva. *Cont. Lens J.*, **3**, 19–22

Poggio, E. and Abelson, M. (1993) Complications and symptoms in disposable extended wear lenses compared with conventional soft daily wear and soft extended wear lenses. *CLAO J.*, **19**, 31–39

Poggio, E., Glynn, R., Schein, O. *et al.* (1989) The incidence of ulcerative keratitis among users of daily-wear and extended-wear soft contact lenses. *N. Engl. J. Med.*, **321**, 779–783

Sankaridurg, P. R., Sweeney, D. S., Sharma, S. *et al.* (1999) Adverse events with extended wear of disposable hydrogels: results for the first 13 months of lens wear. *Ophthalmology*, **106**, 1671–1680

Schein, O., Glynn, R., Poggio, E. *et al.* (1989) The relative risk of ulcerative keratitis among users of daily-wear and extended-wear soft contact lenses. *N. Engl. J. Med.*, **321**, 773–778

Schein, O., Buehler, P., Stamler, J. *et al.* (1994) The impact of overnight wear on the risk of contact lens-associated ulcerative keratitis. *Arch. Ophthalmol.*, **112**, 186–190

Skotnitsky, C., Sweeney, D. F., Keay, L. and Holden, B. A. (1999) Patient responses and attitudes to 30 night continuous wear of high *Dk* silicone hydrogel lenses and attitudes to refractive surgery. *Optom. Vis. Sci.*, **76**, S214

Smith, R. and MacRae, S. (1989) Contact lenses: convenience and complications. *N. Engl. J. Med.*, **321**, 824–826

Spring, T. F. (1974) Reaction to hydrophilic lenses. *Med. J. Aust.*, **1**, 449–450

Suchecki, J. K., Ehlers, W. H. and Donshik, P. C. (1996) Peripheral corneal infiltrates associated with contact lens wear. *CLAO J.*, **22**, 41–46

Terry, R., Schnider, C., Holden, B. *et al.* (1993) CCLRU standards for success of daily and extended wear contact lenses. *Optom. Vis. Sci.*, **70**, 234–243

van Cranenburgh, B. (1999) What do practitioners think about continuous-wear lenses? *Optician* **217**, 36–37

Zantos, S. (1984) Management of corneal infiltrates in extended-wear contact lens patients. *Int. Cont. Lens Clin.*, **11**, 604–610

Ziegler, D. (1997) Maintaining profitability in these competitive times. *Cont. Lens Spectrum.*, **12**, 29–32

Index

Note: page numbers in *italic* type refer to figures and tables.

Other books in the series

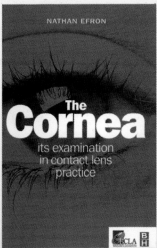

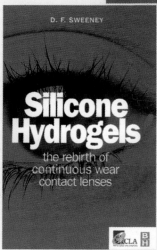

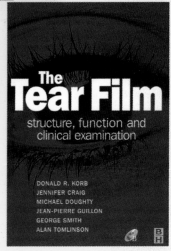

Contact Lens & Anterior Eye

Official Journal of the British Contact Lens Association

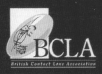

BCLA
British Contact Lens Association

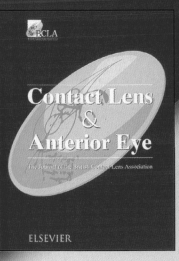

To promote excellence in contact lens research, manufacturing and clinical practice

Editor-in-Chief:
T. Buckingham, *Bradford, UK*

Contact Lens & Anterior Eye is a research-based journal covering all aspects of contact lens theory and practice, including original articles on invention and innovations, as well as the regular features of:

- Case Reports
- Literary Reviews
- Editorials
- Instrumentation and Techniques
- Dates of Professional Meetings

ISSN: 1367-0484   4 issues per year

An Invitation to Submit your Paper

Contact Lens & Anterior Eye is the Official Journal of the British Contact Lens Association.

Please visit the journal webpage for further details: **http://authors.elsevier.com/journal/clae**

Manuscripts may be submitted to:
Dr Terry J. Buckingham, Editor-in-Chief
Contact Lens & Anterior Eye, PO Box 15, Guiseley
Leeds LS20 8YH, UK
E-mail: terry.j.buckingham@btopenworld.com

Please visit the journal web page for further details

www.elsevier.com/locate/clae

All members of the BCLA receive free online access to the journal as part of their membership package, for more information and to register please visit

www.bcla.org.uk

SCIENCE @ DIRECT

ELSEVIER SCIENCE